Forensic and Clinical Applications of Solid Phase Extraction

FORENSIC
SCIENCE AND MEDICINE

Steven B. Karch, MD, SERIES EDITOR

FORENSIC AND CLINICAL APPLICATIONS OF SOLID PHASE EXTRACTION

Michael J. Telepchak, BS, MBA
Thomas F. August, BS, MS
and
Glynn Chaney, MS, TC(NRCC)

UNITED CHEMICAL TECHNOLOGIES INC.,
BRISTOL, PA

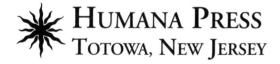

HUMANA PRESS
TOTOWA, NEW JERSEY

Production Editor: Mark J. Breaugh.

Cover design, layout, and photography by Mark K. Connelly.

For additional copies, pricing for bulk purchases, and/or information about other Humana titles, contact Humana at the above address or at any of the following numbers: Tel.: 973-256-1699; Fax: 973-256-8341; E-mail: humana@humanapr.com or visit our website: http://humanapress.com

E-ISBN: 1-59259-292-9

Library of Congress Cataloging-in-Publication Data

Forensic and clinical applications of solid phase extraction / edit-
    ed by Michael J. Telepchak, Thomas F. August, and Glynn Chaney.
      p. cm. -- (Forensic science and medicine)
    Includes bibliographical references and index.
    ISBN 0-89603-648-0 (acid-free)
    1. Chemistry, Forensic.   I. Telepchak, Michael J. 1955- II. August, Thomas F.
    III. Chaney, Glynn IV. Series.
    [DNLM: 1. Forensic Medicine. 2. Chemistry, Analytical. 3.
  Toxicology.   W 750 F7123 2004]
  HV8073.F558 2004
  614'.13--dc22

  2003018154

Preface

It is hoped that the soup-to-nuts approach used in organizing *Forensic and Clinical Applications of Solid Phase Extraction* will provide the reader with a good basis for developing the types of customized extractions that will need to be developed to solve the practical problems associated with the analytical chemistry of toxicological problems.

There are books in which solid phase extraction (SPE) is summarized and reviewed either independently or as part of some other field of endeavor. However, the present work is different in that it is designed to be used as a laboratory reference manual in a variety of forensic environments. It is also designed to provide a comprehensive review of the principles that affect the outcome of novel extractions that researchers may wish to perform.

Along with sections of history, theory, and chemistry, a significant number of applications, troubleshooting, and appendices have been included to provide reference tables and helpful data related to forensic analysis. The applications have been grouped by drug types and matrices.

As we review the history of SPE and look at its application to very selective extractions, one may reach the conclusion that SPE is being purported as a cure-all. This is not the case. Rather, it is a powerful tool that seems to excel in separating specific compounds from very complex matrices, and its improvement makes it extremely useful for extracting both neutral drugs and polar metabolites. A good rule of thumb is that the dirtier the matrix and more polar the compounds, the more likely SPE will be the best choice for sample preparation.

Michael J. Telepchak, BS, MBA
Thomas F. August, BS, MS
Glynn Chaney, MS, TC(NRCC)

Dedication

To my wife and family, and all the people who did not get my time and attention while this project was ongoing.

To Christine Makai, my administrative assistant, for all the typing and organizing she did and for tolerating me through this process.

To Ellen Smith, my administrative assistant, for all the typing and organizing she did.

To Earl Brookins, UCT's graphic specialist, for all the drawing and redrawing he has done for this project and for helping to convert all of my thoughts in drawings.

To UCT for allowing me all of the time and necessary resources to make this project a reality, thereby making all this information available to its readers.

Michael J. Telepchak

Contents

Acknowledgments

The following is a list of people who directly and indirectly contributed to this work. I am sure that there are many more whom I have not mentioned and I apologize to them for any omissions.

KATHY RYMUT • Hartford Hospital, Hartford, CT

LISA O'DELL • REO Agency, Denver, CO

CHET KITCHENS • Merck & Co., West Point, PA

CHRISTINE MOORE • US Drug Testing, Chicago, IL

GERALD LONG • Quintiles, Atlanta, GA

BRUCE GOLDBERGER • University of Florida, Gainesville, FL

DAVID DARWIN • NIDA, Baltimore, MD

JONATHAN OYLER • NIDA, Baltimore, MD

LAUREEN MARINETTI • Montgomery County Medical Examiner's Office, Dayton, OH

MICHELE GLINN • Michigan State Police, Lansing, MI

FRED HOUSE • Michigan State Police, Lansing, MI

JOSEPH SAADY • Medical College of VA Department of Pathology, Richmond, VA

DENNIS CROUCH • Center for Human Toxicology, University of Utah, Salt Lake City, UT

JOSEPH TOUCHSTONE • Hospital of the University of Pennsylvania, Philadelphia, PA

ALLEN RAY • Texas Agricultural and Mechanical University, College Station, TX

ROBERT MACKENZIE • Michigan Department of Agriculture, East Lansing, MI

RANDALL STONE • Las Vegas Metro Police Forensic Lab, Las Vegas, NV

JOHN D'ASARO • United Chemical Technologies Inc., Bristol, PA

GUY PURNELL • Philadelphia Medical Examiner's Office, Philadelphia, PA

FRANK CAPUTO • Philadelphia Medical Examiner's Office, Philadelphia, PA

DAN ANDERSON • LA County Coroner's Office, Los Angeles, CA

JOSEPH CRIFASI • St. Louis University Forensic Toxicology Lab, St. Louis, MO

STEVEN KOLLMAN • County of San Mateo, Redwood City, CA

LEON GLASS • United Chemical Technologies Inc., Bristol, PA

MARC LEBEAU • Federal Bureau of Investigation, Washington, DC

KATHRYN KALASINSKI • AFIP, Rockville, MD

PHIL DIMSON • SPEware, Los Angeles, CA

MICHAEL SMITH • US Army Drug Testing Lab, Washington, DC

MARILYN HUESTIS • NIDA, Baltimore, MD

MATT LAMBING • University of North Carolina Medical Examiner, Chapel Hill, NC

BRIAN BRUNELLI • Quest Diagnostics, Atlanta, GA

DAVID ENGELHART • Cuyahoga County Medical Examiner, Cleveland, OH

JERRY PRUETT • Mayo Clinic, Rochester, MN

JOEL CHARLESON • Mayo Clinic, Rochester, MN

CRAIG PERMAN • 3M, Minneapolis, MN

DAVID WELLS • Sample Prep Solution Co., Minneapolis, MN

Chapter 1

Introduction to Solid Phase Extraction

Solid phase extraction (SPE) is a broad term used to describe the separation technique in which liquids contact modified solid surfaces and a component of the liquid adheres to the solid. In a separate step, the solid releases the component. This solid usually consists of an inert core covered with unique hooks that remove the targeted material from the starting liquid. SPE manufacturers pack these active solids into various containment devices such as plastic columns.

1.1 History

A timetable of historic events that led to the discovery of SPE in 1974 is presented in Table 1, with a strong emphasis on sample preparation. It has been widely believed that Tswett's 1906 work represents the advent of chromatography. Thanks to the research of Dr. Joseph Touchstone of the University of Pennsylvania, however, we can see that a very early form of pre-chromatography can be traced all the way back to 23 AD (1–9), although the number of written articles was limited. Interest in various chromatographic phenomena grew in the 1800s, resulting in Tswett's publication in 1906. Developments in chromatography moved quickly ahead during the 1900s until, today, new publications have become too numerous to list.

Modern SPE originated in 1974, when three researchers, Drs. Reginald Adams, Thomas Good, and Michael Telepchak, were working on high-performance liquid chromatography (HPLC) applications for clinical laboratories. Specialty HPLC column packings were being tested and evaluated for specific steroid applications. Inadvertently, some of the C18 column packing material fell into the urine sample being tested. On testing the sample it was discovered that the steroids of interest were missing. Further testing demonstrated that the steroids were bonded to the column packing

From: *Forensic Science and Medicine:*
Forensic and Clinical Applications of Solid Phase Extraction
Edited by: M. J. Telepchak, T. F. August, and G. Chaney © Humana Press Inc., Totowa, NJ

Table 1
The Development of Chromatography and SPE

Date	Event	Scientist	Reference
23 and 79 AD	Papyrus and gallnuts	Pliny	
1855	Paper chromatography	F. F. Runge	*1*
1861	Paper chromatography	F. Goppelstroeder	*2*
1891	Paper chromatography	C. F. Schonbein	*3*
1892	Paper chromatography	E. Fischer and E. Schmidmer	*4*
1893	Column chromatography	L. Reed	*5*
1897	Column chromatography	D. T. Day and C. Engler/E. Albrecht	*6* *7*
1906	First publication on the chromatographic separation method	M. S. Tswett	*8,9*
1931	"Rediscovery" of chromatography	R. Kuhn and E. Lederer	*10,11*
1941	Liquid/liquid: classical first description of liquid/liquid partition chromatography	A. J. P. Martin, R. L. M. Synge Consden et al.	*12* *13*
1941	Gas-solid adsorption chromatography	G. Hesse et al.	*14*
1950	Thin-layer chromatography	J. G. Kirchner and G. J. Keller	*15*
1952	First description of gas-liquid partition chromatography	A. T. James and A. J. P. Martin	*16*
1959	Modern paper chromatography	F. Cramer	*17*
1962	Supercritical fluid chromatography	E. Klesper et al.	*18*
1962	Diatomaceous earth extraction column		
1963	High-performance liquid	L. Halasz and C. S. Horvath	*19*
1965	Capillary electrophoresis chromatography	S. Hjerten et al.	*20*
1966	First publication on high-pressure liquid chromatography	C. S. Horvath S. R. Lipsky	
1971	Densitometry	J. C. Touchstone	*21*
1974	Toxi Tube®	Ansys	
1974	First reported use of solid phase extraction	R. Adams T. Good M. Telepchak	
1974	Hydrophobic columns		
1978	Countercurrent chromatography	I. A. Sutherland Y. J. Ito	*22*
1978	First publication on SepPak[(r)]	W. Mitchell and P. Rahn	*23*
1980	Overpressured thin-layer chromatography	H. Kalasz et al.	*24*

Table 1 (*continued*)
The Development of Chromatography and SPE

Date	Event	Scientist	Reference
1980	Ion-exchange columns		
1986	Copolymeric solid phase extraction	M. Telepchak	
1987	Borosilicate glass fibers	Ansys	
1989	Empore technology	3M	
1991	Solid phase dispersion	S. Barker	
1993	Microtiter plates	3M	
1993	Solid phase microextraction	Supelco	

material. Filtering, washing, and resuspending the packing in methanol caused the steroid to be released for analysis.

SPE was done by placing the packing into the sample for several years; this method is still used in certain situations or in difficult applications. As the technique evolved, the material was put into syringe barrels and a variety of holding devices that ultimately resembled the SPE devices seen today.

The development of hydrophobic columns progressed quickly; the first publication on SepPak® cartridges appeared in 1978. In 1980, ion-exchange columns were adopted for sample preparation. In 1986, the first multimodal column (copolymeric phase) was introduced into the forensic market by Telepchak, followed by further developments in SPE through 1994. However, the introduction of copolymeric phases has had the most significant impact on SPE and its application in the separation of many classes of drugs from their biological matrices.

1.2 ADVANTAGES OF SPE OVER LIQUID–LIQUID EXTRACTION

Scientists who relied on liquid–liquid extraction (LLE) in the past have asked why we should consider using SPE in place of liquid–liquid extraction. The following are some reasons to consider SPE in place of LLE.

SPE allows you to use lower sample quantities and lower solvent volumes. Lower sample volumes are possible because higher-efficiency lower-bed volume devices are available and, in specific cases, sample volumes of 100 μL or less can be used. The reduced-volume columns allow elution in smaller volumes of solvent, which can be dried down quickly. Using smaller volumes of solvent is very important today. Lab personnel need to be mindful of solvent usage as it costs more to dispose of solvents today than it does to buy them. This is especially true in the case of chlorinated hydrocarbons.

For the most part, SPE allows for shorter sample extraction times. This is especially true when back-extractions are required (1). In SPE the analyst can switch from organic solvents to aqueous solvents and back to organic solvents in a matter of 15 minutes. This is not the case in liquid–liquid extraction.

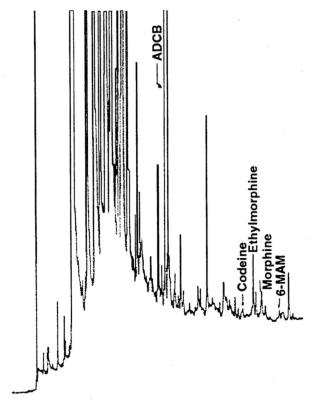

Fig. 1. A liquid–liquid extraction of opiates from urine.

Biological samples are notoriously dirty; injecting them with minimum cleanup onto very sensitive and expensive instruments makes very little sense. SPE has been shown to significantly increase gas (GC) and liquid chromatography (LC) column life while reducing the downtime on equipment like gas chromatography and liquid chromatography mass spectrometers (GCMS and LCMS) for source cleaning.

SPE recoveries should exceed 90% absolute recovery. If you don't get that kind of recovery you are not adjusting other parameters (such as solubility, pH, and solvent strength) correctly. Liquid–liquid extraction not only has trouble achieving high recovery on a reliable, reproducible level but also, the more extractions you need to do, the more of your sample you lose. SPE, on the other hand, actually concentrates your sample on the column and allows for reproducible results at very low levels of analytes.

LLE is a general technique that extracts many compounds, whereas SPE gives the analyst the ability to extract a broad range of compounds with increased selectivity.

SPE can be automated quite easily with a variety of currently available equipment.

Figures 1–5 show a progression of chromatograms from extractions, which will demonstrate the improvements made in extractions over the past 10 years. Figure 1 shows a liquid–liquid extraction of opiates from urine. Notice the high level of impurities and the low recoveries of the opiates in this extraction.

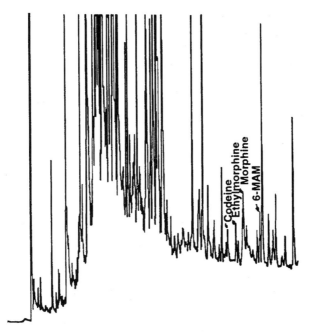

Fig. 2. An extraction of opiates from urine using C18 SPE column.

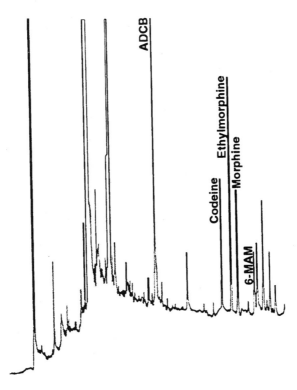

Fig. 3. An extraction of opiates from urine using high-efficiency copolymeric SPE column.

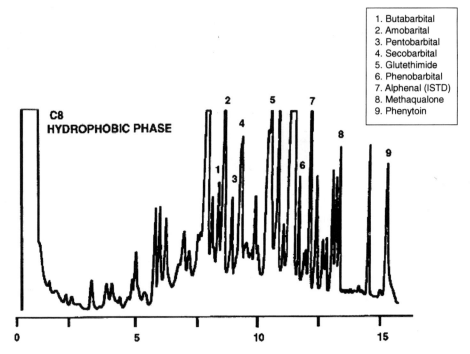

Fig. 4. An extraction of barbiturates from urine using C8 SPE column.

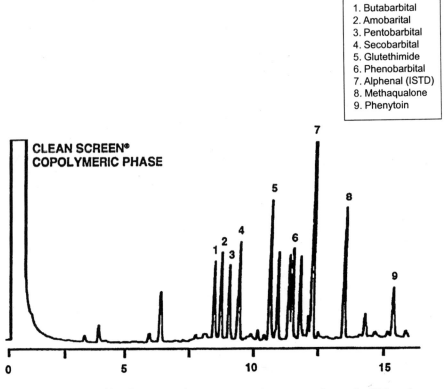

Fig. 5. An extraction of barbiturates from urine using a copolymeric SPE column.

Figure 2 shows the same extraction done on a C18 bonded phase SPE column. Even though the recoveries of opiates are better, there is little if any improvement in the removal of background interference. The compounds of interest are still buried in the interferences. If you are going to rely on your GC, LC, or mass spectrometer to resolve the problems of background noise, remember that continuing to put dirty extracts on an expensive instrument will result in extra downtime, loss of sensitivity, and possible instrument damage.

Figure 3 shows the same extraction again, only this time on a high-efficiency copolymeric extraction column. Notice both improved recovery and elimination of a significant amount of background interference.

Figure 4 shows an extraction of barbiturates from urine using a C8 bonded phase extraction column. Notice that there is still a significant amount of interference even though recovery is acceptable.

Figure 5 shows the same extraction on a copolymeric SPE column. Notice the absence of the background interferences.

Differences in the cleanup approach in these examples are worth noting. In Figures 4 and 5 the ion-exchange on the copolymeric SPE column is used to hold back ionic interferences, allowing the drugs to come off cleanly. In Figures 1–3 the ion-exchanger is used to retain the drugs while the other impurities are worked off the column. Then the drugs of interest are eluted off cleanly. This should be a reminder to try different approaches to the cleanup as you develop your SPE skills.

1.3 LIQUID–LIQUID EXTRACTION

Compounds of interest are extracted from complex matrices by addition of organic and aqueous solvents. Acidic analytes are soluble in organic solvents at acidic pHs because they are not ionized. To improve extract cleanliness, acids are back-extracted into aqueous solvents by ionizing them (pH change). In fact, compounds are usually partitioned between organic and aqueous solvents several times to improve extract cleanliness, which can result in analyte loss during each extraction step (lower recovery). The reverse is true for basic analytes: at alkaline pH, basic compounds are more soluble in organic solvents than in aqueous ones and may be extracted through a change of pH (Figures 6–8).

The following equations describe the mechanism of liquid–liquid extraction (Wu et al. Clin. Chem. 40:216–220, 1994).

$$K_o = C_o / C_A$$

$$E = K_o V / (1 + K_o V)$$

Where K_O = distribution constant
C_O = concentration in organic phase
C_A = concentration in aqueous phase
E = efficiency
V = organic/aqueous phase ratio.

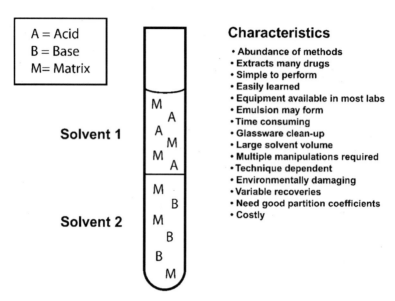

A = Acid
B = Base
M = Matrix

Solvent 1

Solvent 2

Characteristics

• Abundance of methods
• Extracts many drugs
• Simple to perform
• Easily learned
• Equipment available in most labs
• Emulsion may form
• Time consuming
• Glassware clean-up
• Large solvent volume
• Multiple manipulations required
• Technique dependent
• Environmentally damaging
• Variable recoveries
• Need good partition coefficients
• Costly

Fig. 6. A diagram of the mechanism of liquid–liquid extraction.

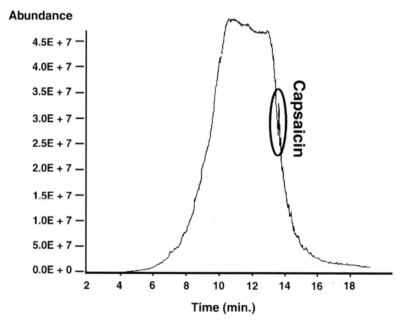

Fig. 7. Liquid–liquid extraction of mace from the sweatshirt of a suspected assailant.

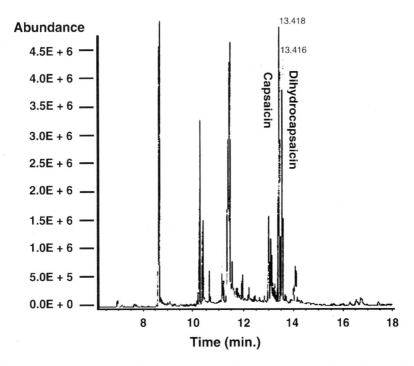

Fig. 8. The extraction of mace from the sweatshirt of a suspected assailant using a high-efficiency copolymeric SPE column.

1.4 DIATOMACEOUS EARTH EXTRACTIONS

The extraction principle used in diatomaceous earth columns (Figure 9) is a modified hybrid liquid–liquid extraction in which the aqueous portion of the sample acts as an immobilized stationary phase. This mechanism became a bridge for future development in SPE. The aqueous sample is poured into the column, which is prepacked with an inert matrix of large surface area and sometimes contains a buffer to adjust the pH of the sample. The added organic solvent interfaces with the sample. Water and impurities—such as pigments, particulate matter, and other polar compounds—are retained in the matrix on the immobilized aqueous sample and later adsorbed to the diatomaceous earth. The compounds of interest partition into the organic mobile phase and pass freely through the column.

This technology, which worked effectively in demonstrating the mechanism, was eventually developed into bonded or solid phase extraction. Although it is novel and effective, the drawback of this technique is that the volumes of solvent must be exact to produce the desired effect; 10 mL too little of solvent and the recovery drops off significantly, 10 mL too much of solvent and the dirt can be carried off the column with the analytes of interest.

Table 2 gives a procedure for extraction of theophylline from serum or plasma using diatomaceous earth columns (also *see* Figures 10, 11).

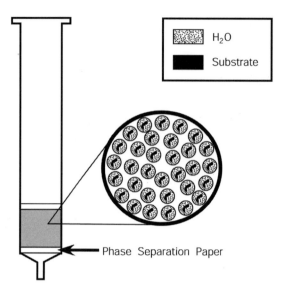

H₂O

Substrate

Phase Separation Paper

Fig. 9. A diagram showing the structure of a diatomaceous earth column.

Table 2
Extraction of Theophylline from Serum or Plasma
Using Diatomaceous Earth Columns

1. Add 50 µL of the internal standard solution (β-Hydroxyethyl theophylline, 100 µL, in 0.5 *M* phosphate buffer at pH 5.0) to the columns.
2. Add up to 250 µL of the serum sample to the columns.
3. Add 3 mL of dichloromethane-isopropanol (90:10) extraction solvent to the columns; wait 5 min for complete elution.
4. Collect the eluants; evaporate to dryness.
5. Reconstitute with 100 µL of methanol.

1.5 BONDED PHASE EXTRACTION

Compounds of interest are retained from complex matrices on a solid support (e.g., silica) to which one or more functional groups have been permanently attached. If nothing were bound to the silica support the separation mechanism would be adsorption. Alkyl groups provide hydrophobic interaction mechanisms, polar groups-ion-exchange, and copolymeric phases-combinations of the above. Compounds are eluted with various solvents of different polarities. More than one set of interactions is usually involved, so it is important to remember need to know what mechanisms are in operation. Figure 11 shows a typical extraction using a C18-bonded phase extraction column.

Caution: Remember that this technique is not designed to be miniature column chromatography. It has been referred to as digital chromatography, step chromatography, and stop-and-go chromatography, the idea being that the compounds should not be constantly moving down the column.

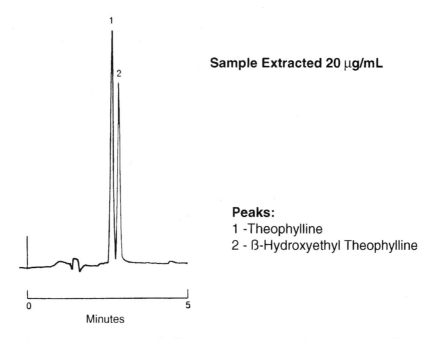

Sample Extracted 20 µg/mL

Peaks:
1 -Theophylline
2 - ß-Hydroxyethyl Theophylline

Fig. 10. The extraction of tyeophylline from serum or plasma using a diatomaceous earth SPE column.

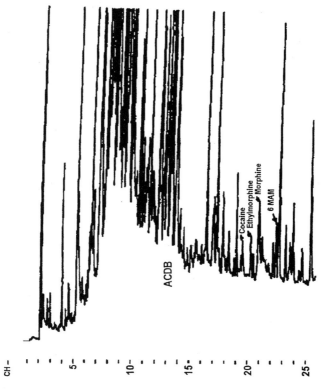

Fig. 11. The extraction of opiates from urine using a C18 SPE column.

Table 3
SPE Method for Opiates in Urine Using a C18 Column (Reversed Phase Separation)

1. COLUMN CONDITIONING STEPS
    a. Wash column with 2 × 3 mL of methanol.
    b. Wash column with 2 × 3 mL of water.
    c. Wash column with 2 × 5 mL of water adjusted to pH 9.5 with NH₄OH.
2. SAMPLE ADJUSTMENT STEPS
    a. Adjust 10 mL of urine to pH 9.5 with 1 mL of saturated NH₄CL and NH₄OH.
    b. Vortex, centrifuge, and discard the precipitate.
3. SAMPLE ADDITION
    a. Add the urine to CLEAN-UP® column CEC18111 at a rate of 1.0 mL/min.
4. COLUMN WASH
    a. Wash column with 2 × 5 mL of distilled water.
5. DRY COLUMN
    a. Pull dry air at >1.0 mL/min through the column for 15–30 min.
6. ELUTION STEPS
    a. Elute column with 2 × 750 µL of 50:50 dichloromethane-acetone.
    b. Evaporate to dryness.
7. DERIVATIZE
    a. Derivatize with 1% trimethylchlorosilane (TMCS) in N,O-bis(trimethylsilyl)tri-fluoroacetamide (BSTFA).
8. INJECTION
    a. Inject 1.0 µL onto GC with nitrogen phosphorous detection (NPD).

In SPE, compounds should be retained and released-although this is an ideal situation, which is not always attained, changing the elution solvents can help approach the ideal situation in all cases.

A typical Solid Phase Extraction (SPE) procedure is outlined in Table 3.

1.5.1 Hydrophobic Extraction Columns

Hydrophobic or reversed phase is the mechanism that partitions a non-polar analyte functional group from a polar matrix or solvent. The non-polar group is attached by "Van Der Waal's" or dispersive forces to the sorbent until a more favorable solvent will carry the analyte off the sorbent. Figure 12 shows a typical syringe barrel configured C18 bonded SPE column. Figure 13 shows an example of hydrophobic bonding. Figure 14 shows and example of a hydrophobic phase.

This sorbent is composed of a silica backbone bonded with hydrocarbon chains. It is used to extract compounds, which exhibit non-polar or neutral characteristics out of complex matrices. The C18 phase is the most widely used for non-polar interactions because of its non-selective nature; C18 will extract a large number of compounds with differing chemical properties. To enhance selectivity, manufacturers offer a wide range of hydrophobic sorbents, from C2 to C30. Multiple chain configurations are available for some sorbents (e.g., butyl vs t-butyl). Endcapped or unendcapped sorbents are available for all chain lengths. Table 4 gives examples of typical analytes and the washed and Elution solvents of hydrophobic phases. Table 5 gives the varied functional groups that can be attached to silica to give a hydrophobic sorbent.

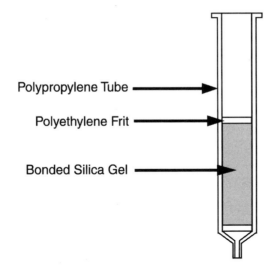

Fig. 12. A typical syringe barrel configuration of an SPE column.

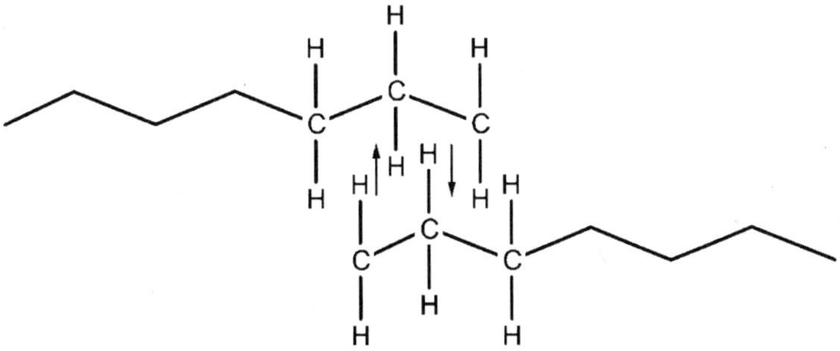

Fig. 13. An example of hydrophobic bonding.

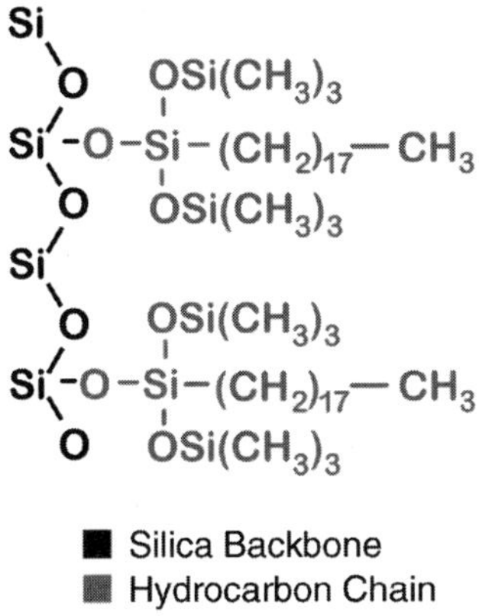

■ Silica Backbone
▨ Hydrocarbon Chain

Fig. 14. An example of a hydrophobic phase.

Table 4
Typical Analytes and Wash and Elution Solvents of Hydrophobic Phases

Analytes[a]	Washes	Elutions
Alkanes	Aqueous,	
Alkenes	usually with	Nonpolar
Aromatics	some polar	to
Neutral compounds	Organic solvents	polar organic

[a]Typical compounds that can be extracted using hydrophobic columns.

Table 5
Hydrophobic Sorbents and Structures

Sorbent	Structure
C2 ethyl	$SiCH_2CH_3$
C3 propyl	$Si(CH_2)_2CH_3$
C4 n-butyl	$Si(CH_2)_3CH_3$
iC4 isobutyl	$SiCH_2CH(CH_3)_2$
tC4 tertiary butyl	$SiC(CH_3)_3$
C5 pentyl	$Si(CH_2)_4CH_3$
C6 hexyl	$Si(CH_2)_5CH_3$
C7 heptyl	$Si(CH_2)_6CH_3$
C8 octyl	$Si(CH_2)_7CH_3$
C10 decyl	$Si(CH_2)_9CH_3$
C12 dodecyl	$Si(CH_2)_{11}CH_3$
C18 octadecyl	$Si(CH_2)_{17}CH_3$
C20 eicosyl	$Si(CH_2)_{19}CH_3$
C30 tricontyl	$Si(CH_2)_{29}CH_3$
Cyclohexyl	SiC_6H_{11}
Phenyl	SiC_6H_5

Compounds are retained by non-polar interactions from polar solvents or matrix environments (*see* Figure 15) they are bound by dispersion forces/van der Waals forces. Elution, or disruption of the nonpolar interactions is achieved by solvents or solvent mixtures with sufficient non-polar character. Some polar solvents, such as acetonitrile have enough non-polar characteristics to disrupt non-polar binding and cause elution of a compound from the sorbent. Methanol can be used as well, although it should be noted that methanol would take off both polar and non-polar analytes of interest and causes interferences.

1.5.3 Unendcapped vs Endcapped Columns

Bonded phases are manufactured by the reaction of organosilanes with activated silica. During the polymerization reaction of carbon chains to the silica backbone, a very stable silyl ether linkage forms. Unendcapped columns (Figure 16) allow hydroxyl sites to remain, thus making these columns slightly hydrophilic.

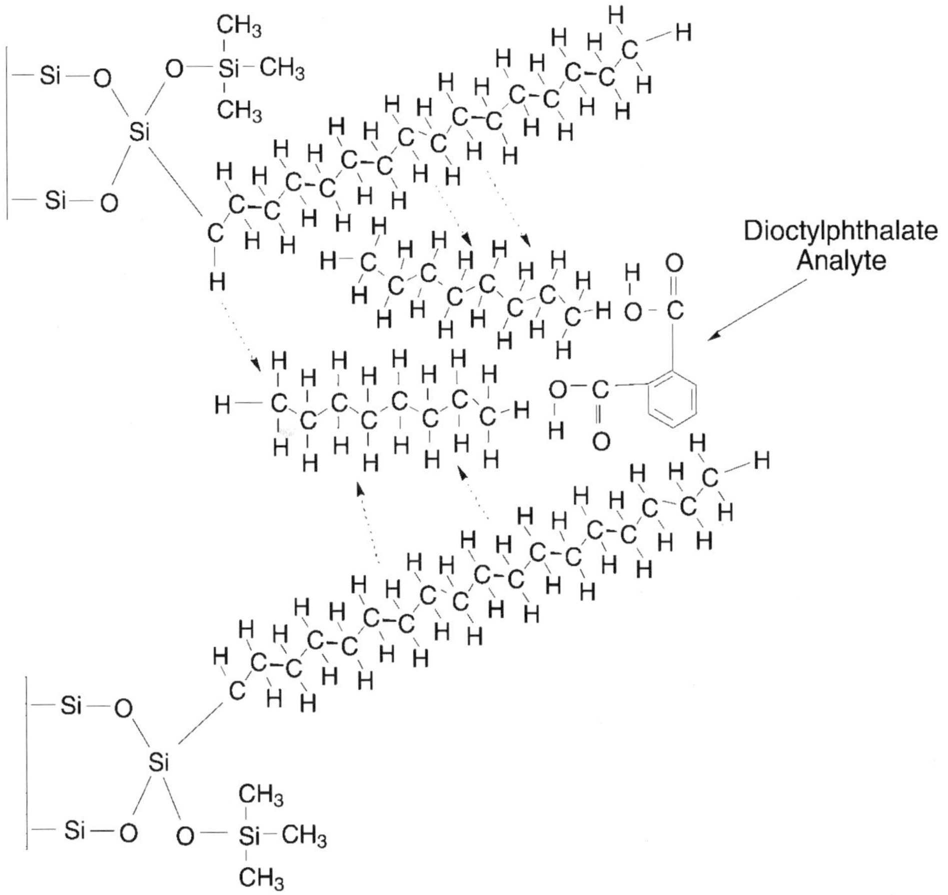

Fig. 15. The mechanism of hydrophobic interaction.

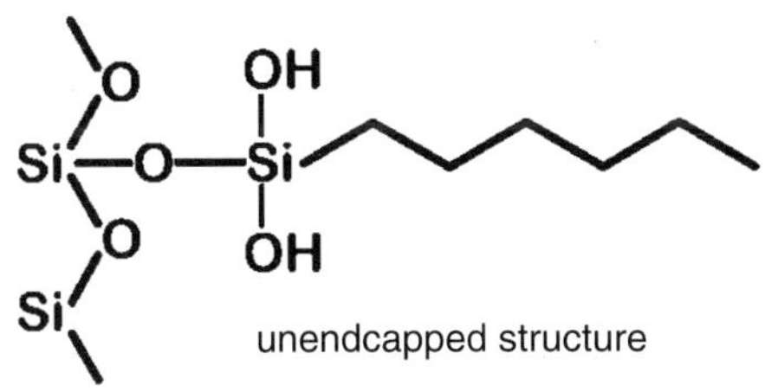

unendcapped structure

Fig. 16. The structure of an unendcapped structure site.

To decrease this slight polarity, these hydroxyl sites are deactivated. Proprietary bonding techniques ensure that these sites are 100% reacted, leading to a complete endcapping. Because there are no hydroxyl sites left, our endcapped columns (Figure 17) are more hydrophobic than our unendcapped columns.

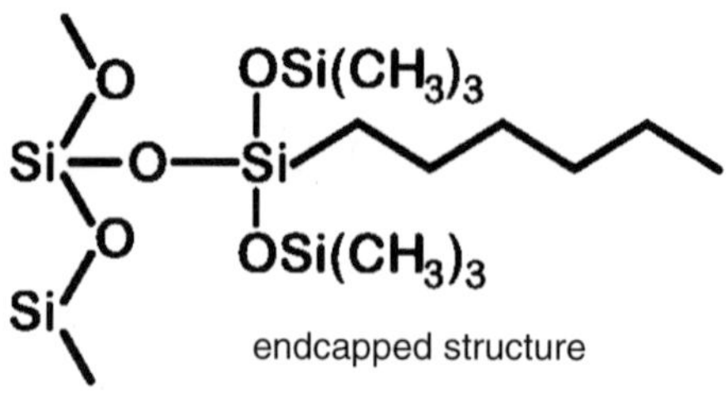

Fig. 17. The structure of an endcapped extraction column.

Table 6
Typical Analytes and Wash and Elution Solvents of Hydrophilic Phases

Analytes[a]	Washes	Elutions
R-OH, R-SH	Nonpolar organic	Polar organic
R-NH$_2$	solvents	solvent
R$_2$-NH	e.g., hexane/ethyl acetate (80:20)	Usually with
R$_3$-N	methylene chloride	some aqueous

[a]Typical compounds that can be extracted using hydrophilic columns

Table 7
Hydrophilic Sorbents and Structures

Sorbent	Structure
Silica	SiOH
Diol	Si(CH$_2$)$_3$OCH$_3$CHOHCH$_2$OH
Cyanopropyl	Si(CH$_2$)$_3$CN

Note: If un-ionized, ion-exchange sorbents can be used as hydrophilic (polar) sorbents.

1.5.4 Hydrophilic Extraction Columns

A hydrophilic sorbent is composed of a silica backbone bonded with carbon chains containing polar functional groups. Groups, which will possess such polarity, include amines, hydroxyls, and carbonyls. Table 6 gives examples of typical analyes and the wash and elution solvents of hydrophilic phases. Table 7 gives examples of hydrophilic sorbents and their structures. Figure 18 shows the structure of a hydrophilic extraction sorbent. In this case the sorbent is a diol phase.

1.5.5 Mechanism of Hydrophilic Bonding

Compounds are retained on hydrophilic sorbents through polar interactions, including hydrogen bonding, pi–pi or dipole–dipole interaction. These types of interactions occur when a distribution of electrons between individual atoms in functional groups is unequal, causing negative and positive polarity. Compounds typically extracted on a hydrophilic column include analytes that have polar groups, including amines, hydroxyls and carbonyls. Elution is performed by strong polar solvents. Figure 19 shows the mechanism of a hydrophilic extraction.

1.5.6 Ion-Exchange Principles

Along with structural data, ionization data is probably the most useful data you have to help you in doing solid phase extraction on charged compounds.

Although the following review is very fundamental, the principles reviewed apply directly to solid phase extraction in terms of weak and strong ion-exchange packings. Since the majority of drugs that you will encounter will be weak acids or bases these principles of ionization will have direct bearing on how well you can get an extraction column to perform in the ion-exchange mode.

1.5.6.1 pH

Water, as you recall, dissociates to form hydronium ions and hydroxide ions.

$$2 \, H_2O \rightleftharpoons [H_3O^+] + [OH^-]$$

In water this dissociation occurs in only a very small amount. (10^{-7} moles/L) in one liter of water). This means there are 10^{-7} mol of hydrogen ions and 10^{-7} mol of hydroxyl ions.

The chemical shorthand for 10^{-7} mol of hydrogen ions is pH 70. At pH 7.0 the concentration of hydrogen ions and hydroxyl ions are equal and in equilibrium with un-ionized water molecules. This equilibrium point, pH 7.0, is referred to as neutral on our measurement scale.

Referring to the Brönstead-Lowry theory, an acid is a substance that donates a hydrogen ion to an acceptor substance, called a base. The relative strength of acids is determined by the extent to which they dissociate in water. The dissociation of strong acids such as $HClO_4$, HNO_3, H_2SO_4, HCl, HBr, and HI in water is virtually complete. A typical strong acid-base reaction is that of hydrochloric acid (HC1) with water shown in the following equation.

$$HCl \, (aq) + H_2O \, (l) \rightleftharpoons H_3O^+ \, (aq) + Cl^- \, (aq)$$

In this reaction, HCl, the acid, donates a hydrogen ion (H^+, a proton) to a water molecule, the base. The products of the reaction are a hydronium ion (H_3O^+) and a chloride ion (Cl^-).

Weak acids on the other hand dissociate to a much lesser extent. The extent of the dissociation of any weak acid in water is indicated by the magnitude of its acid dissociation constant (K_a), which is the equilibrium constant for the dissociation reaction for that acid.

The reaction for a typical weak acid is that of acetic acid, as shown in the following equation.

$$CH_3COOH \, (aq) + H_2O \, (l) \rightleftharpoons H_3O^+ \, (aq) + CH3COO^- \, (aq)$$

In this reaction, an acetic acid molecule (CH_3COOH) becomes an acetate ion (CH_3COO^-) when it donates a proton to a water molecule, forming a hydroxium ion (H_3O^+). This dissociation occurs only to the extent of 1%.

Table 8
Acid Dissociation Constants
for Some Weak Acids at 25°C

Acetic acid	1.7×10^{-5}
Boric acid	5.8×10^{-10}
Chloroacetic acid	1.4×10^{-3}
Crotonic acid	2.0×10^{-5}
Formic acid	1.8×10^{-4}
Hydrogen carbonate ion	4.8×10^{-11}
Dihydrogen phosphate ion	6.2×10^{-8}
Hydrogen phosphate ion	1.7×10^{-12}
Hydrogen sulfite ion	5.6×10^{-8}
Propionic acid	1.4×10^{-5}

The acid dissociation constant expression for CH_3COO^- is shown as follows.

$$K_a = \frac{[H_3O^+]\,[CH_3COO^-]}{[CH_3COOH]}$$

The square brackets [ ] indicate the molar concentration (mol L-1) of the species in the brackets.

Table 8 demonstrates the expected degree of ionization for some weak acids. The degree of ionization of your compound is directly related to the structure of the compound and the pH at which you do your extraction. This will ultimately affect the recovery of your drug. Figures 20 and 21 show the titration curves of the pK_a for acidic and neutral dugs and for basic drugs. The pK_a is the pH midway up the deflection in the titration curve. It is extremely important to know the pK_a of your compound. If multiple pK_as exist, be sure to use the extreme values to adjust your elution solvents. Keep in mind that to get approximately 100% ionization you must be 2 full pH units above the appropriate pK_a of the compound for acids 2 full pH units below for basic drugs.

1.5.6.2 pK_a

pK_a can be defined as the pH at which the analyte is 50% ionized (equilibrium), pKa is a very important concept in the ion-exchange mode of solid phase extraction and directly affects the extraction of the compounds of interest. Acidic compounds are negatively charged above their pK_a. Basic compounds are positively charged below their pK_a. A comprehensive listing of drug pK_a values is included in Appendix G.

Table 9 is a useful summary of various elements of ion-exchange extraction concepts. If you understand the summary you will be able to move around in the area of ion-exchange SPE very easily.

1.5.7 Ion-Exchange Extraction Columns

An ion-exchange sorbent is composed of a silica backbone bonded with a carbon chain terminated by a negatively or positively charged functional group. Ion-exchange interactions occur between a sorbent that carries a charge and a compound of opposite

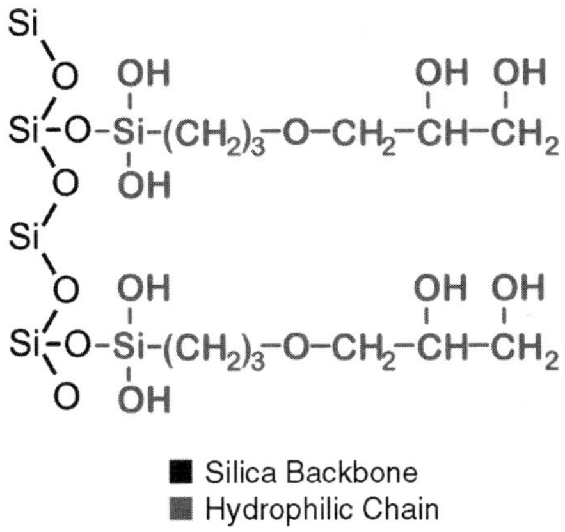

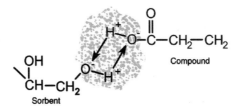

Fig. 18. The structure of a hydrophilic extraction column.

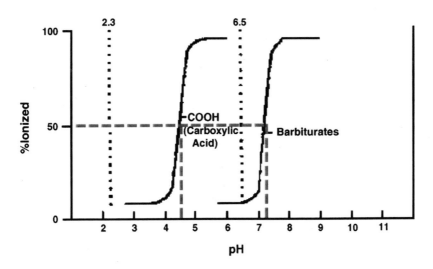

Fig. 19. The mechanism of hydrophilic interaction.

Fig. 20. The titration curves of the pK$_a$'s for acidic and neutral drugs.

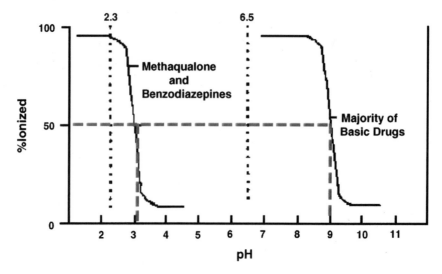

Fig. 21. The titration curves of the pK$_a$'s for basic drugs.

Table 9
Ion-Exchange Extraction Concepts

	Anion-Exchange Sorbent		Cation-Exchange Sorbent	
	Goal	pH	Goal	pH
Wash	To promote bonding between sorbent and analyte	>Analyte pK$_a$ or <Sorbent pK$_a$	To promote bonding between sorbent and analyte	<Analyte pK$_a$ or >Sorbent pK$_a$
Elution	To disrupt bonding between sorbent and analyte	<Analyte pK$_a$ or >Sorbent pK$_a$	To disrupt bonding between sorbent and analyte	>Analyte pK$_a$ or <Sorbent pK$_a$

Percent of Compound in Ionic State					
		pH units away from pK$_a$			
Functionality	Ionization State	2 < pK$_a$	1 < pK$_a$	At pK$_a$	1 < pK$_a$	2 < pK$_a$
Acid	Anionic (−)	1	9	50	91	99
Base	Cationic (+)	99	91	50	9	1

charge. This electrostatic interaction is reversible by neutralizing the sorbent and/or analyte. Ion-exchange bonds can also be disrupted by introduction of a "counter-ion" to compete with the analyte for binding sites on the sorbent.

1.5.8 Mechanism of Ion-Exchange Bonding

Compounds are retained on the sorbent through ionic bonds. Therefore it is essential that the sorbent and the analyte to be extracted be charged. Generally, the number of molecules with charged cationic groups increases at pH values below the molecules pK_a value. The number of molecules with charged anionic groups decreases at pH values below the molecule's pK_a value. To ensure 99% or more ionization, the pH should be at least two pH units below the pK_a of the cation and two pH units above the pK_a of the anion. Elution occurs by using a solvent to raise the pH above the pK_a of the cationic group or to lower the pH below the pK_a of the anion to disrupt retention. At this point, the sorbent or compound will be neutralized.

1.5.9 Types of Ion-Exchange

Ionic interactions occur between charged sorbent and analyte of opposite charge. The pH is manipulated to ionize analytes functional group. Ionic bonds are strong and retain analytes. Hydrophobic interferences can be washed away with organic solvents. Polar interferences can be removed with aqueous or weak aqueous/organic washes. Elution solvents contain stronger counter-ions or bring about changes in pH.

Ionic/hydrophobic analytes can be eluted by simultaneously disrupting both interactions. There are basically three types of ion-exchange mechanisms. (1). Cation exchange, (2). Anion-exchange, and (3). Copolymeric mixed-mode ion-exchange. Figure 22 shows a dichotomous key that can be used to determine which ion-exchange column is the best for your application. Table 10 shows a list of common ion-exchange sorbents and their structures. Table 11 shows typical analytes, washes, and elution solvents for ion-exchange bonding.

1.5.10 Cation Exchange Extractions

Cation-exchange sorbents are negatively charged while basic analytes are manipulated to carry a positive charge. Opposites attract, forming strong bonds. Common cationic sorbents are benzenesulfonic acid (strong), propylsulfonic acid (strong), and carboxylic acid (weak).

Analytes extracted on cation exchange packings are positively charged. This can be amine-containing compounds or positively charged metal ions. Typical applications include basic drugs, catecholamine, pharmaceuticals, herbicides, and the like. These extractions are normally done out of aqueous matrices. A basic elution solvent is used to neutralize the analyte.

Figure 23 shows an example of a cation exchange phase.

1.5.11 Anion-Exchange Extractions

Anion-exchange sorbents are positively charged, whereas acidic analytes are manipulated to carry negative charges. Again, opposites attract forming strong bonds. Typical anion-exchange sorbents include primary, secondary amine (weak), aminopropyl (weak), diethylamino (weak), and quaternary amine (strong). Typical

Table 10
Ion-Exchange Sorbents and Structures

Sorbent	Structure	pK$_a$
Anion-exchangers		
Aminopropyl (1 amine)	$Si(CH_2)_3NH_2$	9.8
N-2-aminoethyl (2 amine)	$Si(CH_2)_3NH_2^+(CH_2)_2NH_2$	10.1, 10.9
Diethylamino (3 amine)	$Si(CH_2)_3NH+(CH_2CH_3)_2$	10.6
Quaternary Amine (4 amine)	$Si(CH_2)_3N+(CH_3)_3$	Always charged
Cation Exchangers		
Propylsulfonic Acid	$Si(CH_2)_3SO_3H$	<1
Benzenesulfonic Acid	$Si(CH_2)_2SO_3H$	Always charged
Carboxylic acid	$SiCH_2COOH$	4.8

Notes: In an un-ionized state, these sorbents are hydrophilic (polar) sorbents. In the case of weak ion-exchangers, neutralization can occur on either the sorbent or the analyte of interest. Either will disrupt the bond of the desired compound. In the case of strong ion-exchangers, neutralization can occur only on the analyte.

Table 11
Typical Analytes, Washes,
and Elution Solvents for Ion-Exchange Bonding

Analytes[a]	Washes	Elutions
Anions	Organic solvent or aqueous buffer at pH that allows the ion to remain charged	Organic solvent and aqueous buffer at pH that would neutralize the ion
Cations	AND/OR at a low ionic strength AND/OR at a weak concentration	AND/OR at a high ionic strength AND/OR at a strong concentration

[a]Typical compounds that can be extracted using ion-exchange.

analytes extracted include phosphates, carboxylic acids, and sulphonic acids (cations). Applications of the anion-exchange include phosphates, acidic drugs, organic acids, vitamins, and the like.

These extractions are normally done out of aqueous matrices. Acidic elutions are used to neutralize the analytes of interest.

Figure 24 shows an example of an anion-exchange phase.

1.5.12 Copolymeric Ion-Exchange

Copolymeric ion-exchange sorbents have both hydrophobic and ionic retention mechanisms. They consist of silica backbones with both reverse phase and ion-exchange functionality. They can be applied to acidic, neutral, and basic analytes.

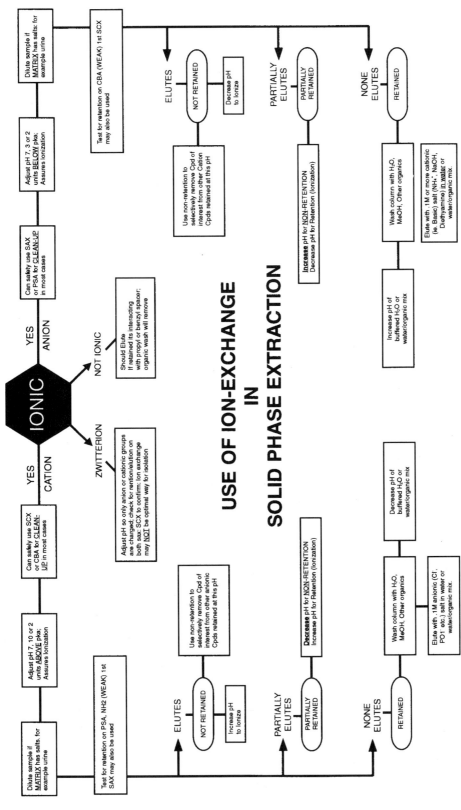

Fig. 22. A dichotomous key that can be used to determine which ion-exchange column is best for your application.

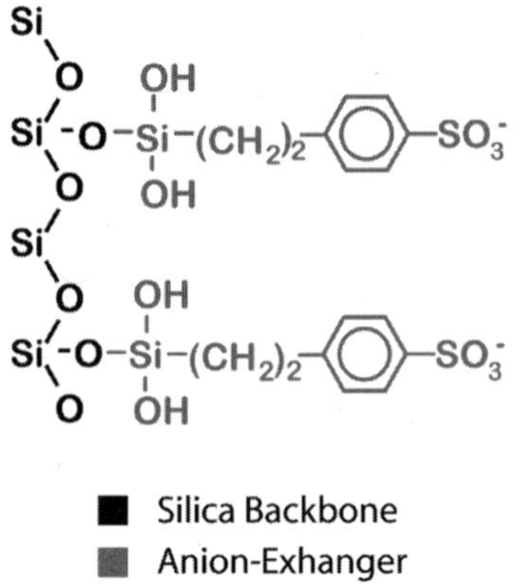

Fig. 23. An example of he structure of a cation-exchange phase.

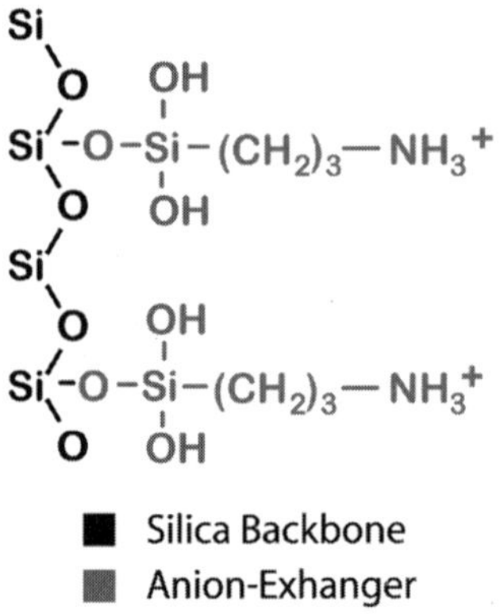

Fig. 24. An example of the structure of an anion-exchange phase.

These materials have found a lot of use in drug abuse applications, where wide ranges of components need to be extracted in a single procedure. Selective elution allows for the removal of interferences. This technique allows for the fast back-extractions on the column. Acids, neutrals, polar compounds, and bases can be class separated on a single column. These extractions are normally done in aqueous systems using selective washes. Elution solvents are solvent mixtures of organic solvents with acids or bases added. This provides for superior sample clean up.

Figures 25 and 26 show the chemical structures of two popular sorbents used for copolymeric ion-exchange.

Although most ion-exchange occurs out of aqueous systems ion-exchange can be accomplished out of organic solvents such as methanol or ethyl acetate, as long as the analyte can be pH adjusted to make it ionic.

1.5.13 Specialty Anion-Exchange Columns

Ion-exchange columns possess charged functional groups, which allow analytes to bind upon sample application. Prior to column use, these groups require counter-ions at these charged sites. The standard counter-ion for cation exchangers is the

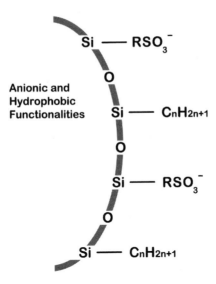

Fig. 25. An example of a cationic copolymeric ion-exchange.

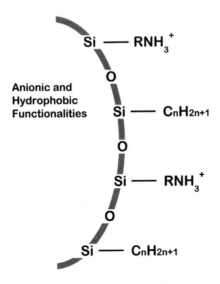

Fig. 26. An example of an anionic copolymeric ion-exchange.

hydronium ion and for anion-exchangers is the chloride ion. From time to time during sample application, a charged analyte is not strong enough to displace the counter-ion and therefore does not bind to the column. In cases such as these, a weaker counter-ion is required. Two such columns with weaker counterions—quaternary amine with acetate counter-ion and quaternary amine with hydroxide counter-ion—are commercially available. In terms of strength, the acetate ion is stronger than the hydroxide

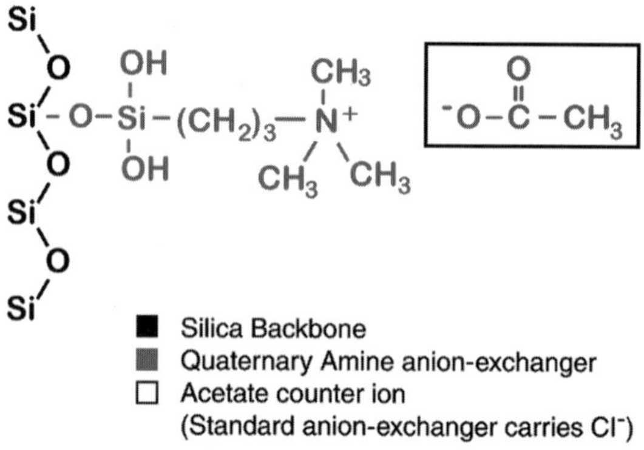

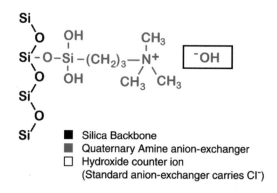

Fig. 27. An example of an acetate counter-ion on an anion-exchange.

Fig. 28. An example of a hydroxide counter-ion on an anion-exchanger.

ion. Figure 27 shows an example of an acetate counterion on the anion-exchanger and Figure 28 a hydroxide counter-ion on the anion-exchanger.

Table 12 lists relative counter-ion selectivities.

1.5.14 Ion-Exchange Issues

Ion-exchange is most frequently done in aqueous systems. However, ion-exchange can also be done effectively out of an organic solvent system. The major key to success in ion-exchange is being certain you are far enough away from the pK_a to get 100% elution or retention. It is sometimes difficult to measure pH in organic solvents but it can be done. When measuring pH in aqueous systems use a pH meter instead of pH paper, as the range of the paper is probably too broad to depend on.

The pH of a solution may not be what you think it is. A common error is to adjust pH upward using ammonium oxide (NH_4OH) in an attempt to reach pH 11.0–12.0. If the NH_4OH is old or if there is less than half a bottle left, the NH_3 will evaporate and the best you will be able to do is pH 8.0–9.0. This will show up as two problems: (1) variable recovery from run to run (2) loss of recovery of the analyte of interest. The

Table 12
Relative Counter-Ion Selectivity

Strong Cation Exchanger		Strong Anion-Exchanger	
Cations		Anions	
Ba^{2+}	8.7	Benzene Sulfonate	500
Ag^{2+}	7.6	Citrate	220
Pb^{2+}	7.5	I⁻	175
Hg^{2+}	7.2	Phenate⁻	110
Cu^{2+}	5.3	HSO	85
Sr^{2+}	4.9	ClO	74
Ca^{2+}	3.9	NO	65
Ni^{2+}	3.0	Br⁻	50
Cd^{2+}	2.9	CN⁻	28
Cu^{2+}	2.9	HSO⁻	27
CO^{2+}	2.8	BrO	27
Zn^{2+}	2.7	NO_2	24
Cs^{2+}	2.7	Cl⁻	22
Rb^+	2.6	HCO_3	6.0
K^+	2.5	IO_3	5.5
Fe^{2+}	2.5	Formate	4.6
Mg^{2+}	2.5	Acetate⁻	3.2
Mn^{2+}	2.3	Propionate⁻	2.6
NH^{4+}	1.9	F⁻	1.6
Na^+	1.5	OH⁻	1.0
H^+	1.0		
Li^+	0.8		

Larger numbers reflect greater ability of the ion to displace other ionic materials from the bonded surfaces.

solution to this problem is to buy smaller bottles of NH_4OH so it doesn't stand on the shelf for extended periods of time and to prepare solutions only for what you expect to use that day.

In preparing solutions such as methylene chloride/isopropanol/ammonium hydroxide, add the ammonium hydroxide to the isopropanol first, and then add the mix to the methylene chloride. If you do not do it in this fashion you may get a separation of the solvents into two layers. Of all the problems chromatographers have with ion-exchange the pH of the elution solvents is the problem 90% of the time. This is especially true when compounds like morphine or benzoylecgonine (whose pK_a is above 9) are extracted on strong cation exchange columns.

When using ion-exchangers, capacity is not determined purely by the organic loading of the phase, although it is related to it. When determining how much compound an ion-exchanger will hold, you need to know what its milliequivalence is. This is a calculation of the charge-to-mass ratio of the packing material.

Milliequivalent and millimole calculations can be seen in Appendix D.

1.5.14.1 Strong Ion-Exchangers vs Weak Ion-Exchangers

Strong ion-exchangers are charged across the entire pH range. Therefore, the only neutralization that can be done to release a compound is the neutralization of the charge on the compound itself. When you put a strong acid or base on a strong anion or cation exchanger you have no way to break the ionic bond since both sorbent and analyte are always charged. In this situation your compound simply goes on and never comes off.

For this reason we usually use weak ion-exchangers on strong acids and bases. Weak ion-exchangers are only charged in a given pH range and can be neutralized to release strong anions and cations. When using weak ion-exchangers with weak acids or bases, we can choose to neutralize either the compounds themselves or the packing depending on what conditions we hope to achieve in the final elution.

1.5.15 The Use of Copolymeric Bonded Phases to Enhance the Recovery and Selectivity of Drugs of Abuse and Their Metabolites

Previous attempts to extract drugs of abuse from a single aliquot of urine have met with various obstacles. When hydrophobic phases such as C18 or XAD-2 are used, all three classes of drugs are eluted together, exhibit poor extraction efficiencies when selectively eluted, or require matrix optimization for each class, precluding a single extraction. Unfortunately, the nonspecific nature of these materials causes the eluate to contain many other urinary constituents that often interfere with the compounds of interest.

These interferences are readily observed on a gas chromatograph when nonselective detection is used. The most common sample preparation method for extracting all classes of drugs from one aliquot of urine is liquid–liquid extraction. The drawbacks to this procedure include long analysis times, the need for large solvent volumes, and low drug recovery.

The sample preparation method described in this booklet uses a copolymeric bonded phase column to extract acidic, neutral, and basic drugs from a single aliquot of urine. Following sample preparation, the extract were analyzed by a variety of analytical techniques, including wide-bore capillary gas chromatography (CG) with flame ionization detection, NPD detection, and GC mass spectroscopy. The extracts were clean, detection limits were at least 100 ng/mL, and recoveries generally exceeded 93% for all drugs at urine concentrations of 100 to 1000 ng/mL.

The concept of copolymeric bonded silicas for sample preparation has pioneered a new generation of hybrid extraction sorbents. The column used in this work was designed to be both hydrophobic and ionic, thus providing several primary retention mechanisms. By matrix and sorbent manipulations, drug classes can be quantitatively isolated, then selectively eluted for chromatographic analysis.

The concept of solid phase sample preparation is one consisting of two unique events: the retention of the compound of interest on the extraction column followed by the selective elution of the compound in a purified, concentrated state. Until now, a single bonded moiety has had the responsibility of both retaining the compound of interest and offering a selective elution profile. A trade-off of recovery versus selectivity was encountered.

New bonding techniques allow for the placement of copolymers on the silica particle. This surface is useful in that one bonded moiety can be used for the retention of the compound out of the matrix, while the other bonded moiety can be used for extremely selective elution profiles.

1.5.16 Copolymeric Bonded Phases for Drug Abuse Testing

Analytical demand for more efficient, robust and clean extraction of drugs from biological matrices led to the development of copolymeric mixed-mode sorbents (Table 13). SPE columns that are true copolymeric sorbents are those containing hydrophobic and ion-exchange functional groups uniquely polymerized to a silica substrate, and not simply two or more packings physically blended together. The design and quality provide superior sample clean up, recovery and reproducibility. Table 14 shows typical analytes, wash solvents, and elution solvents used with copolymeric phases.

Mixed-mode separations allow maximum selectivity for extraction of acids, neutrals, and bases. This selectivity is ideal for both screening and confirmation analysis for virtually all drug categories. CLEAN SCREEN DAU, THC and GHB columns are used extensively by forensic and clinical chemists for applications including postmortem investigations, criminal investigations, urine drug testing, athletic drug testing, racing laboratories, therapeutic drug monitoring, medical drug screening. Using this new technology, one can utilize several different chemical characteristics of compounds to be isolated to reproduce very clean extractions.

If performing extractions out of viscous matrices such as tissue or horse urine, the XtrackT high-flow/gravity flow columns are used. The CLEAN SCREEN DAU chemistry is available in this larger particle size.

Copolymers allow for the extraction and "back-extraction" on the same column with nothing more than a change of solvents. The chemistries for making highly specific copolymeric phases have been developed over the past several years and have yielded some unique results. In essence, what has been done is to use copolymers to enhance and improve on mixed mechanisms that have been known for quite some time. In the past, these mixed mechanisms have been looked at as somewhat problematic rather than being exploited as additional tools for improved selectivity and recovery.

1.5.17 Copolymeric Extraction Columns
(Ion-Exchange with Hydrophobic Character)

This sorbent is composed of a silica backbone with two types of functional chains attached: an ion-exchanger or polar chain and a hydrophobic carbon chain. These copolymeric phases are produced in a way that allows for equal parts of each functional group to attach to the silica backbone. This polymerization technique yields reproducible bonded phases and unique copolymeric chemistries, which allow the controlled use of mixed-mode separation mechanisms. This type of dual chemistry is beneficial especially when one is looking for both a neutral and a charged compound. This is common when a neutral parent drug metabolizes and becomes a charged compound.

Figure 29 shows an example of a copolymeric phase containing a weak anion-exchanger and a hydrophilic phase. Table 15 shows a list of commercially available

Table 13
Typed of Mixed Mechanisms

Type of phase	Mechanisms
Hydrophobic phases, endcapped	Normal and reverse phase adsorption
Hydrophobic phases, unendcapped	Normal and reversed phase adsorption
Polar phases, endcapped	Selective adsorption
Polar phases, unendcapped	Normal and reverse phase adsorption
Hydrophilic ion-exchange phases	Ion exchange Normal and reversed phase adsorption
Hydrophobic ion-exchange phases	Ion exchange Normal and reversed phase adsorption
Copolymeric Phases	
	Selective
Hydrophilic copolymers	normal phase
Hydrophobic copolymers	reverse-phase
Endcapped copolymers	adsorption, ion-exchange

Table 14
Typical Analytes, Washes, and Elution Solvents of Copolymeric Phases

1. Analytes[a]	2. Washes	3. Elutions
Cations/anions Alkanes Alkenes Aromatics	a) Aqueous to disrupt hydrophilic interactions b) Methanol to disrupt residual hydrophobic and hydrophilic interferences	a) Organic, possibly with some aqueous to elute hydrophobically bound analytes b) Aqueous buffer with a pH that would neutralize ionically bound analytes or an aqueous with high ionic strength or a solvent with a counter-ion that would bind to sorbent.

[a]Typical compounds that can be extracted using copolymeric columns.

copolymeric phases and the functional groups attached. Other copolymeric phases are available, but these are the more common ones.

Figure 30 shows an example of an amine-containing compound and its interaction with a copolymeric cation exchanger. Notice that there are three different mechanisms capable of interacting with the compound, (1) adsorption, (2) reverse phase, and (3) ion-exchange.

Table 15
Copolymeric Sorbents and Structures

Sorbent	Structure	pKa
Benzenesulfonic Acid (BCX2) strong cation exchange column	$Si(CH_2)_2SO_3H$	Always charged
Propylsulfonic acid (PCX2) strong cation exchange column	$Si(CH_2)_3 SO_3H$	<1
Carboxylic Acid (CCX2) weak cation exchange column	$Si(CH_2)_2 COOH$	4.8
Quaternary amine (QAX2) strong anion exchange column	$Si(CH_2)_3 N^+(CH_3)_3$	Always charged
Aminopropyl (NAX2) weak anion-exchange column	$Si(CH_2)_3 NH_3^+$	9.8
Cyanopropyl (CNP2) Hydrophilic exchange column	$Si(CH_2)_3CN$	
Cyclohexyl (CYH2) Hydrophobic exchange column	$Si(CH_2)$	

Each copolymeric sorbent also contains a carbon chain approximately equal to a C8 chain.

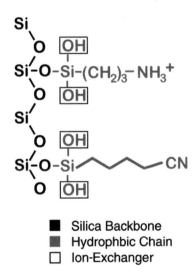

■ Silica Backbone
■ Hydrophbic Chain
□ Ion-Exchanger

Fig. 29. An example of the structure of a copolymeric ion-exchanger.

1.5.17.1 Mechanisms of Copolymeric Extraction

A sample composed of a theoretical neutral parent drug and its charged (acidic) metabolite is applied at a pH of 6.0 (Figure 31). At this pH, many amine groups are positively charged. Since the column is also positively charged, compounds with this chemistry (cations) are repelled. Depending on the pKa of the metabolite, carboxylic

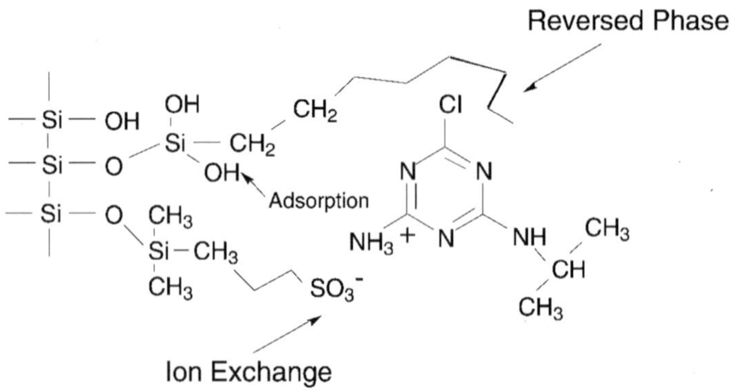

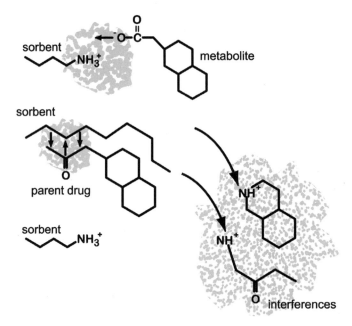

Fig. 30. An example of an amine-containing compound and its interaction with a copolymeric cation-exchanger.

Fig. 31. A neutral drug and its acidic metabolite are applied to a copolymeric anion-exchange column.

acid groups may be negatively charged, allowing the metabolite to bond to the positively charged sorbent. Since the column also possesses a hydrophobic chain, the neutral parent drug also bonds to the column. Water or a weak aqueous buffer (pH 6.0) washes away hydrophilically bound interferences (Figure 32).

The column is then dried, taking care to free the column of any residual aqueous phase that would interfere with elution of neutral drugs.

In elution 1 the hydrophobically bound neutral parent drug is eluted with a solvent of minimal polarity, such as hexane/ethyl acetate, 80:20 (Figure 33). In elution 2 (Figure 34) the final elution employs an acid to neutralize the charge of acidic analytes. Ionic interaction is released, and analytes are eluted in an appropriate solvent mixture.

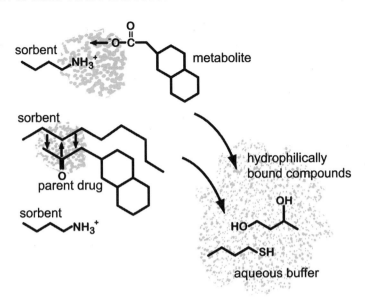

Fig. 32. Hydrophilically bound compounds are washed of the column.

1.5.17.2 Mechanism of CLEAN SCREEN

When a sample is loaded onto the column at pH 6.0, many carboxylic acid functionalities present in the sample are not ionized. This creates an attraction between the column and both sample compounds of interest and interferences. At this pH, ibuprofen is not ionized but instead is attracted to the sorbent by both adsorption and hydrophobic interactions. At the same time, drugs with amine functionalities such as methamphetamine, adsorb onto the column via both hydrophobic and ionic attraction (Figure 35). The column can then be washed with water or weak aqueous buffers at or below pH 6.0 without risking loss of the analytes.

Cationic analytes bound to the column can be eluted after another drying step. The drying steps are necessary to remove water that would have prevented the water-immiscible elution solvents from optimally interacting with the analytes.

After drying the column, it is possible to elute the hydrophobically bound analytes using solvents of minimal polarity such as methylene chloride or a hexane/ethyl acetate mixture (elution 1 [Figure 36]). Cationic analytes will remain bound to the column. Many compounds of intermediate polarity and potential interferences will also remain on the column. The majority of these potential interferences can be removed by using a methanol wash, which at this point elutes off everything that is not ionically bound (Figure 37).

To elute the cationic analytes, an organic solution with a high pH (between 11.0 and 12.0) should be used. A methylene chloride-isopropanol-ammonium hydroxide mixture will simultaneously disrupt these ionic interactions and successfully elute the desired compound (elution 2 [Figure 38]). By using this diluted-strength elution solvent instead of MeOH/ammonium hydroxide 98:2, some of the more ionic and polar interferences will remain on the column allowing only the desired analytes to elute (Figure 37).

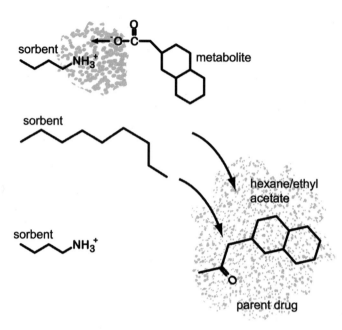

Fig. 33. The neutral parent compound is eluted off the column.

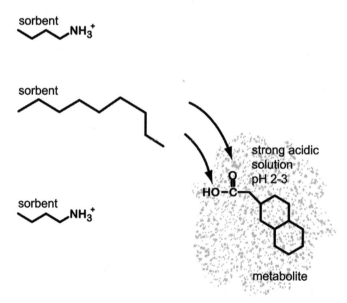

Fig. 34. The acidic metabolite is eluted from the column.

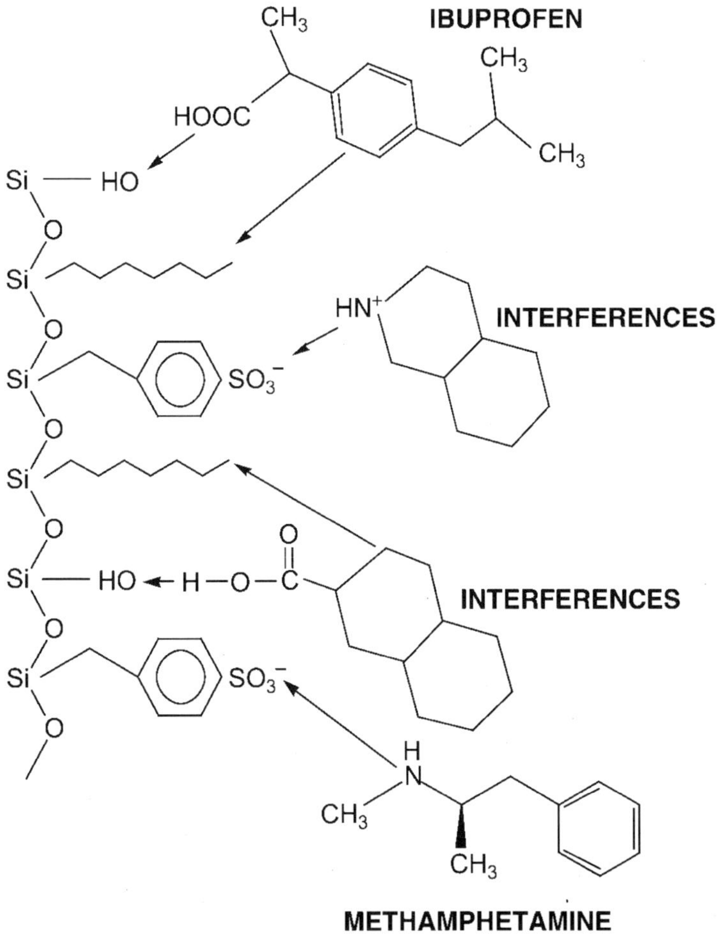

Fig. 35. A basic drug sample is loaded onto a copolymeric cation-exchange column.

1.5.17.3 Clean-Thru Tips

Clean-Thru provides the first SPE cartridge system that eliminates sample carryover from the vacuum manifold lid. The technology consists SPE columns with a disposable tip that attaches to the end of each column. This system was designed in order to meet the strict requirements that the Substance Abuse and Mental Health Services Administration certification has placed on laboratories to address the problem of cross-contamination between samples. Clean-Thru tips provide a completely disposable system that eliminates any contact between the sample, or wash solvents and the extraction apparatus. The continuous passage of the sample through the system provides a direct, accurate route to waste or collection vessels. As each extraction is completed, the column and tip are discarded as a unit. Clean-Thru eliminates concerns about sample residue remaining in the extraction system.

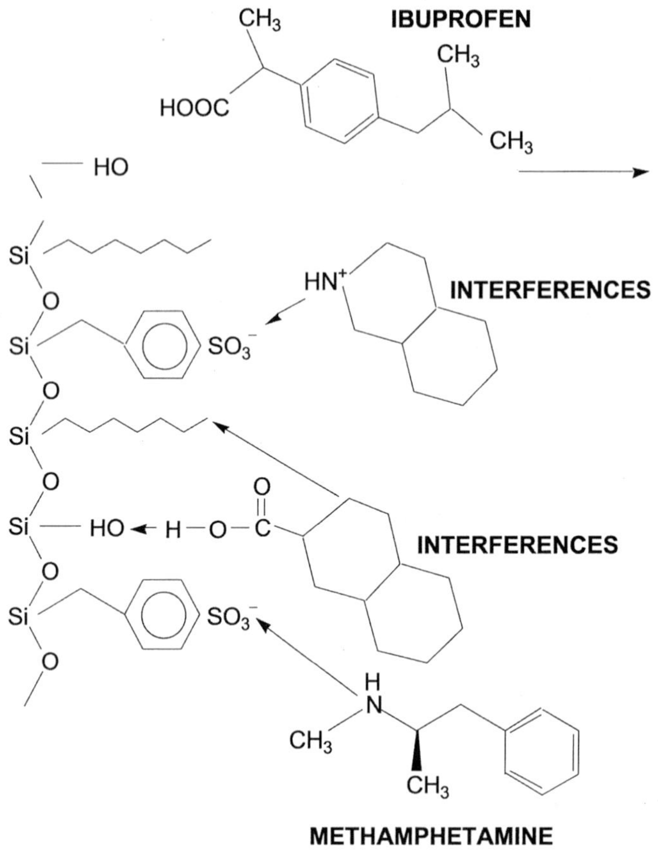

Fig. 36. Hydrophobically bound analytes are eluted with minimal polarity solvents.

1.5.17.4 Reduced Solvent Volume Extraction Columns

Reduced solvent volume (RSV) extraction columns are microbed-packed columns that offer the advantages of disc technology yet maintain the proven track record of our conventional SPE columns.

RSV columns use 75% less solvent than traditional packed columns. Less solvent means faster extractions, higher throughput and less waste disposal, which translates into significant savings in both time and money. Results demonstrate that therapeutic and abused drugs in urine and blood matrices can be extracted with cleanliness, high recoveries and consistent reproducibility by using the RSV extraction column.

RSV columns are available in both 3-mL and 10-mL configurations. These columns can be used with vacuum manifolds or positive pressure, as well as with conventional automated extraction equipment.

Table 16
Advantages of Reduced Solvent Volume Extraction

75% Reduction in total liquid volumes
- Lower cost per extraction
- Faster extraction times
- Less disposal cost
- Increased automated throughput

50% reduction in eluate volume
- Faster dry-down times
- Reduced exposure to organic solvents

Superior flow characteristics
- Less flow restriction from matrix proteins or particulates
- More reliable for automated processing

High capacity
- Greater linear range

Table 17
Solvent Reduction

Analyte	Solvent usage—RSV SPE columns	Solvent usage—traditional packed columns	% solvent reduction
Barbiturates	4.25 mL	18 mL	76%
Benzoylecgonine	4.65 mL	19 mL	76%
THC-COOH	4.85 mL	16.4 mL	73%
Phencyclidine	5.15 mL	19 mL	70%

UCT product CSDAUA*83.

The advantages of RSV columns are summarized in Table 16. The solvent reduction possible with this apparatus is given in Table 17.

Capacities are as follows:
- 91% (n4) for 1000 ng/mL
- 90% (n2) for 3000 ng/mL
- 91% (n4) for 4000 ng/mL

There is no analyte breakthrough at 1000 ng/mL and less then 0.2% analyte breakthrough at 3000 and 4000 ng/mL levels.

Recoveries are in linear ranges exhibiting 85% recoveries in urines.

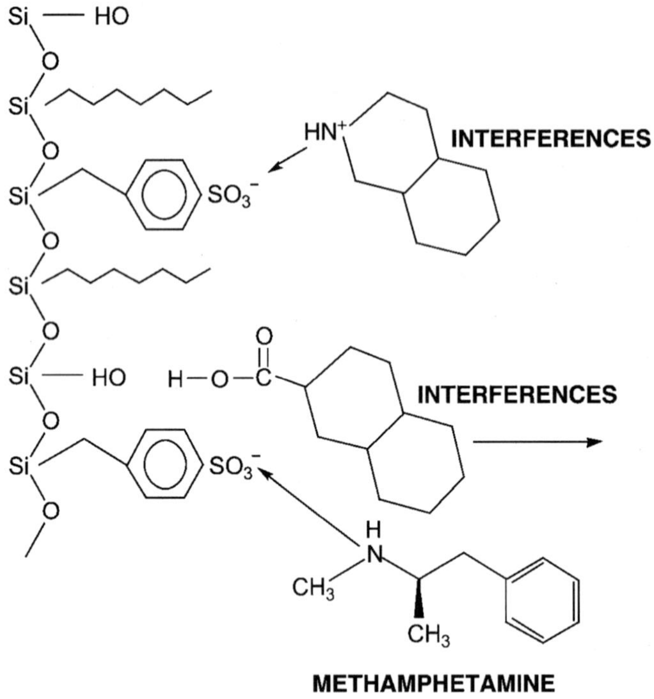

Fig. 37. Interferences are removed using a methanol wash.

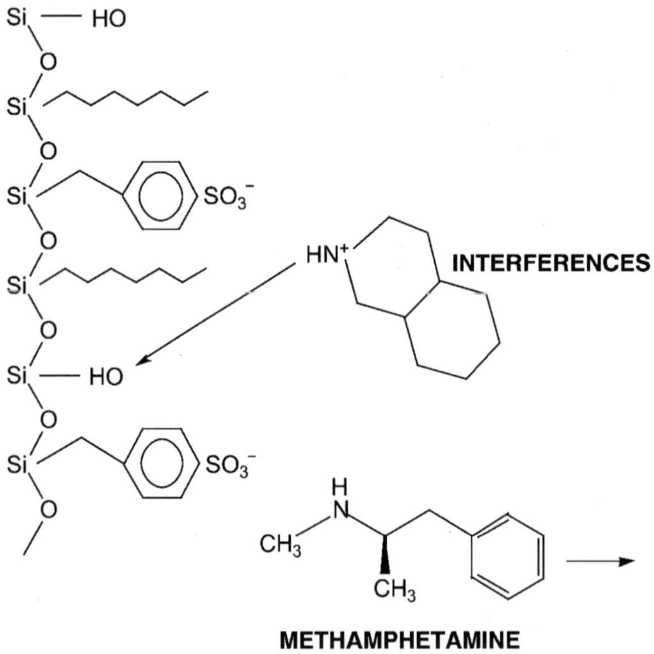

METHAMPHETAMINE

Fig. 38.

REFERENCES

[1]Runge, F. F. "Der Biddungstrieb der Stoffe," Verenschlaulicht in Selbstaqndiggewachsenen Bedern. Sebsterlag Oranenberg, Germany, 1855.

[2]Gopplestroeder, F. Verk Naturforsch. Ges. Basel 3:268, 1861.

[3]Schonbein, C. F. Verk Naturforsch. Ges. Basel 3:249, 1861.

[4]Fischer, E. and Schmidmer, E. Annalen 272:156, 1892.

[5]Reed, L. Proc. Chem. Soc. 9:123, 1893.

[6]Day, D. T. Amer. Phil. Soc. 36:112, 1897.

[7]Engler, C. and Albrecht, E. Z. Angew. Chemie 889, 1901.

[8]Tswett, M. S. Ber. Stoch. Bat. Geo. 24:384, 1906.

[9]Ibid., Ber. 64:1349, 1906.

[10]Kuhn, R. and Lederer, E. Naturwiss. 19:306, 1931.

[11]Ibid., 24:384, 1906.

[12]Martin, A. J. P. and Synge, R. L. M. Biochem. J. 35:1358, 1941.

[13]Consden, R., Gordon, A. H., and Martin, A. J. P. Biochem. J. 38:224, 1944.

[14]Hesse, G., Eilbrecht, H., Reichender, F. Liebigs Ann. Chem., 546 (1941).

[15]Kirchner, J. G., Keller, G. J. J. Am. Chem. Soc. 72:1867, 1950.

[16]James, A. T. and Martin, A. J. P. Biochem J. 50:679–690, 1952.

[17]Cramer, F. Paper Chromatography. London: Macmillan, 1959.

[18]Klesper, E., Carwin, A. H., Turner, D. A. J. Org. Chem. 27:700, 1962.

[19]Hjerten, S., Jerstedt, S., and Tiselius, A. Anal. Chem. 11:211, 1965.

[20]Halasz, I., Horvath, C. Anal. Chem. 35:499, 1963.

[21]Touchstone, J. C., Levine, S. S., and Muraweck, T. Anal. Chem. 43.

[22]Sutherland, I. A. and Ito, Y. J. High Res. Chrom., Chrom Commun. 171, 1978.

[23]Mitchell, W. and Rahn, P. Drug and Cosmetics Ind. 123(5):56–57, 1978.

[24]Kalasz, H. Nagg, J., Tyihak, E., and Mincsovics, E. J. Liquid Chrom. 3:845, 1980.

[25]Singh, K., Ashraf, M., Granley, K. J., Mishra, U., andMadhusudanarao, M. Chrom. 473:215–226, 1989.

Chapter 2

Silica-Based Solid Phase Extraction

Estimates have shown silica gel to be the base material for 90% of extraction columns manufactured. The other 10% of materials used for SPE are alumina, carbon, Fluorosil®, and synthetic polymers.

Synthetic polymers include polystyrene divinyl benzene (PSDVB), polystyrene divinyl pyrrolidone (PSPVP), and dimethyacryloxymethyl naphthalene divinyl benzene (DMN-DVB), and mixtures of these compounds to obtain the desired characteristics.

Silica gel is an amorphous, highly porous, partially hydrated form of silica (SiO_2, a substance made from the two most abundant elements on earth, silicon and oxygen). In fact, 55% of the earth's surface consists of either silica (silicon dioxide) or silicates (silica combined with metal oxides). Most of the silica found naturally is not significantly hydrated and can be in crystalline or amorphous forms. It is a simple material to characterize chemically and physically.

Silica gel has a number of distinctive properties that make it an ideal base material. It is easily made, at minimal cost, and is uniform in its properties. Silica gel has a rigid backbone, which shows little if any swelling or shrinking in a broad range of solvents. It can be cleaned easily prior to use for high-sensitivity work. Ion-exchangers on silica backbones recover quickly from changes in pH or solvent types. The hydroxyl groups on silica allow a large variety of different functional groups to be added for increasing selectivity. These various characteristics have a significant impact on how well the bonded phase packing performs as an extraction device.

The silica used for SPE extraction columns is essentially porous and noncrystalline, with the general formula $SiO_2 \times H_2O$. Water is chemically available in nonstoichiometric amounts, forming the silanol groups (SiOH). The silanol groups are the polar groups through which other organic moieties are bonded. We will discuss the unique properties of the silanol groups in detail later in this chapter.

From: *Forensic Science and Medicine:*
Forensic and Clinical Applications of Solid Phase Extraction
Edited by: M. J. Telepchak, T. F. August, and G. Chaney © Humana Press Inc., Totowa, NJ

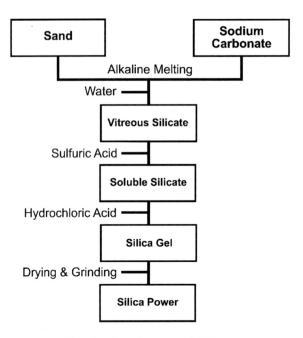

Fig. 1. Manufacture of Silica.

Amorphous silica gel does not carry the same hazard of silicosis encountered with crystalline silica. Even though the silica is nonhazardous, when working around any product that may be suspended into the air, analysts are advised to use proper respiratory protection, especially when working with particles 10 µm size or smaller.

The safe working pH range of silica is 2.0 to 9.0. Below pH 2.0, Si-C bonds of derivatized material can be cleaved; above pH 9.0, silica is slowly solubilized into silicate.

The kinetics of the dissolution of silica are slower at atmospheric pressure than at the high pressures used in HPLC, and the residence time of any elution solvent is measured in terms of minutes, not hours. Therefore, the dissolution of silica gel in not a problem in SPE as it is in HPLC. If you are getting a white precipitate you may want to check your preliminary column wash to see if it is strong enough to remove any unbound polymers from the column. Also check to see if you have buffer salts that may be insoluble in your elution solvents.

2.1 THE MANUFACTURE OF SILICA GEL

Silica gel has been manufactured by a variety of methods. It was originally made from sand by alkaline melting with sodium carbonate to produce sodium silicate solution. On standing under controlled conditions, sodium silicate solution will form silica gel (Figure 1). This process is termed the Patrick process (1919) and was developed by the US Army after World War I to produce commercially an inexpensive replacement or addition to the charcoal adsorbent in gas masks.

Tetraethoxysilane → **Polyester** → **Silica Gel**

$$m[Si(OC_2H_5)_4 + nH_2O \overset{EtOH}{\underset{HCl}{\rightarrow}} [C_2H_5O)_2nSiOn)m + {}_2mmC_2H_5OH$$

$$[(C_2H_5O)_4 nSiOn]m \overset{H_2O}{\rightarrow} n(SiO_2)m + {}_2mmC_2H_5OH$$
$$NH_4OH$$
$$Cyclohexane$$
$$EtOH$$

Fig. 2. Synthesis of high-purity silica gel.

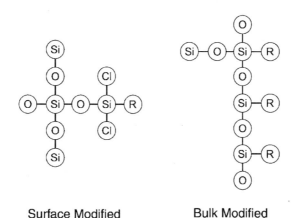

Surface Modified　　　Bulk Modified

Fig. 3. Modified silicas.

　　The current method for the synthesis of high-purity (i.e., chromatographic grade) silica gels includes the polymerization of tetraethoxysilane to form silica gel molecules (Figure 2). By introducing additional alkoxysilanes into the polymerization process you can create bulk-modified silicas where the bonded phase is polymerized not just on the surface but also throughout the silica copolymers (Figure 3).

2.2 SILANOL GROUPS

　　Silanol (Si-OH) groups must cover the surface of the silica for the silica to be useful for the preparation of SPE materials. The silanol groups are the points of attachment for the bonding of various chemistries onto silica. Figure 4 shows several different types of silanols available for bonding. Amorphous silica, with its porous, highly disordered structure, bears all three types of silanols (Figure 5).

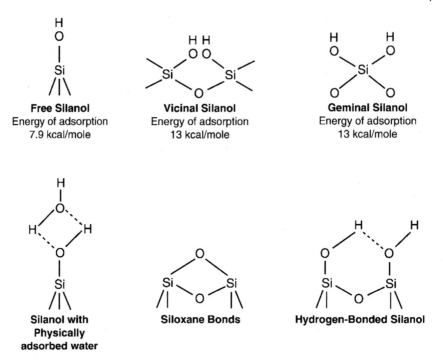

Fig. 4. Types of silanols on silica.

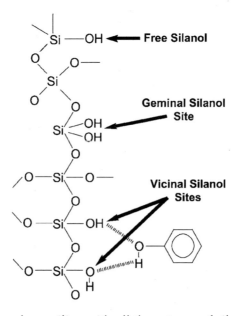

Fig. 5. Amorophous silica with all three types of silanol groups.

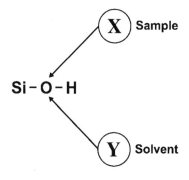

Fig. 6. Silanol and analyte interaction on silica.

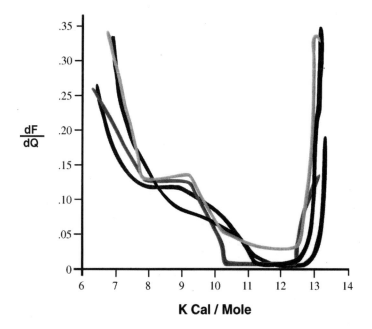

Fig. 7. Energy of adsorption on silica gel.

The silanol concentration of completely hydroxylated silica is about $9/\mu mol/m^2$. Because of steric considerations, only about 50% of these can be bonded, giving a maximum bonding density of about 4.5 $\mu mol/m^2$.

The silanol group can absorb compounds onto the silica surface by hydrogen bonding (Figure 6). A free silanol group has energy of absorption of 7.9 kcal/mol. Geminal and vicinal silanol groups have energies of absorption of 13 kcal/mol (Figure 7). The strong energies of absorption for these groups leads to strong, sometimes irreversible bonding of compounds onto the silica surface. This factor limits the effectiveness of raw silica as a sorbent, especially for normal phase separations. Bonded phase sorbents are able to limit the silanol group interactions of the silica backbone by attaching a blocking group commonly referred to as an endcap. Table 1 shows a summary of characteristics of silica gel that make it so viable for use in SPE.

Table 1
Summary of Bonded Phase Packing

- Most SPE column packings use silica gel as a backbone.
- Silica (SiO_2) is essentially porous and noncrystalline (amorphous).
- Silica gel has hydroxyl groups termed silanol groups.
- Silanol groups are the polar groups through which other functionalities can be attached.
- The nature of silanols has a direct effect on extractions.
- Free hydroxyl groups have an energy of absorption of 7.9 kcal/mol.
- Vicinal and geminal silanols have high energies of absorption (>13 kcal/mol), which may lead to irreversible adsorption.

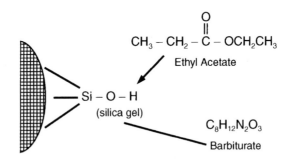

Fig. 8. Silica gel shapes and adsorption, liquid/solid.

The primary differences seen in recovery in many SPE sorbents can be attributed to the effectiveness of the endcapping process. The most efficient bonded phase is one that has the minimum number of hydroxyl groups unreacted and, consequently, the maximum surface coverage. Owing to the steric hindrance from the bonded moiety itself only a proportion of the silanol groups can be bonded, and there was little that could be done in the past to avoid this problem. Current technologies have overcome this problem and there are encapped packings available now that exhibit negligible absorption due to free hydroxyls. Keep in mind, however, that this does not eliminate minor absorptive effects due to the oxygen in the siloxane structure (Si–O–Si). Figure 8 shows the hydroxyl site on the adsorption column.

2.3 SILICA GEL SHAPES AND SIZES

Silica comes in two basic shapes: irregular (Figure 9) and spherical (Figure 10). For the purposes of bonded phase extraction, there appear to be no significant differences between irregular particles and spherical particles. These terms are basically self-defining.

Silica also comes in two consistencies: porous and pellicular. Porous silicas are used most frequently in SPE because of their high surface area and capacity. In porous silica up to 97% of the surface can be internal, leading to a large amount of surface area. Pellicular silicas (ones with solid cores and porous surfaces) are used predominantly in HPLC because of their efficient mass transfer capability.

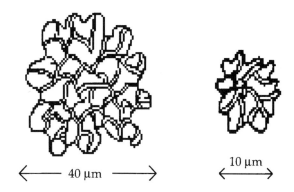

Fig. 9. Irregular silica particles of 40 μm and 10 μm.

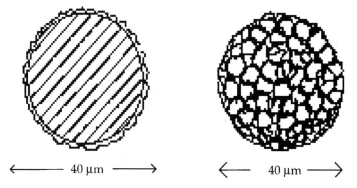

Fig. 10. Pellicular and porous spherical silica particles of 40 μm diameters.

Table 2
Particle Size and Pore Diameter

Silica shape	Particle range (μm)	Pore diameter (in Å)	Type of application
Irregular	5–20	60	Analytical
	40–60	60	SPE
	60–90	60	SPE
	90–125	60	Preparative
	120–200	60	Process
Spherical	5	120, 200, or 300	
	10	120, 200, or 300	
	15	120, 200, or 300	
	15	120, 200, or 300	
	25	120, 200, or 300	
	50	120, 200, or 300	

Diatomaceous earth (diatoms) is a natural source of silica and has been used in earlier forms of sample cleanup techniques.

All silicas used in contemporary SPE are synthetically manufactured and available in a variety of particle sizes and pore diameters. Table 2 shows particle size distributions and pore diameters for irregular and spherical silicas.

2.4 PARTICLE SIZE

Particle sizes directly affect the flow characteristics of a SPE column and attention must therefore be given to both the average particle size and the particle size distribution.

The average particle size for most SPE columns is between 40 μm and 60 μm. Smaller particles do not improve the extraction efficiency. Larger particles give better flow characteristics but there have been reports that recoveries may drop off at lower sample concentrations. At the present time it has not been determined whether this is due to the larger particles or the increased flow rate that accompanies them.

In addition to the average particle size, the particle size distribution is an important consideration in SPE. It would be ideal if every particle in the tube had exactly the same particle size and composition; however, the economics of accomplishing this would make it impractical. Therefore, the particles in SPE columns are of various sizes. Even if the reported particle size is 50 μm the actual particle sizes may be anywhere between 5 μm and 100 μm depending on how well the material is processed. The narrower the particle size ranges, the better the consistency flow from column to column. Fine particles, or "fines" (i.e., particles smaller than the actual distribution), will increase resistance to flow, whereas larger particles may reduce the efficiency of extraction.

Figure 11 A–C illustrates particle size analysis of several silica gels using a Coulter multisizer analyzer. Silica gel A has a distribution centered around 36–40 μm. This is a relatively narrow cut with very few smaller (fines) or larger particles. Silica gel B has a larger mean value, at 60 μm. This silica has no fines or larger particles. Silica gel C has a distribution centered on 50 μm. Notice the amount of larger and smaller particles outside the distribution. The relatively small number of larger particles will not affect the efficiency of the extraction. The smaller particles (fines) may clog the frits and impede sample flow through the column.

Another concern is that the process of automating column packing may affect the actual particle distribution of the final product. Figures 12 and 13 illustrate the particle size distribution during the steps of automated packing in a machine. Note that the particle distribution was fractured on the final step (placing of the frit on the top of the SPE column). This particular batch of columns had flow problems.

2.5 SURFACE AREA OF SPE SORBENTS

The surface area of a porous solid is equal to the sum of its internal and external surface areas. The external surface area corresponds to the geometric surface of particles per gram of silica. In general, the surface area of silica tends to vary inversely with the pore size, so that the larger the pore size, the smaller the surface area. The surface area of silica used for SPE ranges from 400 m^2/g to about 550 m^2/g.

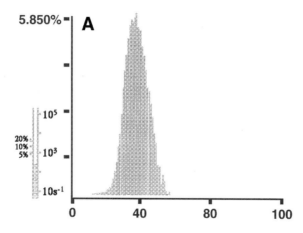

Fig. 11A. Particle size distribution silica gel A.

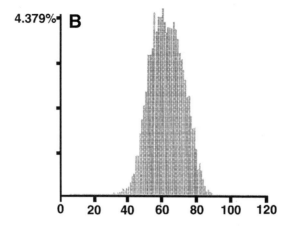

Fig. 11B. Particle size distribution silica gel B.

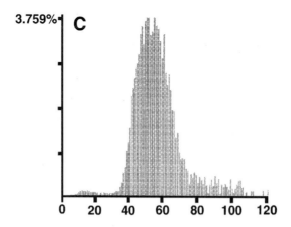

Fig. 11C. Particle size distribution silica gel C.

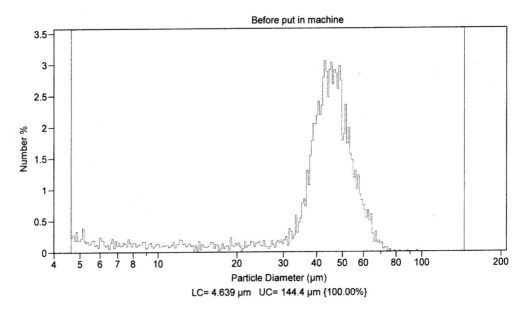

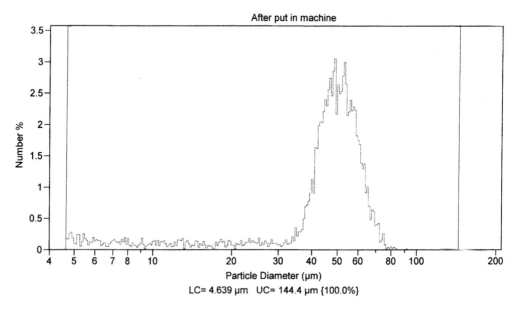

Fig. 12. Particle size analyses of silica before and after it was added to an automatic filling machine.

2.6 POROSITY

A pore is a cavity or channel connecting with the surface of a solid. Figure 14 shows two types of pores that connect with the surface. The spaces or interstices between particles are voids rather than pores. A pore that does not connect with the surface is

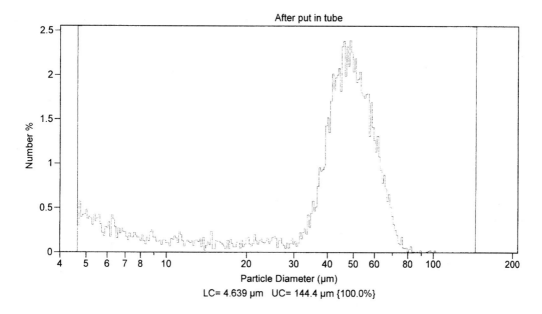

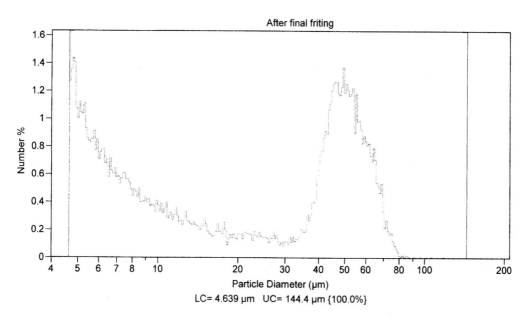

Fig. 13. Particle size analyses of silica as it was filled into tubes by an automatic filling machine.

called a closed pore or an internal void and will not contribute to the porosity or specific surface area. Pores that connect with the surface at one location are called terminal pores. Pores that connect on the surface at two or more locations are called continuous pores. Continuous pores exhibit better mass transfer than terminal pores (Figure 15).

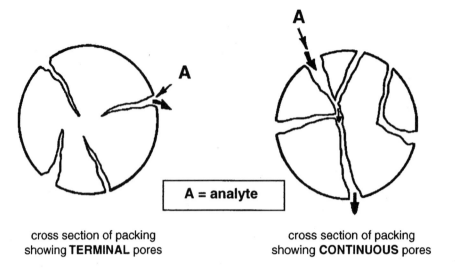

Fig. 14. The difference between continuous and terminal pores.

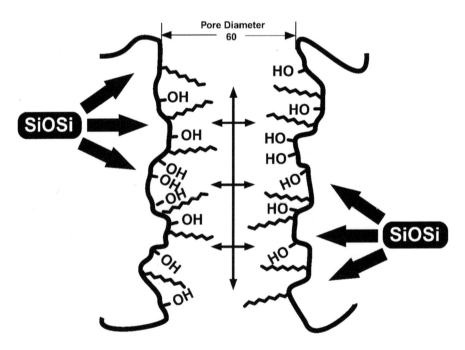

Fig. 15. The internal surface of a continuous pore.

More than 97% of the specific surface area is internal surface area because of the pores. Therefore, the particle diameter has little importance with regard to the surface area. The surface area of silica gels depends mainly on the pore size and pore volume.

Pore sizes cover a range of several orders of magnitude. The average pore size diameter useful for SPE is 60 Å. Pores of 100 Å seem to work as well. The advantage of larger-size pores for SPE has not yet been demonstrated, and manufacturers of silica gel have not been able to consistently manufacture reproducible pore diameters of 50 Å.

2.7 METAL CONTENT OF SILICA GEL

Silica gel contains impurities on processing. These impurities include alkali metals, calcium, magnesium, and trivalent metals such as alumina and iron (1).

Although small amounts of these impurities can be tolerated, their levels must be carefully controlled. Metal ions present on the silica surface at trace levels can form sites of nonspecific absorption with high activities. These sites also may facilitate the dissolution of silica when it comes into contact with solvents. A significant source of metals may be in the grinding of the silica gel to smaller particles. In most cases the manufacturing process will reduce the metal content of the bonded silica.

REFERENCE

[1]Hocky, J. Chem Indust. Jan. 9: 57, 1965.

The Chemistry of Bonded Silicas

3.1 ORGANOSILANES

The matrix of a silica gel particle consists of a core of silicon atoms joined with oxygen atoms by siloxane bonds (silicon-oxygen-silicon bonds). On the surface of each molecule exists uncondensed hydroxyl groups that gives silica its polar properties. It is these hydroxyl groups that

Organosilane reagents can react to form the bonded phases. The following chapter will review organosilanes, how they are made and the types of functional groups that can be attached.

3.2 SYNTHESIS OF ORGANOSILANES

Organosilanes are the primary building blocks used to manufacture surface-modified silicas. Organosilanes can be synthesized by two different synthetic pathways. The first route is hydrosilation, which is the reaction of an alkene with chlorosilane in the presence of a platinum catalyst. Hydrosilation reactions are very energetic and require initiation and constant monitoring. The second pathway is via a Grignard reagent, which an alkyl magnesium halide (Grignard reaction) is reacted with tetrachlorosilane in a dry solvent such as ether. Grignard reaction tend to have low yields and produce salts that can complicate the purification of the final product. Figure 1 shows the general equations for each of these reactions. Figure 2 shows the synthesis of phenethyltrichlorosilane by both synthetic pathways. Figure 3 illustrates the synthesis of 2-(4-chlorosulfonylphenyl) ethyltrichlorosilane; a common reagent used in the synthesis of silica based cation exchangers.

From: *Forensic Science and Medicine:*
Forensic and Clinical Applications of Solid Phase Extraction
Edited by: M. J. Telepchak, T. F. August, and G. Chaney © Humana Press Inc., Totowa, NJ

Hydrosilation Reactions

$$H - SiCl_3 + CH_3(CH_2)_{15}CH_2 = CH_2 \xrightarrow{Pt} CH_3(CH_2)_{16} - CH_2SiCl_3$$

Grignard Reactions

$$CH_3(CH_2)_{16} - CH_2MgCl + SiCl_4 \longrightarrow CH_3(CH_2)_{16} - CH_2SiCl_3 + MgCl_2$$

Fig. 1. Synthesis of chlorosilanes.

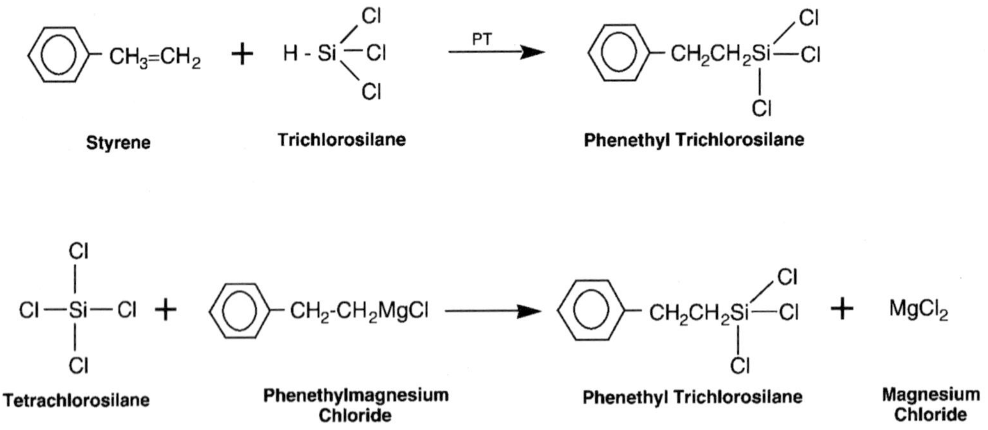

Fig. 2. Synthesis of phenethyltrichlorosilane.

It is recommended that you do not try these reactions without significant experience in these types of chemistry. In both cases, the starting materials and the finished products are low-boiling flammable reagents that are acidic and reactive in nature. The reaction itself is highly exothermic, thus increasing the hazardous nature of the synthesis. These reagents are water-sensitive and react with the slightest amount of water.

3.3 Silane Reactivity

Silanes allow the formation of a Si–O–Si bond on the surface of the silica. These bonds are more hydrolytically stable across a wider pH range than Si–O–C bonds. Two types of Silanes are commonly used for bonded phases: chlorosilanes and alkoxysilanes. They differ in rates of reaction and types of reaction.

$$R–SiCl_3 > RSi(OCH_3)_3 > Rsi(OCH_2CH_3)_3$$

Trichlorosilane > Trimethoxysilane > Triethoxysilane

Chlorosilanes are more reactive than alkoxysilanes. Chlorosilanes react almost immediately upon contact with reactive groups. Alkoxysilanes on the other hand react slower than their corresponding chlorosilanes but can be used in situations in which

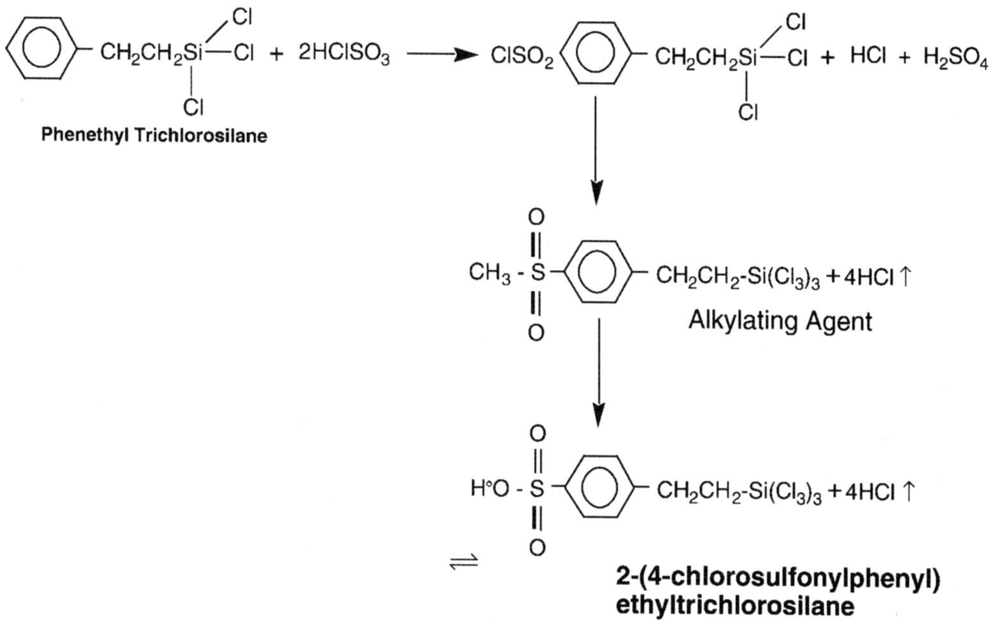

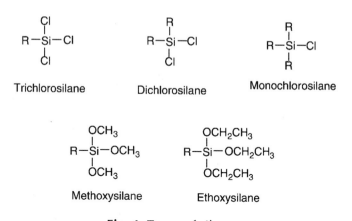

Fig. 3. Synthesis of 2-(4-chlorosulfonylphenyl) ethyltrichlorosilane.

Trichlorosilane   Dichlorosilane   Monochlorosilane

Methoxysilane   Ethoxysilane

Fig. 4. Types of silanes.

an additional reactive functional group is required (i.e., amines) or in instances where chloride ions are to be avoided. Figure 4 shows a series of typical silanes. The type of substution on the Silane can have a significant effect on the bonded phase produced.

Monochlorosilanes are traditionally used for lightly loaded sorbents or for endcapping active sites (Figure 5).

The brush type of bonded phase shields the hydroxyl groups by sterically hindering the coverage of the two adjacent hydroxyl groups. These hydroxyl groups have become the site for silica erosion by acid or base attack.

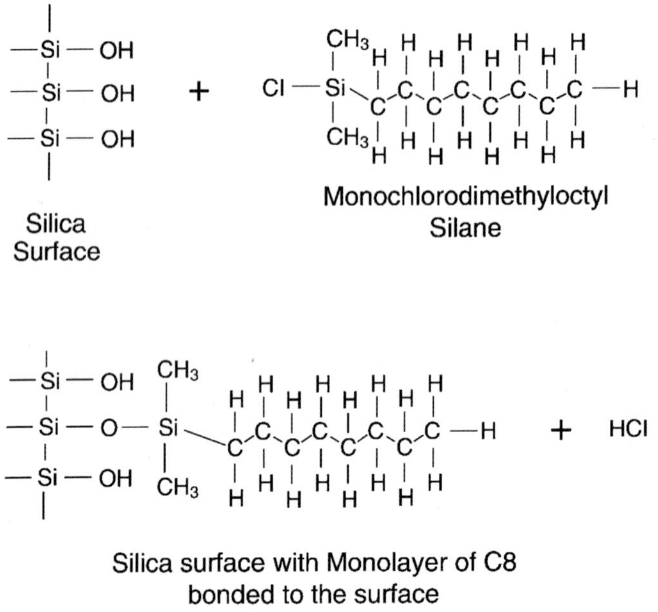

Fig. 5. Synthesis of C8 bonded monofunctional phase.

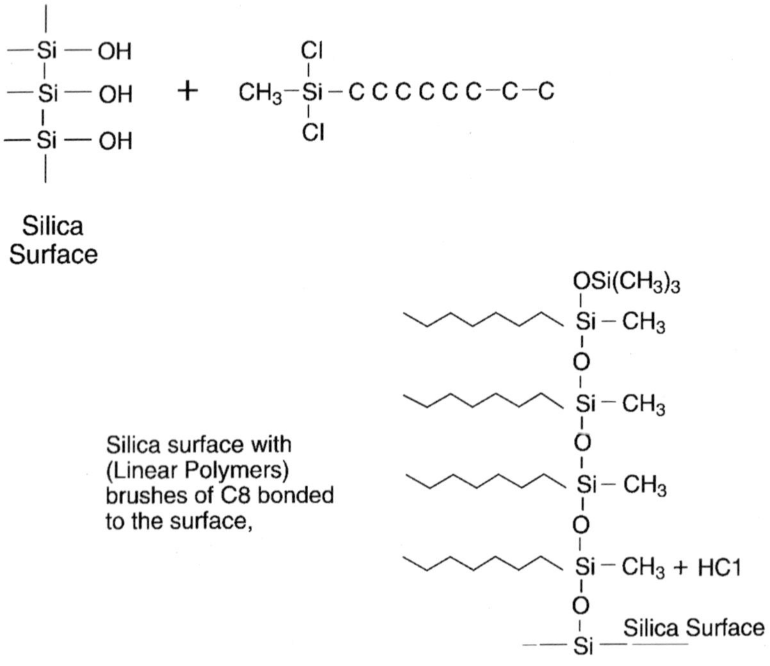

Fig. 6. Difunctional phase.

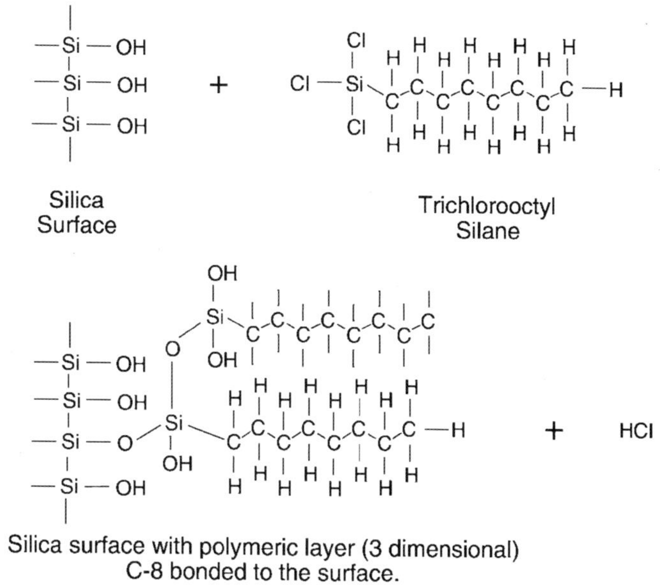

Fig. 7. Synthesis of C8 bonded trifunctional phase.

Dichlorosilanes are used to form traditional brush compounds (linear polymers). In the presence of water this type of reaction can result in cross-linking thus producing a polymeric type of sorbent (Figure 6). Linear polymers especially from this process are difficult to synthesize and are not commercially available.

Trichlorosilanes are used to form polymeric compounds (three-dimensional polymers) (Figure 7). This polymeric reaction has a multi-layered character; hence the term "bulk" phase. Water is added to the reaction mixture to produce cross linkages that build layers of polymerized functional groups.

The corresponding alkoxysilanes are used when the chemical group (R) is an amine (NH_3), an ionic compound (e.g., chlorine), or another active site. Table 1 shows a list of organosilanes availiable commercially, available as modifying reagents.

These reagents can be used by individuals wishing to manufacture their own SPE sorbent materials. The user must be made aware, though, that having the proper reagents is only a small part of the process. You are better advised to seek commercially available packings to use in SPE.

Table 1
Surface-Modifying Reagents

A wide range of polar and non-polar silanes, which may be used to modify the surface of substrates such as glass, silica, alumina and transition metals, is commercially available. Such treatment allows differential polar or hydrophobic interactions. The surface may be treated to decrease wettability or increase adhesion of the polymer to glass, silicon or metals. Such adhesion promotion renders functionalized reagents of critical importance in the electronics and building industries. Below are representative samples of our extensive product line of surface-modifying agents, grouped by class. Many mono- and difunctional silyl reagents are not listed, they find application where a monolayer surface is preferred.

PETRARCH®

Class	Functionality	Part No.	Chemical name
Hydrophobic	C2	E6350	Ethyltrichlorosilane
		E6380	Ethyltriethoxysilane
Hydrophobic	C3	P0800	n-Propyltrichlorosilane
		P0810	n-Propyltrimethoxysilane
Hydrophobic	C4	B2850	n-Butyltrichlorosilane
		B2856	n-Butyltrimethoxysilane
Hydrophobic	C6	H7332	n-Hexyltrichlorosilane
		H7334	n-Hexyltrimethoxysilane
Hydrophobic	C8	09830	n-Octyltrichlorosilane
		09835	n-Octyltriethoxysilane
Hydrophobic	C10	D3795	n-Decyltrichlorosilane
Hydrophobic	C12	D6220	n-Dodecyltrichlorosilane
	D6221		n-Dodecyltriethoxysilane
Hydrophobic	C18	09750	n-Octadecyltrichlorosilane
		09775	n-Octadecyltriethoxysilane
		09780	n-Octadecyltrimethoxysilane
		PS200	Glassclad 18
Hydrophobic	C20	E6240	n-Eicosyltrichlorosilane
Hydrophobic	C22	D6217	n-Docosyltrichlorosilane
Hydrophobic	C30	T2188	n-Triacontyldimethylchlorosilane

Category	Functional group	Chemical name	Catalog no.
Hydrophobic	Phenyl	Phenyltrichlorosilane	P0280
		Phenyltriethoxysilane	P0320
Hydrophobic	Tridecafluorooctyl	(Tridecafluoro-1,1,2,2-Tetrahydrooctyl)-1-trichlorosilane	T2492
		(Tridecafluoro-1,1,2,2-tetrahydrooctyl)-1-triethoxysilane	T2494
Reactive	Acryl	3-Acryloxypropyltrichlorosilane	A0396
		3-Acryloxypropyltrimethoxysilane	A0397
Reactive	Allyl	Allyltrichlorosilane	A0560
		Allyltriethoxysilane	A0564
		Allyltrimethoxysilane	A0567
Reactive	Bromo	3-Bromopropyltrichlorosilane	B2615
		3-Bromopropyltrimethoxysilane	B2620
Reactive	(Chloromethyl)phenyl	(p-Chloromethyl)Phenyltrichlorosilane	C3277
		(p-Chloromethyl)Phenyltrimethoxysilane	C3277.4
		1-Trimethoxysily1-2-(p,m-chloromethyl)-phenylethane	T2902
Reactive	Chloromethyl	Chloromethyltrichlorosilane	C3280
		Chloromethyltriethoxysilane	C3281
Reactive	Chloroethyl	2-Chloroethyltriethoxysilane	C3150
Reactive	Chloropropyl	3-Chloropropyltrichlorosilane	C3291
		3-Chloropropyltrimethoxysilane	C3300
Reactive	Epoxy	3-Glycidoxypropyltrimethoxysilane	G6720
Reactive	Iodopropyl	3-Iodopropyltrimethoxysilane	17750
Reactive	Isocyanate	3-Isocyanatopropyltriethoxysilane	17840
Reactive	Phosphino	2-(Diphenylphosphino) ethyltriethoxysilane	D6110
Reactive	Vinyl	Vinyltriacetoxysilane	V4800
		Vinyltrichlorosilane	V4900
		Vinyltriethoxysilane	V4910
		Vinyltrimethoxysilane	V4917
Reactive	Mercapto	3-Mercaptopropyltrimethoxysilane	M8500
		3-Mercaptopropyltriethoxysilane	M8502
Polar/reactive	Amide	n-(Triethoxysilylpropyl)Urea	T2507
Polar/reactive	Amino	3-Aminopropyltriethoxysilane	A0750
		3-Aminopropyltrimethoxysilane	A0800

(continued)

Table 1 (*Continued*)
Surface-Modifying Reagents

A wide range of polar and non-polar silanes, which may be used to modify the surface of substrates such as glass, silica, alumina and transition metals, is commercially available. Such treatment allows differential polar or hydrophobic interactions. The surface may be treated to decrease wettability or increase adhesion of the polymer to glass, silicon or metals. Such adhesion promotion renders functionalized reagents of critical importance in the electronics and building industries. Below are representative samples of our extensive product line of surface-modifying agents, grouped by class. Many mono- and difunctional silyl reagents are not listed, they find application where a monolayer surface is preferred.

PETRARCH®

Class	Functionality	Part No.	Chemical name
Polar/reactive	Carbomethoxy	A0700	n-(2-Aminoethyl)-3-Aminopropyltrimethoxysilane
Polar/ reactive	Carboxylic acid	C2905	2-(Carbomethoxy)Ethyltrichlorosilane
		T2913	n-[(3-Trimethoxysilyl)Propyl]Ethylene-diamine Triacetic Acid, Trisodium Salt
Polar/reactive	Cyano	C3555	3-Cyanopropyltrichlorosilane
		C3555.3	3-Cyanopropyltriethoxysilane
Polar/reactive	Chlorosulfonyl	C3355	2-(4-Chlorosulfonylphenyl) ethyltrichlorosilane
		C3360	2-(4 Chlorosulfonylphenyl) ethyltrimethoxysilane
Polar/ reactive	Pyridine	T2907	2-(Trimethoxysilyl)Ethyl-2-Pyridine
Polar/reactive	Pyrrole	T2923.5	n-(3-Trimethoxysilylpropyl)Pyrrole
Polar/ reactive	Quaternary	09745	n-Octadecyldimethyl-1-(3-trimethoxysilyl)propyl] ammonium chloride
	T2925		n-Trimethoxysilylpropyl-n,n,n-trimethyl-ammonium Chloride

PETRARCH is a registered trademark of United Chemical Technologies, Inc., Bristol, PA.

62

Chapter 4

Bonded Phase Sorbent Synthesis

The reaction to produce a bonded phase is discussed in this chapter.

4.1 Bonding

The generic reaction of a silane bonding to silica gel can be seen in Figure 1. Material A is silica gel. The requirements for silica gel have been previously discussed in Chapter 2, and are summarized as follows:

- Particle distribution: The normal particle distribution is 40-63 (m.
- Porosity = 60 Å
- Surface area = about 500 m^2/g
- Acid washed

The choice of a silane (B) depends on the functional group desired as well as on what kind of surface attachment is needed (monolayer, linear, or three-dimensional polymer). The use of an alkoxysilane may be needed owing to the kind of chemical group (amine), an ionic compound, or another active site requiring attachment.

4.1.1 Step 1: A + B → C

This is the formation of the Si–O–Si bond with the removal of a single Cl atom, which forms HCl. If left as such with active chlorine groups still attached, this bonded silica will react with the first active H^+ donor that comes past it and bond the donor molecule to the column permanently. You may have seen these problems if your compounds go on the column and won't come off. Irreversible reactions can also occur if various functional groups irreversibly bond material to the column material. An example of this is the formation of a Schiff's base by an aldehyde molecule in contact with an amine phase. These phenomena can be used to advantage in the formation of certain covalent-bonded phases, but the sample should not become the phase.

From: *Forensic Science and Medicine:*
Forensic and Clinical Applications of Solid Phase Extraction
Edited by: M. J. Telepchak, T. F. August, and G. Chaney © Humana Press Inc., Totowa, NJ

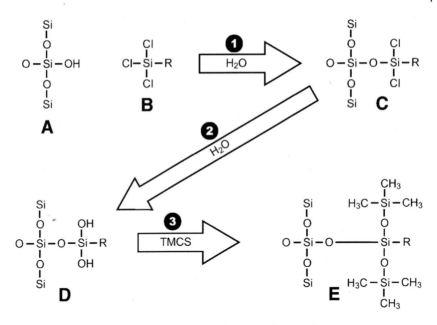

Fig. 1. Silane bonding to silica gel.

4.1.2 Step 2: C → D

This step is the hydrolysis of the remaining active chlorine groups to release HCl and leave hydroxyl groups behind. Material D now represents an unendcapped packing material. The hydroxyl groups will remain and have an adsorption effect on the sample; however, this can be overcome with the addition of a more polar elution solvent.

4.1.3 Step 3

Step 3 is the endcapping reaction and comes into effect when we are trying to eliminate any adsorptive effects from the solid phase extraction packing.

4.2 Functional Groups

Functional group attachment is the primary value of using silanes in the synthesis of SPE sorbents. For many years, people used primarily C18 bonded SPE columns and never tried other functional groups. Unfortunately, the same characteristics that make C18 an excellent HPLC column material also make it an undesirable sample preparation material. C18 lacks selectivity and often recovers a large amount of unwanted material during an extraction.

If a single functional group is attached, the particle is referred to as monofunctional-packing. If two groups such as a C8 and a sulfonic acid are attached, the material is difunctional. These materials have been used for increasing selectivity for specific analytes. Other useful bifunctional combinations are (C8 + amino), (C18 + diol), and (C8 + cyano).

Table 1
Dye Testing for Endcapping Hydrophobic Phases

Dye preparation
  a. Stock solution consists of 100 mg of Azure A (Sigma cat. no. A-6270) in 100 mL of distilled water.
  b. Working solution consists of 2 mL of stock solution diluted with 98 mL of distilled water.
Column preparation
  100 mg of packing into a mL tube.
Condition column
  Two column volumes of methanol.
  Two column volumes of water.
Dye test
  1 mL of working dye solution into each column.
Wash column
  1 mL of distilled water and 1 mL of methanol (there may be slight diffusion of dye).
Dye elution
  1–3 mL of 10% 0.1 N HCl in methanol (dye should wash off the column).

Comments:
  1. Any blue color (pale or dark) indicates unendcapped silanols.
  2. Any packing from which blue color does not elute 100% is rejected as not completely endcapped.
  3. The frits may retain some blue specks suspected to be insoluble dye compounds.

Some attempts to make multifunctional phases are currently being investigated. However, creating phases where several functional species appear gives rise to the problem that groups may neutralize the effect of one another.

Some manufacturers have attempted to create multifunctional phases by physically blending monofunctional phases and packing the mixtures into columns. To do this effectively you need to blend the silicas very efficiently, which usually grinds the particle size down since the particles are abrasives. This creates problems of column clogging. If mixing is not complete, columns are not reproducible from column to column, much less from lot to lot. Grinding also frees up many more OH groups and the packing may take on much more of an adsorptive characteristic.

This does not eliminate the necessity to have lot-to-lot reproducibility of the starting lots you may be mixing. Unless you have much time and a good technique it is recommended that you use a commercial product in which both phases are attached to the same particle as a copolymer. Particle-to-particle reproducibility has been shown to be very good.

4.3 Endcapping

The reaction of trimethylchlorosilane (TMCS) with the free hydroxyls caps them and removes additional adsorptive effects. Even though the free hydroxyls are well endcapped there may be some additional adsorption from the Si–O–Si bonds. This factor may be minimized by endcapping with methylisopropylmonochlorosilane or tertiarybutyldimethylmonochlorosilane. These reagents provide a steric shielding effect and do not allow ready access to the Si–O–Si groups. Table 1 shows a test for checking the effectiveness of endcapping your sorbents.

A useful way of using Si–O–Si groups to your advantage is to wash your column with hexane after you have loaded your sample. This will drive off any aqueous residue remaining. Hexane will wash off only the most nonpolar materials from the column. Polar and ionic compounds will remain.

$MeCl_2$ has enough of a dipole to elute acid and neutral drugs from a hydrophobic or cationic column.

If you prefer not to use chlorinated hydrocarbons, mixtures of hexane and ethyl acetate will work. Ethyl acetate will bring off steroids and similarly polar compounds. Methanol will wash off anything that is soluble in it and is not ionically bound. Methanol is a very good wash solvent to be used before pH adjustment and elution from the column just for that reason. It is not recommended that you use methanol and an acid or base to elute off an ion exchanger simply because you may not want it to bring extraneous material off the column with your analyte of interest. An 80:20:2 mix of $MeCl_2$–IPA–NH_4OH is a very good elution solvent for ion exchangers (1–3).

4.4 CAPACITY

A variety of factors affect capacity and recovery of an SPE column. Extraction capacity, in simple terms, can be defined as the amount of an analyte that a packed bed is capable of retaining from a sample matrix. Specific capacity (C_{sp}), like specific gravity or boiling point, is an intrinsic property in that the capacity per gram does not change as the amount of packing is increased or decreased. In the ideal case, the sample is strongly attracted to the ideal sorbent and the matrix in no way interferes with the extraction mechanisms of the sorbent or the analyte of interest. In this ideal world, the calculation of capacity is simple.

$$C_{sp} = \frac{\text{Amount of material retained}}{\text{Amount of packing used}}$$

$$C_{sp} = \frac{\text{Amount of compound}}{\text{Amount of sorbent B}} = \frac{10 \text{ mg}}{1000 \text{ mg}} = \frac{0.01 \text{ mg}}{1 \text{ mg}} \text{ or } 1\% \text{ capacity}$$

$$C_{total} = [C_{sp} \times \text{grams of packing or total analyte capable of being retained}]$$

4.4.1 Actual Capacity

We might then define actual capacity as total capacity under ideal conditions minus any reduction in capacity due to competition from matrix or other effects.

$$\text{Capacity}_{(ACT)} = C_{total} - C_{int}$$

Capacities calculated in this way usually vary from 1% to 10% based on parameters other than the type of phase or type of analyte under ideal conditions.

Although seemingly fundamental, extracting pure standards out of water and/or spiked into the matrix that is used provides two very valuable pieces of information:

1. It will tell you the maximum extraction efficiency you can achieve under ideal conditions.
2. It will tell you whether the phase you have chosen is the right one for your extraction.

After all, if the phase you have chosen will not extract your sample under ideal conditions, can you imagine it doing better in a real matrix? Analytes extract better out of relatively nonpolar solvent (more water than methanol).

Although these facts are not capacity-related (because no matter how much packing you use, you will still get elution and lower recovery), they can cause problems. How does one deal with this type of situation?

Remember that SPE is both a cleanup tool and a concentration technique. Therefore, whenever you have a sample in methanol or some other polar solvent, dilute it 20:1 with water. The column will now retain the compounds better and reconcentrate them as the sample moves through the column.

4.4.2 Bed Size

We will mention bed size when talking about competitive matrix effects. By running a quick study using neat standards, you can obtain the minimum bed size you require. Typical bed sizes range from 50 mg to 10 grams. The most common are 200–500 mg.

4.4.3 Bed Heights

Unlike HPLC, in which column length increases the resolution, SPE is stop-and-go chromatography; therefore the capacity of a tall, thin column is the same as that of a short, wide column. Since the flow is related to the cross-sectional area of the column, this can be used to your advantage. If the sample flows poorly through a 100 mg bed in a 1-mL tube, try 100 mg in a 6-mL tube. This has the same capacity, but better flow owing to increased cross-sectional area and shortened bed height.

4.4.4 Chain Length Effect

Depending on how polar or ionic your compound is, increasing the chain length of the phase may have a significant effect on its recovery. This is closely related to the degree of ionization of compounds that are discussed under the section on pH. Today's SPE columns can be acquired with chain lengths from C2 to C30.

4.4.5 Loading

Some research has been done to determine the loading effect on recovery (4). The work was done on packings with several different loadings and results were reported. Some polymeric resins, such as polystyrene divinyl benzene, have exhibited high capacities because of their macroporous nature. Unfortunately, most still exhibit leaking and swelling problems. It is expected that these will improve in the future.

4.4.6 Sample Size

Sample size may vary from a 1-gallon drinking-water sample to 100 μL of a concentrated extract. If you put more sample on the column than it has the capacity to hold, your recovery will not be optimum or consistent.

4.4.7 Nature of the Polymer

The nature of the polymeric configuration on the sorbent can have an impact on the ability of the SPE column to perform consistently. Random, linear, and monolayer extraction columns are available. This variety of bonding chemistries will yield distinctly different surface characteristics and the capacity of material will be affected by the structure of the phase. When comparing phases make sure you are always comparing the same phases or chemistries.

4.4.8 Checking Your Analyte's Capacity

1. Make up appropriate dilutions of your compound in distilled water if possible.
2. Condition your extraction column with an appropriate solvent.
3. Add increments of your sample compounds and analyze to determine at what concentration breakthrough occurs.
4. Calculate the C_{sp}.
5. Decide if you have the proper conditions for your extraction.

4.4.9 A Real Example of Calculating Capacity

1. A solution of Azure A blue dye was prepared with a concentration of 0.5 g of dye/L of distilled water (dH_2O).
2. The solution was fed through a weighed amount of sorbent in known quantities until the sorbent, C18, had reached saturation and the blue dye had begun to bleed through. Breakthrough was determined by UV spectrophotometry on the effluent.
3. The following was calculated:

Packing material	mg of blue dye/g of C18	% capacity
1 g CEC18	20	2.0

Sample calculation:

$$C_{sp} = \frac{20 \text{ mg of dye}}{1 \text{ g of packing}} = \frac{20 \text{ mg}}{1000 \text{ mg}} = \frac{0.02 \text{ mg}}{1 \text{ mg}} = 2\%$$

The capacity is 2% (100 mg of the packing under ideal conditions will hold up to 2 mg of the analyte).

Unfortunately, ideal conditions rarely exist anywhere in chromatography and we need to know how to deal with the variables that affect real samples and the capacity of SPE columns.

4.4.10 Recovery

We need to differentiate at this point between capacity and recovery. Capacity has been defined as the amount of analyte that a packed bed is capable of retaining from a sample matrix, and recovery is the actual amount of analyte that is retained and retrieved from the matrix on an extraction device. The optimal situation is one in which the capacity of the columns (in terms of grams of packing) is in excess of the amount of the analyte you are extracting. Excess packing will cost you more in terms of product cost and solvent usage, so you will want to optimize for the smallest amount of sorbents to do the job.

As mentioned earlier, SPE should be a stop-and-go or step type of chromatography in which the sample is totally retained and totally released. Poor choices of matrix solvents, such as methanol extracts, may in fact elute part of your sample and give you the impression of lowered capacity. The capacity of the packing has not changed but you have overidden the mechanism of retention and your recovery will vary. Our experience shows that hydrophobic phases retain analytes better out of polar solvents, whereas normal phase absorbents extract better out of nonpolar solvents.

4.4.11 Solubility

The solubility of your sample in the elution solvent will have a bearing on how much recovery you can achieve. If recovery drops off in $MeCl_{12}$–IPA–NH_4OH try ethyl acetate-hexane, and vice versa.

4.4.12. Sample Matrix

The matrix that contains your analyte is a factor in determining the capacity of your column. The sample matrix can compete with the analyte. Therefore, a sample matrix that contains a large number of compounds or a high level of a specific compound that interacts with the sorbent in a fashion similar to your analyte may reduce the capacity due to competitive interaction. This can occur often in biological samples in which acidic, neutral, and basic compounds all abound.

Solutions to this problem fall into four categories:

1. Increase the bed size to increase the total capacity and overcome the competitive interactions.
2. Change the nature of the sorbent; if you are using a monomeric C18, use a higher loaded polymeric one.
3. Change to a different type of mechanism, such as ion exchange or normal phase.
4. Use coupled columns to filter out unwanted material. A good example is to use a C18 column coupled to an ion exchanger. The C18 adsorbs a lot of organic material that can poison the surface of the ion exchanger, thereby reducing its capacity.

4.4.13 The Right Stuff

Keep in mind that if you pick a phase that does not retain your compound to begin with, there is not much you can do to increase its capacity or make it retain your compound. The quickest way to determine what phase yields the best capacity for your compounds is to extract neat standards on a variety of phases and check the recovery. This should give you rapid insight into what phase—and more importantly, what mechanism—you would want to use. This is an important decision because capacities of reversed phase and adsorption columns are generally greater than those of ion-exchange columns.

Remember that SPE today has become a real science. If you are not getting 90% absolute recovery of your analyte, your method is not optimized.

4.5 ORGANIC LOADING

The organic loading of an SPE column packing will have a direct impact on the capacity of the column. Although other factors may come into play, usually the higher the organic loading, the higher the capacity. Table 2 shows the organic loading on an

Table 2
Organic Loading and Ion-Exchange Capacity

A. Hydrophobic Phases

Packing	Unendcapped	Endcapped
C2	6.1%	6.2%
C3	7.1%	7.8%
C4- Normal	8.0%	9.3%
C4-iso-butyl	8.3%	9.3%
C4-tert-butyl	8.0%	9.2%
C5	9.0%	9.4%
C6		11.0%
C7		9.9%
C8	11.0%	11.2%
C10		16.1%
C12		17.2%
C18	21.7%	21.4%
C20	24.3%	23.7%
C30		20.5%
Phenyl		10.1%
Cyclohexyl		10.7%

B. Anion-Exchange Sorbents

	% Organic loading	Exchange capacity (meq/g)
Primary amine aminopropyl (NAX)	6.1%	0.31
Secondary amine 2-aminoethyl	8.7%	0.32
Tertiary amine diethylamino	8.4%	0.28
Quaternary amine (QAX)	7.1%	0.24

C. Cation Exchange

	% Organic loading	Exchange capacity (meq/g)
Benzenesulfonic acid (BCX)	9.4%	0.32
Propylsulfonic acid (PCX)	8.1%	0.18
Carboxylic acid (CCX)	8.1%	0.17

D. Normal Phase Sorbents

	% Organic loading	Exchange capacity (meq/g)
Silica (Unendcapped)	3.5%	
Diol	9.3%	
Cyanopropyl	6.4%	

Table 2 (*continued*)
Organic Loading and Ion-Exchange Capacity

E. Copolymeric

	% Carbon loading	Exchange capacity (meq/g)
Benzenesulfonate plus C8 (BCX2)	11.8%	0.072
Propylsulfonate plus C8 (PCX2)	14.7%	0.114
Carboxylic acid plus C8 (CCX2)	12.0%	0.105
Quaternary amine plus C8 (NAX2)	13.9%	0.160
Aminopropyl plus C8	12.1%	0.160
Cyanopropyl plus C8	14.0%	0.163
Cyclohexyl plus C8	13.3%	

F. Special Sorbents

	% Carbon loading	Exchange capacity (meq/G)
CSDAU	11.8%	0.08
CSTHC	12.4%	0.180
CSTHCA	10.9%	0.156

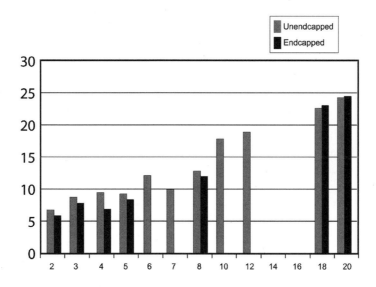

Fig. 2. Organic loading vs carbon chain length.

entire series of modified silicas. Notice that even plain silica (CUSIL) will have some surface contamination that needs to be removed for the most sensitive analyses. These values are specific to these phases. The organic loadings can be varied from around 5% to in excess of 40% or 50% depending on the required application. Milliequivalents can also be manipulated from 0.05 to 1.00 depending on the requirements. Included are the ion-exchange values for the ion exchange sorbents for the Worldwide Monitoring® line of sorbents from United Chemical Technologies, Inc.

Figure 2 illustrates the relationship between percent loading and number of carbon atoms.

4.6 The Relationship Among Recovery, Cleanliness, and Selectivity

This section demonstrates the relationship among recovery, selectivity, and cleanliness using hydrophobic sorbents. It demonstrates that the sorbent carbon chain length affects analyte recovery. It shows that sorbents possess specificity toward certain compounds. In addition it shows that extract cleanliness is a function of carbon chain configuration and that that sorbent capacity is directly related to organic loading and carbon chain length.

4.6.1 Extraction Efficiency and Sample Matrix CLEAN-UP

In this example, the CLEAN-UP® extraction columns were prewashed with 3 mL of 50:50 hexane-ethyl acetate before conditioning with 3 mL of methanol, 3 mL of deionized water, and 1 mL of 0.1 *M* phosphate buffer, pH 6.0. The sorbent was not allowed to dry before sample application. Five milliliters of urine were seeded with 50 µL of drug standard at a concentration of 100 ng/mL in methanol. The urine was pH adjusted with 2 mL of 0.1 M phosphate buffer, pH 6.0, and applied to each conditioned column (5).

The column was washed with 3 mL of deionized water and 1 mL of 1.0 *M* acetic acid and dried at maximum vacuum for 10 min. The column was washed with 2 mL of hexane. The analyses were eluted with 3 mL of 50:50 hexane-ethyl acetate into a test tube containing 50 µL of a 100 µg/mL solution of trimipramine as an internal standard. The eluent was dried under nitrogen at 40°C and reconstituted with 100 µL of ethyl acetate. One microliter was injected onto an HP 5890 Series I gas chromatograph equipped with a J & W 15-m megabore DB-17 column and a flame ionization detector. The oven temperature program started at 150°C, held for 0.5 min, increased at a rate of 10°C/min to 195°C, and then ramped at 20°C/min to a final temperature of 260°C, where it remained for 2 min.

Although the following data are in a single matrix, with a single set of compounds and one type of column, this example allows us to visually demonstrate the various concepts we have highlighted in this section. An enormous amount of information can be gained by analyzing these data.

Figure 3 shows the effect of increasing the linear chain length of the bonded phase on the amount of residue that is extracted along with the analytes of choice. Figure 4 shows the similar effect on recovery of the analytes of interest with the same chain length increases. This presents a dilemma of sorts. If we increase the chain length to maximize the recovery of the analytes we drag along many interference peaks, adding a large amount of impurities on our column and our GC-MS source. The practical answer is to find the shortest linear chain length that will yield the required analyte recovery. For barbiturate-type compounds this appears to be around C12.

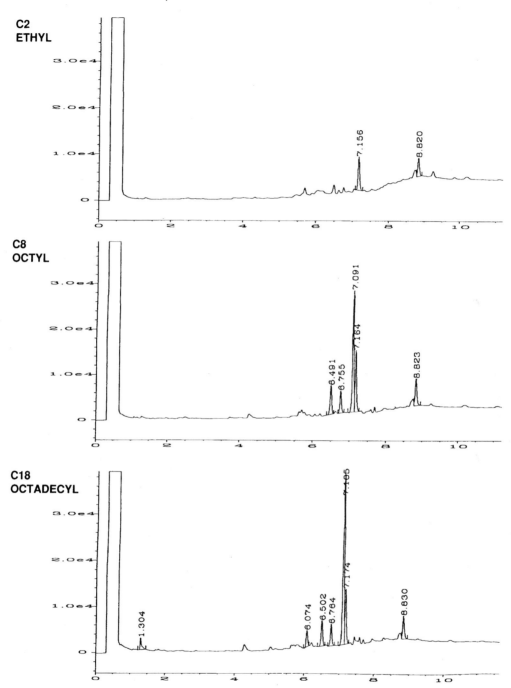

Fig. 3. Normal carbon chain endcapped sorbent extraction of blank urine.

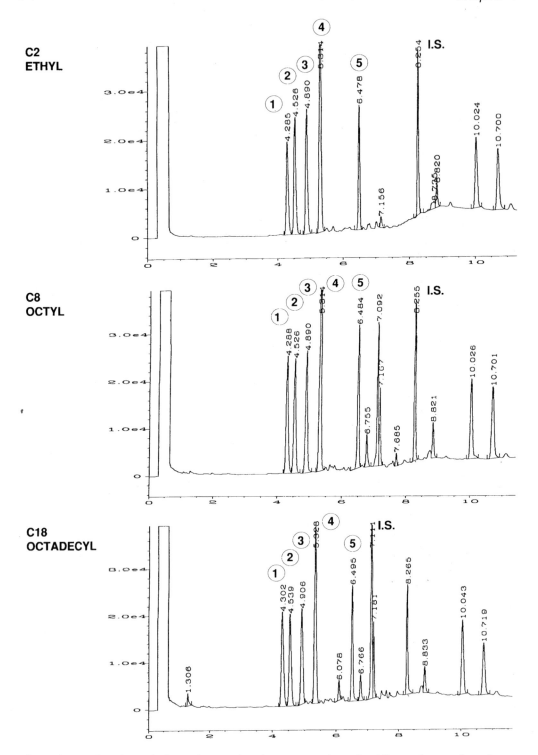

Fig. 4. Normal carbon chain endcapped sorbent extraction of acidic and neutral analytes.

Table 3
Normal Chain Sorbents and Analyte Percent Recovery

	1	2	3	4	5
	Butabarbital	Amobarbital	Pentobarbital	Secobarbital	Glutethimide
C_2	64.8	87.1	88.3	89.3	77.8
C_3	84.0	90.6	91.9	90.8	82.8
C_{n4}	92.9	96.6	97.7	97.6	90.4
C_6	88.0	90.6	91.6	92.0	91.2
C_7	93.4	93.8	94.6	94.3	95.0
C_8	88.8	89.8	90.4	89.8	91.4
C_{10}	86.8	87.7	89.0	88.4	94.0
C_{12}	106.8	107.5	107.2	108.6	108.6
C_{18}	95.6	94.0	93.6	96.2	98.3
C_{20}	98.4	99.4	99.4	100.8	97.8

Table 4
Various Chain Configurations and Analyte Percent Recovery

	1	2	3	4	5
	Butabarbital	Amobarbital	Pentobarbital	Secobarbital	Glutethimide
C_{n4}	92.9	96.6	97.7	97.6	90.4
C_{i4}	97.8	103.0	104.1	102.9	93.0
C_{t4}	27.6	73.3	83.8	98.0	70.2
C_6	88.0	90.6	91.6	92.0	91.2
PHY	66.7	91.2	92.8	96.0	96.8
CYH	102.0	104.2	106.3	105.9	106.2

Table 3 shows recovery data on barbiturates extracted on a series of column packing materials where the chain length of the bonded phase varied from linear C2 to C20. Table 4 shows recovery data on the same drugs on a series of columns packing materials containing various ring and chain configurations.

The next set of data, seen in Figures 5 and 6, demonstrate the effect of isomeric variations of the bonded phase on extraction efficiency. $Cn4$, $Ci4$ were chosen and the same extraction was performed on these phases as on the linear alkanes C2, C8, and C18. The results show what is referred to as effective chain length. This demonstrates that even though the molecular weight and carbon loading are virtually the same, the chain length is shorter for the isomeric C4 compounds and therefore the analyte recovery is affected. A similar effect can be seen with C6 phases in Figure 8 showing the effect of recovery on using linear vs cyclic phases. Using cyclic phases shortens the effective chain length of the phase.

In Figures 5 and 6 an additional effect is seen. Using a tertiary butyl phase results in the surface shielding effect mentioned in Section 4.3. Although this phase did not improve the recovery of barbiturates, it has shown great potential in the clean extraction of large molecules such as DNA and RNA.

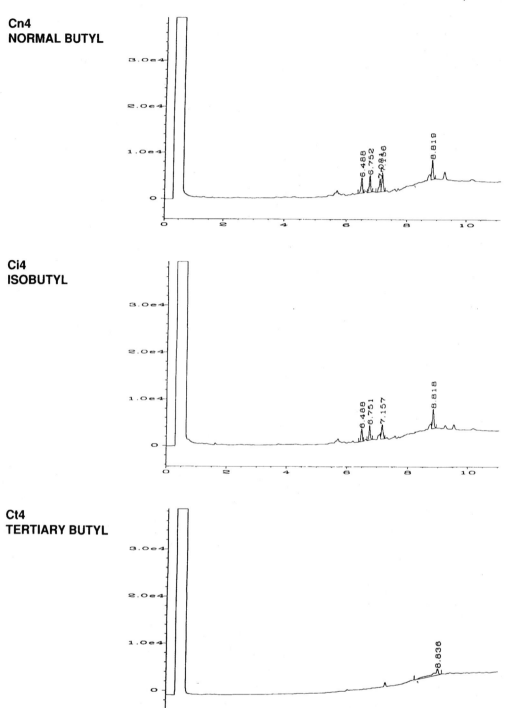

Fig. 5. Isomeric carbon chain endcapped sorbent extraction of blank urine.

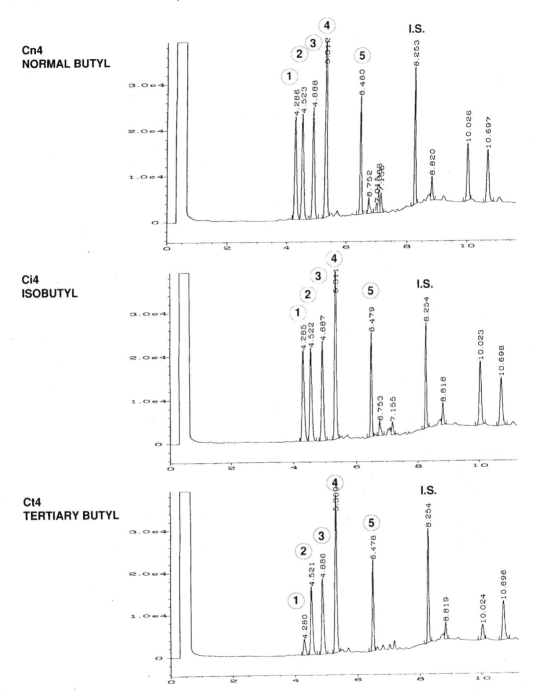

Fig. 6. Isomeric carbon chain endcapped sorbent extraction of acidic and neutral analytes.

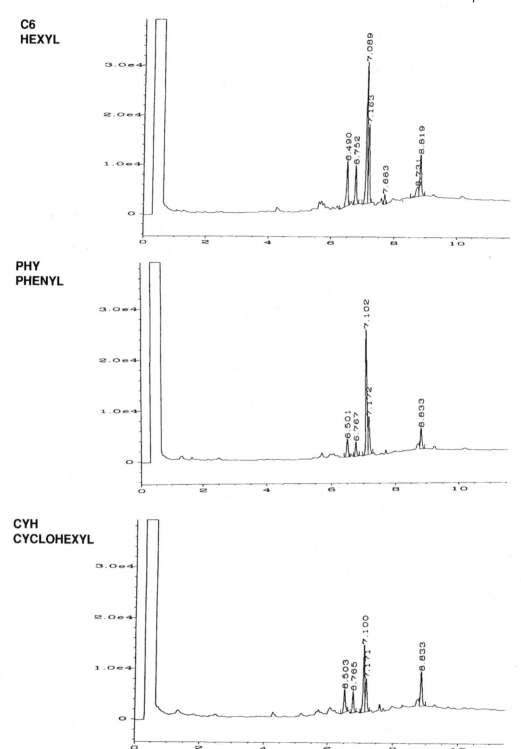

Fig. 7. Six-membered carbon endcapped sorbent extraction of blank urine.

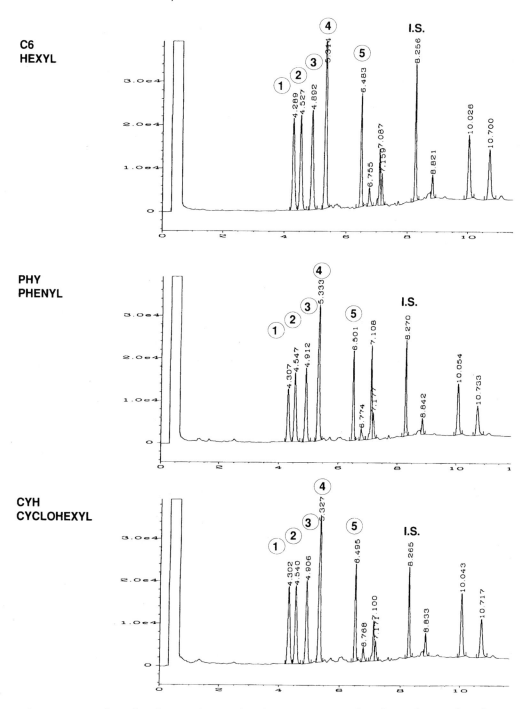

Fig. 8. Six-membered carbon endcapped sorbent extraction of acidic and neutral analytes.

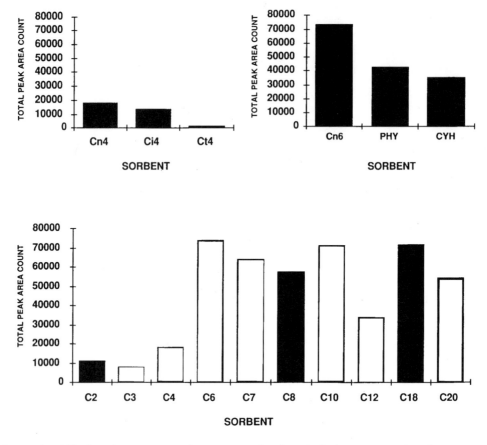

Fig. 9. Qualified endogenous peaks present after bonded phase extraction from a single lot of urine using CLEAN-UP® extraction columns.

In Figures 7 and 8 the effort of configurations can be seen on both analytes and urine blanks extracted on phases containing six carbon atoms. Figure 9 shows quantified endogenous peaks present after extraction from a single lot of urine.

Figures 3–9 and Tables 3 and 4 summarize the data collected in these experiments and are presented to demonstrate the principles of recovery, cleanliness, and selectivity.

In summary, carbon chain length can affect compound recovery. In a simple assay designed to exploit hydrophobic interactions, increasing the carbon chain length results in higher analyte recovery. This is probably due to greater nonpolar interactions between the analyte and the sorbent. Increased carbon chain length of the CLEAN-UP sorbents is reflected by the experimental organic loading results. Retention of urine matrix interference also increases with chain length, as demonstrated by the chromatograms of blank urine extracts from the C2, C8, and C18 CLEAN-UP extraction columns.

Carbon chain configuration also affects matrix cleanup. Extract purity can be enhanced when using nonlinear sorbent isomers. Greater steric hindrance may not allow the larger molecules found in the matrix to bind efficiently to the sorbent.

Analyte geometry may affect recovery when using a sterically hindered isomer. This is clearly indicated by the differences in the butabarbital recovery from the tertiary butyl sorbent, as compared to the normal butyl sorbent.

The polarity of a chain configuration also contributes to recovery and extract cleanliness. A comparison of cyclohexyl and phenyl, both six-membered rings with nearly identical organic loading, shows that the more polar phenyl retains more matrix interferences, yet does not hold the acidic and neutral analytes as well.

The knowledge gained by this study allows the chemist to narrow his or her choices when selecting the best sorbent for a particular application. Although every extraction challenge is different, this information on sorbent matrix and sorbent analyte interaction will facilitate assay development and optimization.

4.7 Alkylation of Drugs at Ion-Exchange Sites on the Surface of SPE Columns

SPE is routinely used in forensic laboratories to extract a wide variety of drugs from body fluids such as urine and blood. SPE has also gained widespread use in pharmaceutical, clinical, and environmental laboratories, particularly since the introduction of copolymeric extraction columns in 1980. A study presented at the Society of Forensic Toxicologists Annual Meeting in Baltimore in 1995 indicated that certain commercially available solid phase extraction columns containing ion-exchange functional groups might cause alkylation of key metabolites back to the parent drug. The resulting alkyl derivatives may lead to reporting errors, especially at or near the SAMSHA cutoff levels. The objective of the study was to determine if alkylation of various drugs was caused by functional groups of the sorbent.

4.7.1 Chemicals

Sodium hydroxide (1 N), glacial acetic acid, and concentrated ammonium hydroxide were purchased from J. T. Baker (Phillipsburg, NJ). HPLC-grade hexane, ethyl acetate, methanol, methylene chloride, isopropyl alcohol, and acetonitrile were obtained from E. M. Science (Hawthorne, NY). Dibasic sodium phosphate (Mallinckrodt, Phillipsburg, NJ), monobasic sodium phosphate, 0.1 N hydrochloric acid (Fisher Scientific, Fairlawn, NJ), and BSTFA in 1% TMCS (Supelco, Bellefonte, PA) were also used.

All analytical standards (benzoylecgonine, D_3-benzoylecgonine, cocaine, D_3-cocaine, norcocaine, codeine, norcodeine, morphine, D_3-morphine, diazepam, nordiazepam, and prazepam) were obtained from Ceroilliant (Austin TX). Working standards of each drug were prepared at 1 and 10 µg/mL by dilution with methanol and were used to spike negative urine.

4.7.2 Sorbent

To determine if the sorbent causes metabolites to convert to their respective alkylated drugs during extraction by solid phase, we used four common copolymeric sorbents, including United Chemical Technologies, Inc. CLEAN SCREEN DAU SPE columns.

Table 5
SPE Procedures

Drug	Sample preparation	Condition	Wash	Elution
Benzoylecgonine Norcocaine	2 mL of urine 2 mL of PB	3 mL of methanol 3 mL of distilled water 1 mL of PB	2 mL of DiH$_2$O 2 mL of 0.1 N HCl 3 mL of MeOH Dry 5 min	3 mL of MC–IPA–AH
Nordiazepam	2 mL of urine 3 mL of AB	1 mL of PB 3 mL of MeOH 3 mL of DiH$_2$O 1 mL of PB	Dry 5 min 2 mL of DiH$_2$O 2 mL of CAN–PB Dry 5 min	3 mL of NH$_4$OH–EA
Norcodeine Normorphine	2 mL of urine 2 mL of AB	3 mL of MeOH 3 mL of DiH$_2$O 1 mL of AB 3 mL of MeOH Dry 5 min	2 mL of hexane 2 mL of DiH$_2$O 2 mL of AB	3 mL of MC–IPA–AH

PB = 0.1 M phosphate buffer, pH 6.0; AB = 0.1 M acetate buffer, pH 4.5; CAN-PB = 0% acetonitrile in 0.1 M phosphate buffer, pH 6.0; NH$_4$OH–EA = 2% ammonium hydroxide in ethyl acetate; MC–PA–EA = methylene chloride/isopropyl/ammonium hydroxide (78:20:2).

Each eluate was spiked with 200 ng/mL of the appropriate external standard and vortexed before evaporating to dryness at 40°C. Derivatization accomplished by adding 50 μL of ethyl acetate and 50 μL of BSTFA (with 1% TMCS), vortex-mixing, and heating at 70°C for 20 min.

Two microliters of derivatized sample was injected splitless onto an HP 5890/5971A GC-MS using an Rtx-1 fused silica capillary column (15 M, 0.25 mm, 0.25 μm). Helium flow was adjusted to 0.55 mL/min. Temperatures for the injector and transfer line were 250°C. Temperature programs were as follows: 150–300°C at 25°C/min (benzoylecgonine); 150–300°C at 20°C/min (norcodeine, normorphine); 150–230°C at 30°C/min, 230–250°C at 10°C/min, then 250–300°C at 25°C/min (norcocaine); 140–250°C at 25°C/min, hold 2 min, then 250–300°C at 25°C min (nordiazepam).

The following ions were monitored using SIM analysis:

Drug	(* Quantitation ion)	Alkylated product	(* Quantitation ion)
Norcodeine	164*, 357, 329	Codeine	371*, 234, 343
Normorphine	415*, 400, 416		
Morphine	429*, 324, 430		
Nordiazepam	341*, 342, 343	Diazepam	256*, 221, 285
Norcocaine	168*, 136, 289	Cocaine	182*, 303, 198
Benzoylecgonine	240*, 361, 256	Cocaine	182*, 303, 198

4.7.3 Sample preparation

Spiked samples were prepared in 2 mL of negative urine at the following levels: 150 ng/mL of norcocaine; 150, 250, 500, and 1000 ng/mL of benzoylecgonine; 300 ng/mL of norcodeine and normorphine; 200, 400, and 1000 ng/mL of nordiazepam. Two milliters of acetate buffer was added to the norcodeine, normorphine, and nordiazepam tubes and 2 mL of phosphate buffer was added to the norcocaine and benzoylecgonine samples (see Table 5).

4.7.4 Column Conditioning and Sample Application

All SPE columns were activated with 3 mL of methanol followed by 3 mL of distilled water and 1 mL of phosphate or acetate buffer (see Table 5). Samples were loaded at 1–2 mL/min.

4.7.5 Column Wash

Interferences were removed with 2 mL of distilled water, 2 mL of either 0.1 *N* HCl, acetonitrile-phosphate buffer, or acetate buffer according to the information from Table 5, and followed by 3 mL of methanol where appropriate (see Table 5). Maximum vacuum was applied for 5 min. Two milliliters of hexane was then added to the nordiazepam tubes before elution.

4.7.6 Analyte Elution

Elution of benzoylecgonine, norcocaine, norcodeine, and normorphine was accomplished by passing and collecting 3 mL of methylene chloride-isopropanol-ammonium hydroxide (78:20:2) through the columns. Three milliliters of 2% ammonium hydroxide in ethyl acetate was used to elute nordiazepam.

4.7.7 Absolute Recovery

Two-milliliter aliquots of negative urine were spiked at various levels and extracted as previously described. Aliquots of blank urine were run through SPE columns (unextracted drug calibrator) and appropriate concentrations of drug, alkylated derivatives, and external standard were then spiked in the eluate before drydown and derivatization. Absolute recoveries were calculated using Equation 1.

$$\% \text{ Recovery} = \frac{\text{ratio of extracted sample}}{\text{ratio of unextracted calibrator}} \times 100 \tag{1}$$

$$\text{Ratio} = (\text{area of drug/area of external standard})$$

4.7.8 Determination of Alkylation Conversion

Equation 2 was used to calculate the absolute amount (ng/mL) of alkylated drug produced and Equation 3 was used to determine the percent (%) of metabolite that converted to the parent drug (i.e., norcodeine to codeine in this example) through alkylation by the sorbent.

$$\text{Alkylated product (ng/mL)} = \frac{\text{ratio of converted alkylated drug} \times [\text{AD}]}{\text{ratio of unextracted alkylated calibrator}} \tag{2}$$

$$\% \text{ Conversion} = \frac{AP \times 100}{[NAD]}$$

(3)

Where

[AD]   = known concentration (ng/mL) of unextracted alkylated (i.e., codeine) calibrator

[NAD] = known concentration (ng/mL) of unextracted nonalkylated (i.e., norcodeine) calibrator

AP   = ng/mL of alkylated product produced

ratio   = (area of drug/area of external standard)

4.7.8.1 Norcodeine to Codeine

Sorbent A shows conversion of norcodeine to 52 ng/mL of codeine (17%), while sorbent C liberated 28 ng/mL of codeine (9%) and sorbent D, 23 ng/mL (8%). Sorbent B did not show any conversion of norcodeine to codeine.

4.7.8.2 Normorphine to Morphine

Sorbent A shows conversion of normorphine to 154 ng/mL of morphine (51%), while sorbent C liberated 35 ng/mL of morphine (12%) and sorbent D, 33 ng/mL (11%). Sorbent B did not show any conversion of normorphine to morphine.

4.7.8.3 Norcocaine to Cocaine

Sorbent A shows conversion of norcocaine to 64 ng/mL of cocaine (42%), while sorbent C liberated 18 ng/mL of cocaine (12%). Sorbents B and D did not show any conversion of norcocaine to cocaine.

4.7.8.4 Benzoylecgonine to Cocaine

Benzoylecgonine did not show any conversion to cocaine at levels <250 ng/mL. Conversion occurred at higher concentrations (500 and 1000 ng/mL) using sorbent A (26% and 29% respectively). Sorbents B and C did not show any conversion of benzoylecgonine to cocaine.

4.7.8.5 Nordiazepam to Diazepam

Nordiazepam shows no conversion of diazepam up to concentrations of 1000 ng/mL on all four sorbents.

A recent review of commercially available packing materials showed that some silica-based materials currently on the market still exhibited such alkylation phenomena; therefore, users are encouraged to check their SPE columns for alkylation prior to use.

It was discussed that the alkylation of drugs may result from certain techniques employed during sorbent manufacturing processes. The SPE columns used in this study are copolymeric, and thus contain both ion-exchange and hydrophobic functional groups. The ion-exchange portion is typically $R-SO_2-OH$ and could convert during specific manufacturing processes to an alkyl sulfonate agent. If conversion were taking place during the extraction procedure, the binding site(s) of the drug would associate with the converted alkyl sulfonate groups of the sorbent. In the process, an alkyl group is added to the analyte containing a derivatizable group.

Table 6
Alkylation of Drugs on Sorbent A

	Sorbent A			
Drug	Concentration (ng/mL)	Drug % recovery	Alkyl derivatives (ng/mL)	Alkyl derivatives (% recovery)
Norcodeine	300	46.3	17.3	52
Norcocaine	150	54	42	63.5
Normorphine	300	55	51.2	154
Nordiazepam	200	82	0	0
	400	104	0	0
	1000	113	0	0
Benzoylecgonine	150	88	0	0
	250	86	0	0
	500	76	26	26
	1000	79	26	26

Table 7
Alkylation of Drugs on Sorbent B

	Sorbent B			
Drug	Concentration (ng/mL)	Drug % recovery	Alkyl derivatives (ng/mL)	Alkyl derivatives (% recovery)
Norcodeine	300	96	0	0
Norcocaine	150	99	0	0
Normorphine	300	85	0	0
Nordiazepam	200	83	0	0
	400	104	0	0
	1000	104	0	0
Benzoylecgonine	150	86	0	0
	250	92	0	0
	500	93	0	0
	1000	89	0	0

CLEAN SCREEN DAU SPE columns were used.

To determine whether drugs convert to their alkyl derivatives, common drugs (norcodeine, norcocaine, normorphine, nordiazepam, and benzoylecgonine) were selected because they contain various functional groups (hydroxyl, amide, acid, and/ or amine). The alkyl derivatives that would form are: norcodeine to codeine; norcocaine to cocaine; normorphine to morphine; nordiazepam to diazepam; and benzoylecgonine to cocaine. Unextracted calibrators contained known amounts of nonalkylated and alkylated drug as well as deuterated drug. Deuterated external standards were checked for background noise, alkylated ions, and any other isotopic or adverse contribution(s). None were detected. Recovery, amount of conversion and percent conversion of

Table 8
Alkylation of Drugs on Sorbent C

Drug	Sorbent C			
	Concentration (ng/mL)	Drug % recovery	Alkyl derivatives (ng/mL)	Alkyl derivatives (% recovery)
Norcodeine	300	62.3	9.4	28
Norcocaine	150	80	12	18
Normorphine	300	53	12	35
Nordiazepam	200	78	0	0
	400	95	0	0
	1000	90	0	0
Benzoylecgonine	150	89	0	0
	250	86	0	0
	500	86	0	0
	1000	71	0	0

Table 9
Alkylation of Drugs on Sorbent D

Drug	Sorbent D			
	Concentration (ng/mL)	Drug % recovery	Alkyl derivatives (ng/mL)	Alkyl derivatives (% recovery)
Norcodeine	300	91	8	23
Norcocaine	150	98	0	0
Normorphine	300	92	11	33
Nordiazepam	200	83	0	0
	400	88	0	0

nonalkylated drugs and alkyl derivatives were determined using Equations 1–3 (Tables 6–9; Figures 10–13). Sorbent A showed the greatest percent conversion of norcodeine, normorphine, norcocaine, and benzoylecgonine to their alkylated forms. Sorbent C demonstrated the next highest overall conversion, followed by sorbent D. Sorbent B showed no conversion of any drug tested.

Nordiazepam showed no conversion to diazepam on any sorbent tested, suggesting that the amide functional group of nordiazepam is not readily susceptible to alkylation during SPE. At levels below 500 ng/mL, benzoylecgonine showed no conversion on any sorbent, suggesting that the acid functional group is not as susceptible to alkylation as the amine groups of norcocaine, norcodeine, and normorphine. Specifically, using sorbents A and C, the amine of norcocaine methylated to form cocaine, indicating that amines may be easily methylated during use of certain SPE columns. Of all

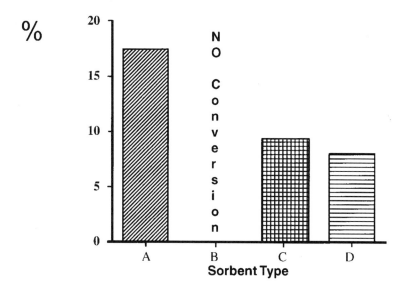

% Formation of Alkyl Derivatives

Fig. 10. Norcodeine to codeine.

the drugs tested, normorphine and norcodeine showed the most alkylation on sorbents A, C, and D. No conversion to morphine or codeine took place using sorbent B. Again, data suggest that the amine groups have higher alkylation ability on three of the four sorbents tested when compared to acid (benzoylecgonine) and amide (nordiazepam) groups.

During routine use of SPE, alkylation of certain drugs can occur and may lead to inaccurate quantitative results. Data indicate that conversion is due to specific processes employed during sorbent manufacturing techniques. These practices are proprietary in nature; however, the derivatization problems associated with them may be avoided by careful selection of SPE columns.

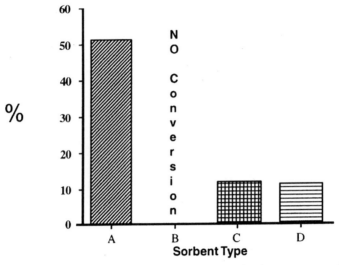

% Formation of Alkyl Derivatives

Normorphine to Morphine

Fig. 11. Normophine to morphine.

4.8 Summary

The preceding three chapters covered many areas of sorbent synthesis. The reader should now be familiar with the following characteristics of solid phase sorbents:

CEC18 Product Characterization
- Material: Silica gel
- Shape: Irregular
- Particle size: 40–60 μm
- Pore diameter: 60 Å
- Bonding: Polymeric
- Phase type: Organic phase
- Carbon analysis by weight: 21%
- Endcapping: Complete

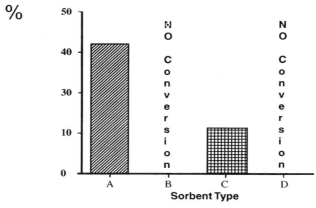

% Formation of Alkyl Derivatives

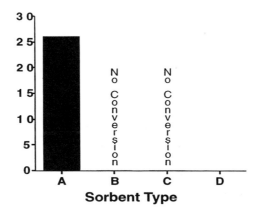

Norcocaine to Cocaine.

Fig. 12. Norcocaine to cocaine.

% Formation of Alkyl Derivatives

Fig. 13.

REFERENCES

[1]Thompson, B. C., Kuzmack, J. M., Law, D. W., and Winslow, J. U. Copolymeric solid-phase extraction for quantitating drugs of abuse in urine by wide capillary gas chromatography. LCGC 7, 10:846–850, 1989.

[2]Heebner, E. T., Telepchak, M. J., and Walworth, D. The use of novel bonded phase absorbents for the extraction of abused drugs from biological matrices. United Chemical Technologies, Inc. 2731 Bartram Rd. Bristol, PA 19007, 1990.

[3]Moffat, A. C., Jackson, J. V., Moss, M. S., and Widdop, B., eds. Clarke's Isolation and Identification of Drugs. London: The Pharmaceutical Press, 1986, pp. 6–34.

[4]Wells, D. A., and Benson Kail, E. Effects of analyte, sorbent and matrix on capacity of solid phase extraction material. 3M I&C Section Research and Development, 3M Center BLDG 209-1C-30, St. Paul, MN 55144,

[5]Fox, D. J., Heebner, E. T., Phillips, T. L., O'Dell, L. A comparative study of the extraction capabilities of various substituted silicas used in bonded phase extraction. United Chemical Technologies, Inc. 2731 Bartram Rd. Bristol, PA 19007, 1990.

Chapter 5

Strategies for the Use of Solid Phase Extraction

In this chapter we discuss four basic strategies used in solid phase extraction (1) filtration, (2) selective adsorption, (3) copolymeric extraction, and (4) immunoaffinity. Most extractions will fall into one of these categories.

5.1 SOLID PHASE EXTRACTION AS A FILTER

One of the first uses of SPE was as a filtration device in pharmaceutical laboratories where scientists were extracting active compounds from fermentation broths. SPE cartridges were used to remove as much of the matrix as possible, allowing active compounds to pass through the columns and to be collected. This technique has evolved into a more sophisticated large-scale type of chromatography, called flash chromatography, used by organic synthetic chemists. Flash chromatography has not found a place in forensic toxicology as yet, so we do not discuss it at this point. Figure 1 shows a graphic demonstration of this type of approach to SPE. The example shown is the isolation of γ hydroxybutyric acid (GHB) from human urine. Urine samples are filtered by a special sorbent that holds interfering substances and allows the analytes of interest to pass through the column to be analyzed. In this case the biggest contaminant is urea, which is effectively removed by the SPE column.

The following describes a forensic application for GHB from human urine that uses SPE as a filtering step followed by additional liquid-liquid extraction techniques.

GHB has become widely known as the "sex drug for the 1990s." In the new millenium, GHB has become popular with college students and club-goers as a mood modulator. Cases of GHB use were rare, but have become numerous over the last two years. On ingestion, it reduces inhibitions and reportedly increases libido. Other popular street names include "scoop" and "liquid ecstasy." This drug has been classified as a date rape drug, along with lorazepam, ketamine, and flunitrazepam.

From: *Forensic Science and Medicine:*
Forensic and Clinical Applications of Solid Phase Extraction
Edited by: M. J. Telepchak, T. F. August, and G. Chaney © Humana Press Inc., Totowa, NJ

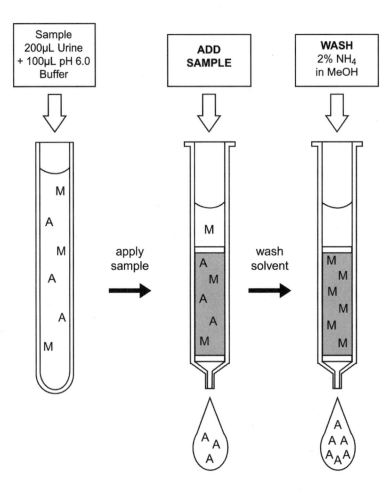

Fig. 1. The use of an SPE column as a filter.

GHB is an endogenous human metabolite structurally similar to the neurotransmitter γ-amino butyric acid (GABA) (1,2). It was first synthesized and used in Europe as an anesthetic, but was later discontinued because this drug was widely sold in health food stores as a weight control drug (functionally similar to L-tryptophan) and to induce the secretion of growth hormone for body building. In 1990 the sale and distribution of GHB was federally banned owing to its potentially harmful effects (3).

GHB is easily synthesized from γ-butyrolactone, a compound that is found in some commercial products. Figure 2 shows the chemical structures of GHB and butyrolactone. The Internet has popularized this drug by giving recipes on how to manufacture it. One particular book claims the drug to be a "natural mood enhancer" (4). In clandestine preparations the concentrations vary significantly, leading to problems with overdosage. Harmful contaminants from low-quality ingredients may also appear. In the 1990s more than 20 deaths in the United States were attributed to the use of GHB, generally in conjunction with alcohol ingestion (5).

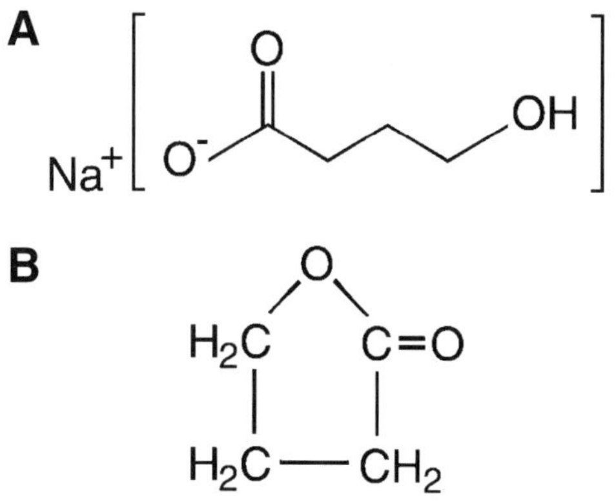

Fig. 2. Chemical structures of **(A)** γ-hydroxybutyric acid and **(B)** butyrolactone.

GHB is a small polar molecule that is very difficult to separate for a qualitative determination. In many methods it is extracted following conversion to butyrolactone and chemically derivatized by silylation (3,6,7). This method allows for the chemical derivatization of the parent compound without the formation of the lactone. Instrumental analysis is performed using gas chromatography/mass spectrometry (GCMS). The method and the sorbent used in the method are patented (U.S. patent no. 6,156,431).

5.1.1 Materials and Methods for GHB Analysis

5.1.1.1 Reagents

Certified American Chemical Society (ACS)-grade hexane, sodium phosphate monobasic, sodium phosphate dibasic, dimethylformamide, ammonium hydroxide, and HPLC-grade methanol and ethyl acetate were all purchased from Mallinckrodt (Phillipsburg, PA). Distilled water was prepared using a millipore purification system, bis (trimethylsilyl) trifluoroacetamide (BSTFA) with 1% trimethylchlorosilane (TMCS) from United Chemical Technologies, Inc. (Bristol, PA).

5.1.1.2 Standards and Solutions

a. GHB sodium salt, was purchased from Aldrich (Milwaukee, WI).
b. GHB-D6 was purchased from Cerrilliant (Austin, TX). The GHB and GHB-D6 were prepared to 0.1 mg/mL in methanol.
c. Prepare the 0.1 M phosphate buffer, pH 6.0, by dissolving 1.70 g of Na_2HPO_4 and 12.14 g of $NaH_2PO_4 \cdot H_2O$ in 800 mL of DI H_2O. Dilute to 1000 mL using DI H_2O. Mix. The solution is stable for at least 1 month.
d. Adjust pH to 6.0 ± 0.1 with 0.1 M monobasic or dibasic sodium phosphate.
e. The $CH_3OH–NH_4OH$ (99:1) is prepared fresh daily.

5.1.1.3 Sorbent

The extraction columns were CLEAN SCREEN ZSGHB020 containing 200 mg of sorbent in a 10-mL column and were manufactured by United Chemical Technologies, Inc.

Table 1
Ions Using SIMS Analysis and Quantitation Ion

RT (min)	Name	Target ion (% of target ion)	Second ion (% of target ion)[a]	Third ion (% of target ion)[a]
5.40	GHB–D6–diTMS	239.2 (100)	240.2 (20)	241.1 (9)
5.43	GHB–diTMS	233.1 (100)	234.1 (19)	235.0 (7)

[a]Observed values.

5.1.1.4 Instrumentation

A Hewlett Packard 5971A Mass Selective Detector, a 7673 Autosampler, and a 5890 Gas Chromatograph fitted with a 30-m, 0.25 mm i.d., 0.25 µm film thickness Rtx-5 (comparable to a DB-5 or HP-5) were from Restek (Bellefonte, PA).

GC conditions		Oven temperature program
Column head pressure	8 psi	Initial temperature 70°C, hold 1.00 min
Injection port temp.	250°C	Ramp to 100°C @15°C/min
Transfer line temp.	280°C	Ramp to 175°C @25°C/min
Split vent flow	50 mL/min	Ramp to 280°C @35°C/min
Septum purge flow	2.6 mL/min	================================
Equilibration time	0.5 min	Total run time = 9.00 min Purge on time
	0.1 min	

Injection Volume 1 µL, Splitless injection
Run time is extended past the elution of the GHB to eliminate any residual BSTFA or urine byproducts.

5.1.2 GC-MS Analysis

The method uses selected ion monitoring (SIM) for three ions for each analyte. The dwell times were set to 30 ms per ion, resulting in 3.62 cycles per second. The most prevalent ions for GHB–diTMS are 147, 233, 148, 149, 204, 143, and 234 *m/z*. The most prevalent ions for GHB–D6–diTMS are 147, 239, 148, 149, 206, and 240 *m/z*. Urea is also derivatized by BSTFA to form a diTMS derivative. It elutes near GHB and has many of the same ions including 147, 148, and 149; therefore, some of the less abundant ions must be used for the SIM analysis. Table 1 lists these ions.

5.1.3 Urine GHB Extraction Procedure Using a ZSGHB020 SPE Column

1. Prepare sample.
   a. To 200 µL of urine add internal standard (GHB-D6) and 100 µL of 0.1 *M* phosphate buffer, pH 6.0.
   b. Mix/vortex.
2. Condition CLEAN SCREEN®GHB extraction column.
   a. 1 × 3 mL of CH_3OH; aspirate.
   b. 1 × 3 mL of DI H_2O; aspirate.

    c. 1 × 0.5 mL 0.1 *M* phosphate buffer, pH 6.0; aspirate.
    Note: Aspirate at ≤3 in. Hg to prevent sorbent drying.
  3. Apply sample.
    a. Place test tubes into vacuum manifold for collection.
    b. Collect both the sample loading and wash.
    c. Decant sample onto column. Aspirate at ~1 in. Hg.
  4. Wash column.
    a. Add 1 mL of CH$_3$OH–NH$_4$OH (99:1) to sample test tube; vortex.
    b. Decant wash onto column.
    Note: Aspirate at ~1 in. of Hg.
  5. Concentrate.
    a. Remove test tubes from vacuum manifold.
    b. Evaporate to dryness at 60°C using a stream of air or nitrogen gas.
  6. Sample Cleanup.
    a. Add 200 μL of dimethylformamide.
    b. Add 1 mL of hexane saturated with dimethylformamide.
    c. Mix by inversion for 5 min.
    d. Centrifuge at 1500*g* for 5 min.
    e. Transfer lower dimethylformamide layer to a clean test tube.
  7. Concentrate.
    a. Evaporate to dryness at 50°C using a stream of air or nitrogen gas.
  8. Derivatize.
    a. Add 100 μL of ethyl acetate and 100 μL of BSTFA (with 1% TMCS).
    b. Mix/vortex.
    c. No heating is required.
  9. Quantitate.
    a. Inject a 1- to 2-μL sample onto GCMS.
    b. Monitor the following ions:
    GHB–diTMS   233*, 234, 235
    GHB–D6–diTMS 239*, 240, 241

5.1.4 Results

The following results show the kind of data that can be routinely achieved by the methodology presented in this section.

5.1.4.1 Chromatography

See Figure 3.

5.1.4.2 Recovery

Five 50 mg/L standards were prepared by adding 10 μg of GHB to 200 μL of drug-free urine. These standards were extracted using the previously described procedure. The internal standard (4 μg of GHB–D6) was added immediately prior to the evaporation of the DMF. Five 50 mg/L unextracted standards were prepared by adding 10 μg of GHB and 4 μg of GHB–D6 to a test tube that was dried at 50°C. All samples were derivatized using the procedure previously described. The recovery was calculated by comparing the area under the curve of the target ion for the extracted and the average of the unextracted standards. The average recovery was 67.2% (range = 76%–58%).

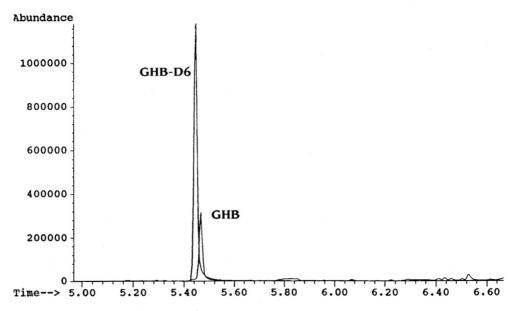

Fig. 3. Chromatogram of the selected target ions showing GHB and GHB-D6 from a 5 mg/L extracted urine standard.

5.1.4.3 Linearity

The assay is linear from 1 to 100 mg/L with the upper range limited by the saturation of the detector. The method could be run with a split injection if higher concentrations need to be quantified.

5.1.4.4 Stability

The diTMS derivatives are stable for more than 7 d at room temperature.

5.1.4.5 Sensitivity

The assay is sensitive to 1 mg/L.

5.1.4.6 Interferences

The only interference identified in this procedure was from urea. It is derivatized along with GHB to form urea–diTMS. Using the SIM ions listed above eliminates the interference.

5.1.5 Summary

This procedure allows for the direct analysis of GHB and eliminates any possibility of forming or extracting γ-butyrolactone (GBL). Conversion to GBL is problematic in forensic analysis where litigation is involved because GHB is a scheduled drug in many states and GBL is not. This method was designed to identify low levels of GHB in urine and requires only 200 μL of sample. Expected concentrations in biological samples may be much higher and therefore a smaller sample size should be used (6). The method utilizes a novel copolymeric sorbent employing SPE as a filter. A sample cleanup step and silylation followed by GCMS analysis is also incorporated

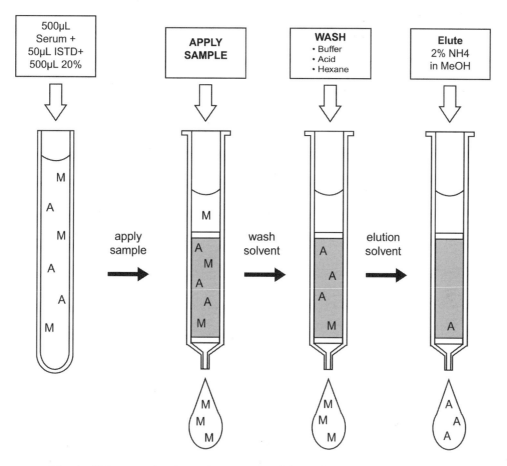

Fig. 4. SPE as a selective adsorption tool for gabapentin serum assay.

into the method. The derivatization with BSTFA with 1% TMCS is accomplished without a heating step, owing to the high reactivity of the BSTFA to the GHB. The derivative is stable for more than a week at room-temperature conditions.

5.2 SPE-SELECTIVE ADSORPTION

A second approach to SPE is to selectively bond the analyte of interest while allowing the matrix to pass through. This is probably one of the more common approaches to SPE. Figure 4 is a graphic demonstration of this approach. The analysis of gabapentin in human serum is presented to illustrate how this sample preparation is performed.

Gabapentin [(1–aminomethyl–1–cyclohexyl) acetic acid] is an anticonvulsant agent used as an adjunctive therapeutic agent in the treatment of seizure disorders not adequately controlled by standard monoanticonvulsant therapy. Adequate drug levels are critical to controlling seizures. Chemically, gabapentin is an interesting drug to isolate because of three functional groups on its molecule an amine group (cationic), a carboxylic acid (anionic), and the ring structure (reversed phase extraction)

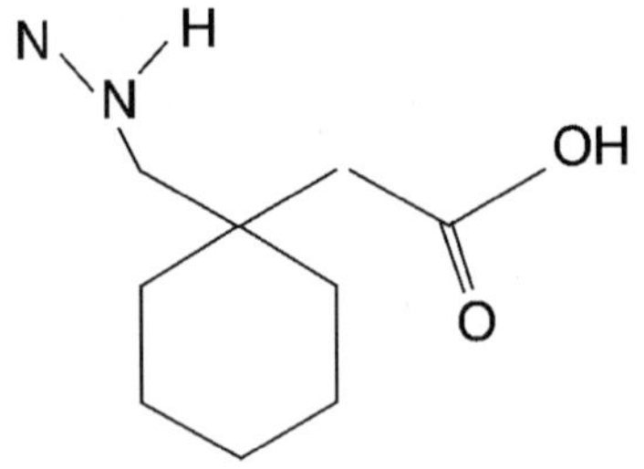

Fig. 5. Gabapentin/Neurontin® [(1-aminomethyl–l–cyclohexyl) acetic acid].

Figure 5 shows the chemical structures of gabapentin and the compound used as the internal standard in this analysis. Section 5.2.1 shows the extraction of gabapentin from serum or whole blood. Section 5.2.2 shows the data from the assay validation for this method.

Presented in this application is a specific and selective gas chromatographic method using a nitrogen-phosphorus detector (1). The selectivity of this method is illustrated in Table 2, which lists compounds found not to interfere with the gabapentin assay from more than 40 drugs screened for potential interference with this method. Figure 6 shows the chromatograms of the serum extracts.

5.2.1 Gabapentin in Serum, Plasma, or Whole Blood for GC or GC-MS Analysis Using a 200-Mg CLEAN-UP C18 Extraction Column

1. Prepare sample.
   a. Place 500 μL of sample, calibrator, or control into a 10 × 25 mm disposable glass test tube and add 25 μL of internal standard (5.0 mg/L).
   b. Vortex tube.
   c. Add 500 μL of 20% acetic acid and vortex tube again.
2. Condition SPE column.
   a. 1 × 3 mL of CH_3OH; aspirate.
   b. 1 × 3 mL of DI H_2O; aspirate.
   c. 1 × 3 mL of 1 N HCl; aspirate.
3. Apply sample.
   a. Load at 1 mL/min.
4. Wash column.
   a. 1 × 3 mL of DI H_2O; aspirate.
   b. 1 × 3 mL of ethyl acetate.
   c. 1 × 3 mL of hexane.
   d. Dry column (5 min at >10 in. Hg or until column is dry).
5. Elute Gabapentin.
   a. 1 × 1 mL of 2% NH_4OH in MeOH.
   b. Evaporate to dryness at 40°C in a water bath.
6. Dervizatize.
   a. Add 50 μL of MTBSTFA + 1 % BDMCS reagent to the residue.
   b. Cap tube and put into a water bath at 70°C for 30 min.
   c. Remove and allow to cool for 5–10 min.
7. Quantitate.
   a. Insert 1–2 μL of the sample onto the chromatograph.

Table 2
Compounds Found Not to Interfere
with Gabapentin Assay

Acetaminophen	Amikacin
Amylase	Amitriptyline
Benzoylecgonine	BUN*
Caffeine	
Carbamazepine	
Chloramphenicol	Cholesterol
Creatinine	Cyclosporine
Digoxin	Disopyramide
Estradiol	Ethosuximide
γ-Hydroxybutyrate	Gentamicin
Glucose	HCG*
LDH*	Lidocaine
Lithium	Methotrexate
m-Hydroxybenzoic acid	NAPA*
Netilmicin	Nortriptyline
p-Aminobenzoic acid (PABA)	Phenobarbital
Phenytoin	Primidone
Procainamide	Quinidine
Salicylate	Theophylline
Thyroxine	Tobramycin
Triiodothyronine	Triglycerides
Uric acid	Valproic acid
Vancomycin	

*Abbreviations: BUN, blood urea nitrogen; HCG, human chorionic gonadotropin; LDH, lactate dehydrogenase; NAPA, n-acetylprocainamide.

5.2.2 Assay Validation

a. Linearity was observed from 0.2 to 30 mg/L.
b. Within-run precision:
   7.0% for 1.1 mg/L ($N = 10$)
   3.4% for 4.5 mg/L ($N = 10$)
c. Between-run precision:
   12% for 1.1 mg/L ($N = 16$) over 3 wk
   5.0% for 4.5 mg/L ($N = 16$) over 3 wk
d. Recovery of gabapentin: Internal standard
   1.0 mg/L: 46%   69% ($N = 10$)
   5.0 mg/L: 57%
   20.0 mg/L: 51%

5.2.3 Summary

A simple, rapid, and selective method for gabapentin is presented that uses a reversed phase separation. Sample chromatograms can be seen in Figure 6. The pH of the sample was used to suppress the ionization of the carboxylic acid group. Ethyl

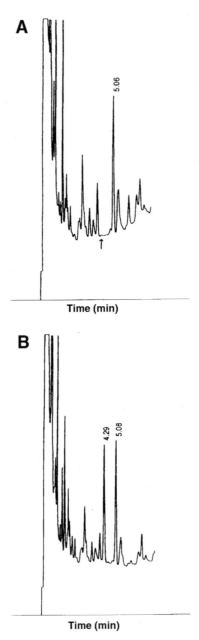

Fig. 6. Gabapentin analysis. Chromatograms of serum extracts: **(A)** Internal standard present (5.06 min). **(B)** Gabapentin 5.0 mg/L (4.3 min) and internal standard (5.08) present.

acetate and hexane were used to wash the matrix away from the sorbent-isolated drug. Gabapentin has a limited solubility in these solvents. Elution at an alkaline pH ionized the acid portion of the drug thus freeing the drug from the sorbent. Increasing the ammonium hydroxide concentration did not improve the recovery of the analyte and could produce ammonium salts, requiring further sample purification.

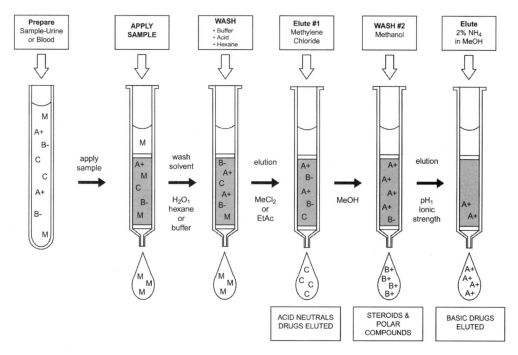

Fig. 7. Copolymeric interaction, forensic drug assay.

The derivatization of gabapentin with MTBSTFA and 1% BDMCS improved the peak shape of the analytes and also increased the molecular weights, thus increasing their retention time on the chromatographic system.

Derivatized gabapentin samples were stable for up to 1 d with a <10% loss due to chemical degradation.

5.3 SPE IN COPOLYMERIC INTERACTION

Figure 7 shows a third approach to SPE, referred to as "copolymeric" or selective extraction. This is a most useful approach in doing class extractions or drug-plus-metabolite extractions in groups of compounds. An example of this type of approach can be seen in the general method used for forensic samples.

The versatility of SPE can be best exhibited by its usage in the separation of a wide variety of drugs using a combination of separation strategies. The widest variety of separations have been developed using the combination of a C8 with a cationic exchanger, usually benzene sulfonic acid. CLEAN SCREEN DAU, Bond Elute Certify®, SPECII®, Isolute®, and NARCII® are a few of the products that currently use this combination and are termed "copolymeric sorbents."

This mechanism works by providing separation of the acid/neutral drugs using reversed phase C8 functionality; the benzene sulfonic acid mechanism works on basic drugs by cation exchange of the amine functionalities. Table 3 lists a variety of drugs that have been extracted by the CLEAN SCREEN DAU extraction column using the method found in sections 5.3.1 and 5.3.2. This method is an example of the kinds of methods that are developed in toxicology laboratories where a general method is used to identify drugs in biological samples for clinical management and toxicological significance. Section 5.3.2 shows the extraction procedure used for forensic drug analysis.

5.3.1 General GCMS Method*

GC-Column:	Selectra® CC-5 or DB-5, HP-5 or equivalent capillary column.
Specifications:	30 m long × 0.25 mm internal diameter × 0.25 μm film thickness
Temperature program:	60°C hold 1 min; increase to 300°C at a rate of 25°C/min; hold for 3 min.
	The total run time is 13.6 min.
Conditions:	The injector temperature is 250°C.
	Ultrapure helium is used as the carrier gas at 30 mL/min flow.
	The transfer line is run at 280°C.
MS Conditions:	The mass spectrometer is run in the total ion mode.
	The photomultiplier voltage is set by the autotune program.

---

*The data for this method were provided by the City of Philadelphia, Department of Public Health—Medical Examiner's Office.

Selectra® is a registered trademark of United Chemical Technologies, Inc. (Bristol, PA). HP 5® is a registered trademark of Hewlett Packard Corporation (Palo Alto, CA). DB-5® is a registered trademark of J & W Scientific Inc. (Folsom, CA). Bond Elute Certify® is a registered trademark of Varian, Inc. (Harbor City, CA). SPECII® is a registered trademark of Ansys (Harbor City, CA). Isolute® is a registered trademark of International Sorbent Technologies, Inc. (Cardiff, UK). NARCII® is a registered trademark of J. T. Baker (Phillipsburg, NJ).

5.3.2 Forensic Drug Analysis for GC or GCMS Using a 200-Mg CLEAN SCREEN Extraction Column (ZSDAU020 or ZCDAU020)

1. Prepare sample
Urine:
   a. To 5 mL of urine add 50–300 μL of 1.0 M acetic acid to adjust sample pH to between 4.8 and 5.5.
Whole blood:
   a. To 2 mL of blood add 8 mL of DI H_2O. Mix/vortex and let stand 5 min.
   b. Add 150–300 μL of 1.0 M acetic acid to adjust sample pH to between 4.8 and 5.5.
   c. Centrifuge for 10 min at 670g and discard pellet.
Tissue:
   a. Homogenize 1 part tissue with 3 parts of DI H_2O.
   b. Centrifuge for 10 min at 670g and discard pellet.
   c. Transfer 10 mL of supernatant to a clean tube.
   d. Add 150–300 μL of 1.0 M acetic acid to adjust sample pH to between 4.8 and 5.5.
2. Condition CLEAN SCREEN extraction column.
   a. 1 × 3 mL of CH_3OH; aspirate.
   b. 1 × 3 mL of DI H_2O; aspirate.
   c. 1 × 1 mL of 0.1 M acetic acid; aspirate.
Note: Aspirate at ≤3 in. Hg to prevent sorbent drying.

Table 3
Some Drugs That Have Been Quantified Using the CLEAN SCREEN Extraction Column

Acepromazine	Etorphine	Naproxen
Acetaminophen	Etorphine–3–glucuronide	Nicotine
Amantadine	Fentanyl	Nordiazepam
Amitriptyline	Floxin	Nubain
Amitriptyline metabolite	Fluoxetine	Oxybutynin
Amphetamine	Furosemide	Oxycodone
Apomorphine	Glutethimide	Pemoline
Azaperone	Glutethimide metabolite	Pentazocine
Azaperone–5–glucuronide	Glycopyrrolate	Phencyclidine
Barbiturates	Hordenine	Phenethylamine
Benzocaine	Hydrocortisone	Phentermine
Benzoic acid	Hydromorphone	Phenylbutazone
Benzoylecgonine	Ibuprofen	l-Phenylcyclohexone
Benzotropine	Imipramine	Phenylpropanolamine
Buspirone	Imipramine metabolite	Phenytoin
Caffeine	Indomethacin	Primidone
Carbamazepine	Ketamine	Procaine
Carisoprodol	Lidocaine	Propionylpromazine
Chlordiazepoxide	Loxapine	Propoxyphene
Chloroquine	Mazindol	Propoxyphene metabolite
Chlorpheniramine	Meclizine	Propranolol
Chlorpromazine	Mefenamic acid	Propylparaben
Chlorpropamide	Meperidine	Quinidine
Clenbuterol	Meprobamate	Quinine
Clonazepam	Methadone	Salbutamol
Cocaine	Methadone metabolite	Salicylic acid
Codeine	Methamphetamine	Strychnine
Cotinine	Methylbenzoate	Temazepam
Cresol	Methylecgoninine	Terbutaline
Cyclobenzaprine	Methyl *p*-aminobenzoate	Tetracaine
Dextromethorphan	Methylphenidate	Tetrahydrocannabinol
		and metabolite
Dextrophan	Methyl salicylate	Theophylline
Diazepam	Methylparaben	Thiopental
Dihydrocodeine	Methyprylon and metabolite	Thioridazine
Diltiazem	Metolazone	Timolol
Diphenhydramine	Morphine	Tranylcypromine
Dipyrone	Morphine-3-glucuronide	Trifluoperazine
Doxepin	*N,N*-Diethyltryptamine	Trimethoprim
Doxepin metabolite	Nalorphine–3–glucuronide	Trimipramine
Doxylamine	Naloxone	Verapamil
Ecgonine		Verapamil metabolite
Ethacrynic acid		

3. Apply sample.
  a. Load at 1–2 mL/min.
4. Wash column.
  a. 1 × 3 mL of 0.1 *M* phosphate buffer, pH 6.0; aspirate.
  b. 1 × 1 mL of 0.1 *M* acetic acid; aspirate.
  c. Dry column (5 min at ≤10 in. Hg).
  d. 1 × 3 mL of hexane; aspirate.
5. Elute acidic and neutral drugs (faction A).
  a. 2 × 2 mL of CH_2Cl_2; collect eluate at ≤5 mL/min.
  b. Evaporate to dryness at ≤40°C.
6. Extract and analyze faction A.
  a. Add 1 mL of hexane and 1 mL of CH_3OH/H_2O (80:20). Mix/vortex.
  b. Centrifuge to separate layers. Aspirate and discard hexane (upper) layer.
  c. Evaporate again to dryness at ≤40°C.
  d. Reconstitute with 100 µL of ethyl acetate and inject 1 to 2 µL onto chromatograph.
7. Wash column.
  a. 1 × 2 mL of methanol; aspirate.
  b. Dry column (5 min at ≤10 in. Hg).
8. Elute basic drugs (fraction B).
  a. 1 × 2.0 mL of methanol–NH_4OH (98:2); collect eluate at 1–2 mL/min.
  Note: Prepare elution solvent daily.
9. Extract and analyze fraction B.
  a. Add 3.0 mL of DI H_2O and 250 µL chloroform to eluate. Mix/vortex 30 s.
  b. Centrifuge to separate phases. Aspirate and discard aqueous (upper) layer.
  c. Inject 1–2 µL of the chloroform layer onto chromatograph.
  Note: Fractions A and B can be combined before analysis and evaporated together.

5.4 THE FUTURE OF SPE

The future of SPE is illustrated in Fig. 8, which shows that immunoaffinity can be used to isolate the analytes of interest. This type of SPE is dependent on the attachment of a biologically active molecule to a matrix surface by the use of an aldehydic silane. This forms a covalent bond with the amine groups of the substrate, allowing for the immobilization of the biomolecule with the surface of a variety of materials.

SPE is a very robust technique; however, what if we could improve on the selectivity of our separations by the use of antibodies, enzymes, peptides, proteins, or the attachment of any biological substrate to pick up our analytes?

This type of technology was introduced many years ago by the gluteraldehyde procedure (1–3) and was used for the immobilization of antibodies for benzodiazepines (4). This immunoaffinity column could pick up most benzodiazepines including their glucuronides. This process could eliminate the acid-base or enzymatic hydrolysis step in conventional SPE procedures.

The only problems with this procedure were in the formation of two Schiff bases in the covalent linkage, making it sterically strained and also susceptible to hydrolysis by various mechanisms. These two limitations represented challenges that limited the effectiveness of this procedure. The recent introduction of a new line of aldehydic silanes (Bio Conext) offers many advantages above the present technologies in ligand

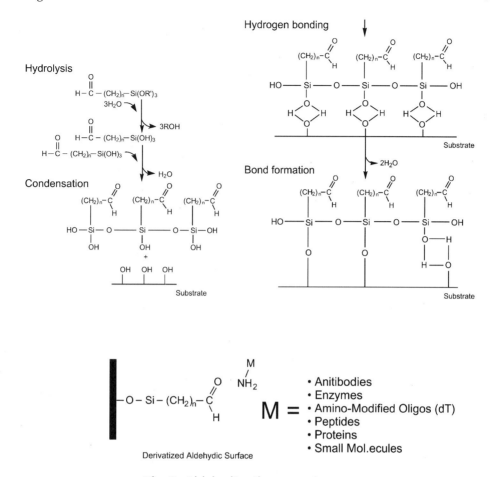

Fig. 8. Aldehydic silane attachment.

immobilization. Aldehydic silanes attach easily to many matrices that contain hydroxyl functions. This includes glass, ELISA plates, silica, plastic beads, metal, agarose, and many polymeric resins. The bonding to primary amines of the substrate creates only one Schiff base attachment. This provides for a more stable linkage that is not sterically hindered. The use of various carbon lengths in the chains from the matrix surface to the biomolecule allow access to active sites and also allow the binding to larger-size molecules.

Figure 8 illustrates the chemistry involved in the attachment of the aldehydic silane to a biologically active substrate. Figure 9 explains, in a step-by-step fashion, an actual synthesis of bonding the aldehydic silane first to the matrix (silica) then to Protein A. Figure 10 illustrates how an immunoaffinity procedure would be performed. The simplicity of the method, along with selectivity and the limitless possibilities for attachment and analysis, illustrate the direction that SPE in the future may take.

Step 1: Attachment of Aldehydic Silane to the Matrix (i.e. Silica)

1. To 25 g of silica gel add 250 mL of hexane and mix for 30 min. Purge the container with dry nitrogen and continue to blanket the reaction with nitrogen to provide an inert environment.

2. Add over the next 2-3 h 7.5 mL of PSX1055 (triethoxy aldehydic silane) in 0.5 mL aliquots.

3. Allow the reaction mix for 5 h.

4. Wash the silica with isopropanol and distilled water.

5. Store the final product in distilled water.

Step 2: Attachment of the Active Substrate

1. Approx 100 mg of the aldehyic silica is placed into a fritted column.

2. This column is washed with five column volumes of pH 7.4 buffer.

3. 3.4 mg of Protein A is added to the column and the column was incubated overnight.

4. The column is washed with pH 7.4 buffer.

Fig. 9. Aldehydic silane bonding.

REFERENCES

[1]Dyer, J. Gamma-hydroxybutyrate: A health-food product producing coma and seizure-like activity. Am. J. Emerg. Med. 9:321–324, 1991.

[2]Chin, M. Acute poisoning from gamma-hydroxybutyrate in California. Wes. J. Med. 156:380–384, 1992.

[3]Andrews, K. Getting the scoop on gamma-hydroxybutyrate or GHB: The new recreational drug. Proceedings of the 49th Annual Meeting of the American Academy of Forensic Sciences, Historical Overview, p. 3, 1997.

[4]Dean, W., Morgenthaler, J., and Fowkes, S. W. GHB: The Natural Mood Enhancer. Smart Publications, 1997.

[5]Sannerud, C. Drug Enforcement Administration. Personal communication, 1995.

SAMPLE PREPARATION

To 2.5 mL of human urine add 2.5 mL of a
0.1 M phosphate buffer.

SAMPLE REACTION

1. Add 5 mL of the sample with buffer
mixture to 250-300 mg of the prepared
aldehydic silica into a column that is fritted
and capped at both ends.

2. Gently shake the tube at room
temparatue for 1-4 h.

3. Allow the tube contents to settle in an
upright position and open the ends of the
column.

SAMPLE ELUTION

1. Wash the immunoabsorbent sample
mixture with 30 mL of water.

2. Elute the analytes of interest with 3 x 1
mL of 90% methanol in water.

3. Analyze the sample.

Fig. 10. Immunoaffinity SPE Procedure.

[6]Gibson, K. Stable isotope dilution analysis of 4-hydroxybutyric acid: An accurate method for quantification in physiological fluids and the prenatal diagnosis of 4-hydroxybutyric aciduria. Biomed. Environ. Mass Spectrom. 19:89–93, 1990.

[7]Stephens, B. and Baselt, R. Driving under the influence of GHB. J. Analyt. Toxicol. 18:357–358, 1994.

[8]Wolf II, C. E., Sady, J., and Pokalis, A. Determination of gabapentin in serum using solid phase extraction and gas-liquid Chromatography. J. Analyt. Toxicol. 20:498–501, 1996.

[9]Neurath, A., and Strick, N. Enzyme linked fluorescent immunoassay using beta-galactosidase and antibodies covalentyly bound to polystyrene plates. J. Virol. Methods 3:155–165, 1981.

[10]Weston, P., and Avrameas, S. Proteins coupled to polyacrylamide beads using glutaraldehyde. Biochem. Biophys. Re. Commun. 45:1574–1580, 1971.

[11]Terynck, T., and Avrameas, S. Polyacrylamide-protein immunoadsorbents prepared with gluteraldehyde. FEBS Lett. 23:24–28, 1972.

[12]Franzelius, C., Ackermann, I., Deinl, I., Angermaier, L., and Machbert, G. Simultaneous extraction of selected benzodiazepines and benzodiazepine glucuronides from urine by immunoadsorption. J. Analy. Toxicol. 22:359–362, 1998.

Chapter 6

Optimizing Solid Phase Extraction Methods

This chapter reviews some of the basic steps required for optimizing additional SPE cleanup steps for forensic samples, and looks at some practical analytical problems and their solutions.

6.1 APPROACHES TO OPTIMIZING METHODS

In methods development there are three basic approaches to the problem:

1. **The intellectual approach:** We proceed to think the problem through to the solution by applying known data and following it to a logical conclusion. Because of the complexity of the subject matter, this works less than 50% of the time.
2. **The shotgun approach:** We screen a large number of phases and solvent combinations and hope to come up with the right combinations. This is also effective only about 50% of the time, depending on how well we guess at the combinations.
3. **The educated approach:** This is the recommended approach to SPE. It requires you to organize your attempt at method development, as well as review your objectives and as much preliminary information as you have on your analyses of interest.

The first step in this recommended procedure is to evaluate the objectives of your work. Establish exactly what it is you are trying to achieve.

- Is it a single or multiple drug extraction?
- Are you doing a low or a high level of detection?
- Is it a qualitative or quantitative analysis?

Once you have defined the objectives you need to define your research parameters and review the chemistry of your procedure, and consider your analyte.

- What is its structure?
- Is it hydrophobic or polar?

From: *Forensic Science and Medicine:*
Forensic and Clinical Applications of Solid Phase Extraction
Edited by: M. J. Telepchak, T. F. August, and G. Chaney © Humana Press Inc., Totowa, NJ

- What functional groups are attached?
- Does it have ionizable groups and if so, what are the pK_as?
- In solvents is it soluble or insoluble?
- Is it free or protein-bound?

Based on the data, choose a mechanism to retain your analyte and then choose the proper bonded phase to attempt separation and choose appropriate wash solvents and elution solvents.

6.2 SOME PRACTICAL ASPECTS OF SPE

6.2.1 Conditioning, Solvation (Wetting)

- Columns are shipped dry, but those with hydrophobic character need to be solvated to interact efficiently and reproducibly with aqueous matrices. Sample capacity is severely reduced on a dry column.
- At low vacuum ($\leq$3 in. Hg) add 1.5 mL of methanol or acetonitrile per 100 mg of sorbent to the sample preparation column. Release the vacuum or begin flushing immediately on completion. The more air that passes through the column before sample loading, the less solvated the sorbent will be.
- Apply deionized or distilled water to remove excess solvent, which will interfere with hydrophobic binding. Use 1 mL of H_2O per 100 mg of sorbent. Momentary high volume (5–8 in. Hg) may be necessary to restart flow.
At $\leq$2.5 in. Hg the column will resist air displacement (vacuum may be left on without drying the sorbent). If the sorbent is accidentally dried, resolvate and reflush.
- When using ion-exchange columns, apply 1 mL of buffer to the column after flushing to ensure that the sorbent pH is optimal for the sorbent analyte interaction desired. Where ion exchange interactions are involved, follow guidelines concerning pK_a, pH, and ionic binding. Use the same vacuum guidelines as described for flushing.

6.2.2 Sample Preparation and Application

- Retention mechanisms may be hydrophobic, polar, or ionic. Add internal standard to the sample if quantitation is desired. Optimize sample application by removing particulates if necessary (by centrifugation or filtering) and/or diluting viscous matrices with water or buffer to ensure proper pH for desired interactions. The analyte and sorbent should be uncharged for optimum hydrophobic retention. On ion-exchange sorbents, analytes must carry the opposite charge of the sorbent anions [–] on anion-exchange sorbents [+]; cations [+] on cation-exchange sorbents [–]. During sample application, the analyte binds by displacing a counter ion on the sorbent.
- Apply sample at a rate of 1 mL/min. Again, a momentary increase in vacuum may be needed to initiate sample flow.
- Be sure to wash the column with the strongest solvent in which the column will be placed during the extraction. This will wash any residual compounds off the column before the sample is applied to the column. This will give you lower background noise in your final analysis.

6.2.3 Washing the Sorbent and Eluting

Ideal washing removes as many interferences as possible while retaining the analyte(s). Ideal elution recovers 100% of the analyte while leaving behind interferences. Make certain your column is dry when changing between aqueous solutions and organic solvents. The easiest way to make sure your column is dry is to pull maximum vacuum on the column for 5 min. Touch the column; if it is at room temperature, it is dry. If it is cold, sorbent is still evaporating off the column.

6.2.4 Hydrophobic and Polar Analytes

The best approach toward using SPE of sorbents is to search for a solvent mixture that will wash the most interferences from the sorbent without loss of analyte. Note that wash pH may greatly affect cleanup and/or recovery. Keep analyte and sorbent pK_a in mind if applicable. Elute with the strongest organic solvent, or by raising the percentage of organic components possibly in combination with a pH change to disrupt binding.

6.2.5 Ion Exchange

Ionic bonds are strong enough to allow the analyte to remain bound while interferences are washed away with high percentages (up to 100%) of polar or nonpolar organic solvents. The pH will also affect sample cleanup. Remember to remain 2 pH units from the relevant pK_a of your analyte and sorbent, both of which need to remain charged for ionic retention. Elute with aqueous buffers containing a stronger counterion than your analyte (classic ion exchange) or by changing pH to disrupt the ionic attraction. Make sure the elution solvent has enough organic character to overcome any adsorption due to the packing material.

6.2.6 Copolymeric Exchange

For ionically bound analytes, use washes of high organic strength to remove interferences retained by hydrophobic (solvent strength-dependent) interactions. If your analyte is also capable of hydrophobic binding, remove polar interferences ionically similar to your analyte by using aqueous or weak aqueous/organic washes while disrupting ionic (pH and ionic strength-dependent) binding. Elute by simultaneously disrupting ionic and hydrophobic interactions.

6.3 The Use of Additional Cleanup Steps with Forensic Samples

With particularly complex samples, even the use of a copolymeric extraction column alone may be insufficient to yield an extract clean enough to give determinant results. In these situations simple wash and back-extractions can be used to render the sample clean enough for analysts.

6.3.1 Example

Smith was an extremely decomposed autopsy case. He died at home and was found about 1 week later and examined. He was negative for drugs except alcohol. The postmortem sample of whole blood was extracted by copolymeric extraction column for the acid/neutral drugs. The problem was that even the extraction using the SPE column left many interference peaks, which make it almost impossible to tell if drugs were present (Figure 1).

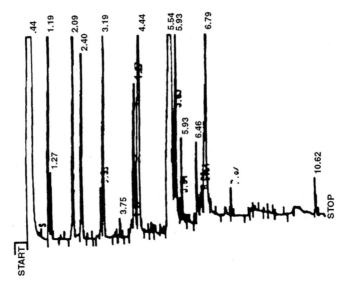

Fig. 1. Chromatogram 1. Sample: Extremely decomposed autopsy case. Preparation: Copolymeric extraction column; DAU bonded phase extraction.

Bonded Phase Extraction	**Additional Cleanup Steps**
1. Sample preparation	*Scheme A*
a. 1 mL of whole blood	
b. 4 mL of DI H$_2$O	7A. Reconstitute with 1 mL of
	MeOH:H$_2$O (80:20)
c. 2 mL of 0.1 *M* phosphate buffer,	8A. Add 1 mL of hexane.
pH 6.0	9A. Mix/vortex for 30 sec.
2. Column preparation WCDAU020:	10A. Centrifuge.
a. 3 mL of MeOH	11A. Aspirate/discard hexane (upper) layer.
b. 3 mL of H$_2$O	12B. Evaporate MeOH to dryness.
c. 1 mL of 0.1 *M* phosphate buffer	
3. Add sample and aspirate.	*Scheme B*
4. Column wash	7B. Reconstitute with 2 mL of 0.1 *N* HCl
a. 2 mL of H$_2$O	8B. Add 1 mL of hexane
b. 2 mL of 0.1 *N* HCl	9B. Mix/vortex for 30 sec.
c. Dry for 5 min.	10B. Centrifuge.
d. Wash 2 mL of hexane.	11B. Aspirate/discard hexane (upper) layer.
e. Turn off vacuum.	12B. Add 2 mL of ethyl acetate.
5. Elute acid/neutrals.	13B. Mix/vortex for 30 sec.
a. 3 mL of hexane/ethyl acetate (50:50)	14B. Centrifuge.
6. Evaporate to dryness.	15B. Transfer ethyl acetate (upper) layer
	and evaporate to dryness.

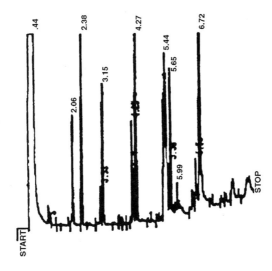

Fig. 2. Chromatogram 2. Sample: Extremely decomposed autopsy case. Preparation: Copolymeric extraction column; DAU bonded phase extraction followed by additional cleanup (Scheme A).

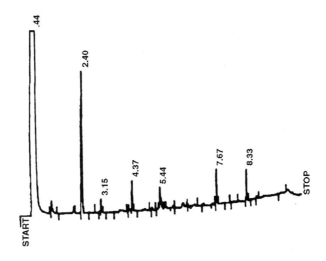

Fig. 3. Chromatogram 3. Sample: Extremely decomposed autopsy case. Preparation: Copolymeric extraction column; DAU bonded phase extraction followed by additional cleanup (Scheme B).

The chromatograms in Figs. 2–5 demonstrate how the additional cleanup step prior to injection ensures the technologists can distinguish trash peaks from decomposition from drug peaks.

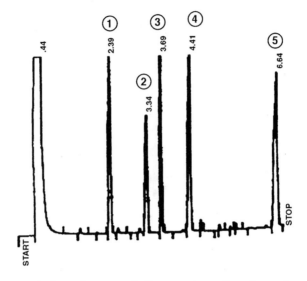

Fig. 4. Chromatogram 4. Sample control. Preparation: Copolymeric extraction column; DAU bonded phase extraction.

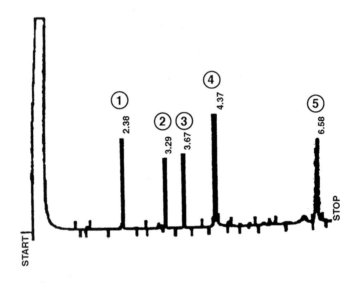

Fig. 5. Chromatogram 5. Serum control. Preparation: Copolymeric extraction column; DAU bonded phase extraction followed by additional cleanup (Scheme A).

6.3.1 The Drugs and Recoveries for the Additional Cleanup Step Are as Follows:

1. Aprobarbital   = 75%
2. Meprobamate   = 71%
3. Glutethimide   = 41%
4. Phenobarbital   = 68%
5. Phenytoin   = 61%

Ibuprofen, acetylsalicyclic acid, and acetaminophen extract better at lower pH sample preparations. It is suggested that one use 1 mL of whole blood, 5 mL H_2O, and 200 µL of 1 N acetic acid. These drugs are also in cleanup steps (scheme B).

Figure 2 shows that using the additional cleanup step shown in Scheme A improves the cleanup slightly, but not much. Figure 3 shows that using the additional cleanup step shown in Scheme B improves the cleanup enough to determine whether or not drugs were present.

Figure 4 shows that the extraction column would extract the drugs from a control if they were present. Figure 5 demonstrates that the additional cleanup step will also recover the drugs from the initial column cleanup eluate if they were present, although the recovery has been reduced by almost 50% due to the additional extraction step. This example should demonstrate that one should not become myopic in an approach to sample cleanup. Often a combination of SPE and an additional cleanup step will yield better results than one or the other.

6.4 FACTORS IN OPTIMIZING ANALYTE RECOVERY

This section reviews variables that are encountered in the laboratory concerning optimization of analyte recovery. In some cases optimal recovery of some analytes may be compromised to meet all your sample requirements. It may be necessary to change the separation conditions to optimize the one analyte that you are concerted with.

6.4.1 Ionization Status and the Mechanism of Separation

A large amount of information has been presented regarding ionization of the analyte of interest when using an ion-exchange mechanism. However, what if we choose to use a hydrophobic mechanism to retain a weak acid? What effect does the pH of the sample have on the recovery of the analyte of interest? Figure 6 shows the structure of ibuprofen, which will be extracted on the C_8 hydrophobic portion of a copolymeric mixed-mode column. Figure 7 shows chromatograms of two samples containing ibuprofen and another drug. When the pH of the sample is lowered from 6.0 to 5.0, the recovery of the ibuprofen increases whereas the other drug recoveries remain relatively unaffected. Why?

The pK_a of ibuprofen is 5.9. This means that as you get close to the pK_a and lower the pH of the separation you are increasing the nonionic molecular form, thus increasing the recovery of the drug on a hydrophobic bonded phase. At the pK_a the drug is 50% ionized and 50% non-ionized. As you lower the pH of an acidic drug you are decreasing the ionization of the analyte. The other drugs must have a pK_a of at least

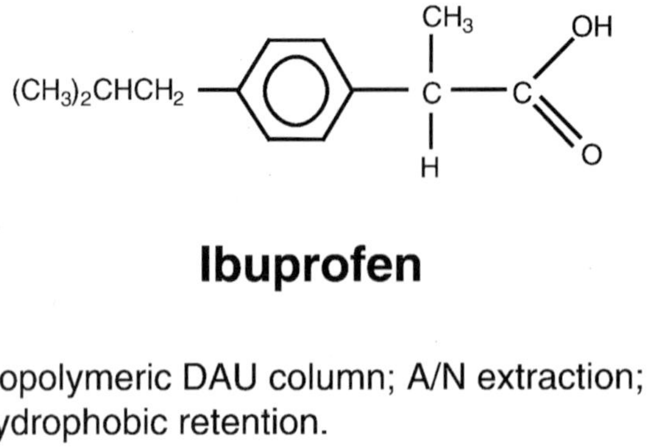

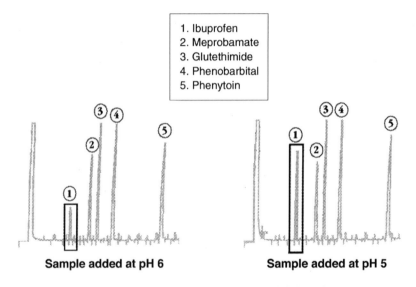

Ibuprofen

Copolymeric DAU column; A/N extraction;
hydrophobic retention.

Fig. 6. Structure of ibuprofen.

1. Ibuprofen
2. Meprobamate
3. Glutethimide
4. Phenobarbital
5. Phenytoin

Sample added at pH 6   Sample added at pH 5

Fig. 7. Sample of pH vs recovery of ibuprofen.

7.0 or better because it remains in its nonionized for, and is not affected by the pH being at 5.0 or 6.0.

Key points:

- Reversed phase or hydrophobic separations require the analyte to be in the nonionized or molecular form.

If the analyte is ionized reversed phase separation will give a lower recovery.

- Ion-exchange separations require the ionic form of the drug.

If the analyte is non-ionized, ion exchange will give lower recoveries.

- It is important to know your analyte's pK_a and to remember what ionization states you need for separation.

6.4.2 Acid/Neutral Drug Recoveries and Changes in Elution Solvents

Figure 8 shows the structure of meprobamate, a polar drug with no ionic character under the conditions of extraction. Figure 9 shows the extraction of ibuprofen and

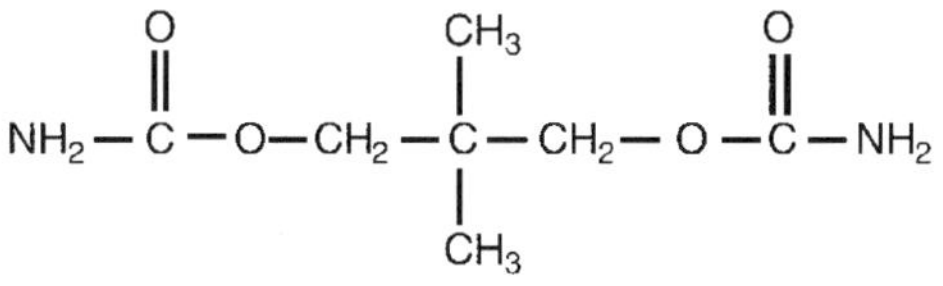

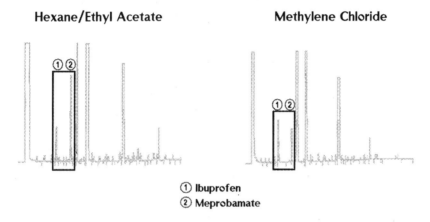

Meprobamate

Polar drug; copolymeric DAU column;
A/N extraction; hydrophobic retention.

Fig. 8. Meprobamate.

Hexane/Ethyl Acetate　　　　**Methylene Chloride**

① Ibuprofen
② Meprobamate

Fig. 9. A/N drug recovery vs changes in elution solvents.

meprobamate using two different elution solvents. How can you explain the differences seen in the recovery of the meprobamate?

Figure 10 shows an abbreviated version of the solvent polarity table. (The complete table is given in Appendix E.) Ibuprofen recovery has been affected very little by the increase in solvent strength from methylene chloride to hexane-ethyl acetate. However, the increase in solvent strength has had an effect on the recovery of the more polar meprobamate.

The energy of adsorption of ibuprofen is most likely below the energy of elution of either solvent, whereas the energy of adsorption of the meprobamate is above the energy of elution of methylene chloride but below the energy of elution of hexane-ethyl acetate.

Key point:

"Like dissolves like." If you see differences in the recovery of your analytes that cannot be explained on the basis of the ionization of the compounds, look at the elution solvents and see if a change in the polarity can have an effect on the recovery of your analytes.

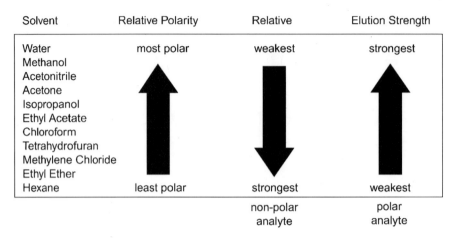

Solvent	Relative Polarity	Relative	Elution Strength
Water Methanol Acetonitrile Acetone Isopropanol Ethyl Acetate Chloroform Tetrahydrofuran Methylene Chloride Ethyl Ether Hexane	most polar least polar	weakest strongest	strongest weakest
		non-polar analyte	polar analyte

Fig. 10. Solvent polarity and elution strength.

Amphetamine
$pK_a = 9.9$

Methamphetamine
$pK_a = 9.9$

Ephedrine
$pK_a = 9.6$

Fig. 11. Amphetamine structures.

6.4.3 Compound Solubility in Elution Solvent and Recovery

The choice of elution solvents also has a significant effect on the recovery of drug classes. Figure 11 shows the structures and pK_a values of amphetamine compounds. Figures 12 and 13 show a series of basic drugs eluted with two different elution solvents. Changing the elution solvent from CH_2Cl_2–IPA–NH_4OH (78:20:2) to ETAC–NH_4OH (98:2) had little effect on most classes of basic drugs. However, recovery of the sympathomimetic drugs such as amphetamines, methamphetamines, phenylpropanolamine, and pseudephedrine decreased significantly. Why?

Since the energy of elution and pH of both elution solvents are correct for these compounds, the only factor to which we could attribute the difference in recovery would be the solubility differences of the sympathomimetics in the elution solvent.

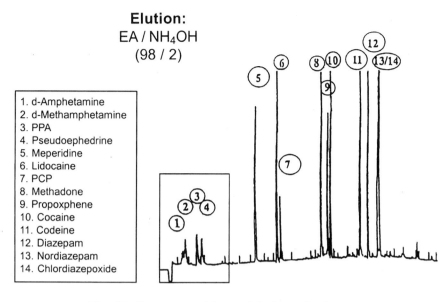

Fig. 12. Recovery without chlorinated solvents.

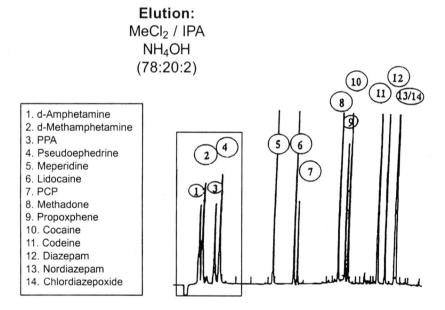

Fig. 13. Recovery with chlorinated solvents.

Apparently, they have a significantly better solubility in the CH_2Cl_2–IPA–NH_4OH than in the ETAC–NH_4OH.

Key point:

"Like dissolves like." Make sure to look at solubility as another factor required for the elution of drugs off the SPE column.

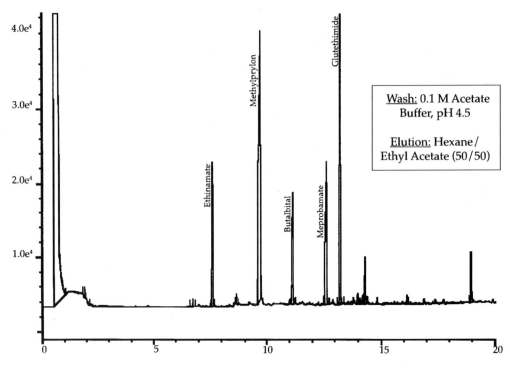

Fig. 14. pH and solvent effects in separation A. Loading pH = 4.5; elution solvent = 50:50 hexane-ethyl acetate.

6.4.4 Changing Variables in Search of Optimum Separation Conditions

Figures 14 through 17 show the results of changing the pH of the analyte solutions and the solvent composition of the elution solvent in an attempt to optimize an extraction method for the drug mixture including:

1. Ethinamate
2. Methylprylon
3. Butalbital
4. Meprobamate
5. Glutethimide

Based on our knowledge of the chemistry of the compounds in the mix and our choice of a hydrophobic extraction column (C18), we make an initial choice of sample conditions with which to apply the compounds on the column and then choose an elution solvent to recover the drugs from the column.

The results of our first attempt at optimizing this method can be seen in Fig. 14. The sample was adjusted to a pH of 4.5 and then applied to the column. The column was washed with a 0.1 *M* acetate buffer at pH 4.5. This is the same pH at which the sample was applied to the column. An elution solvent consisting of 50:50 hexane-ethyl acetate was applied and all five drugs were recovered from the column.

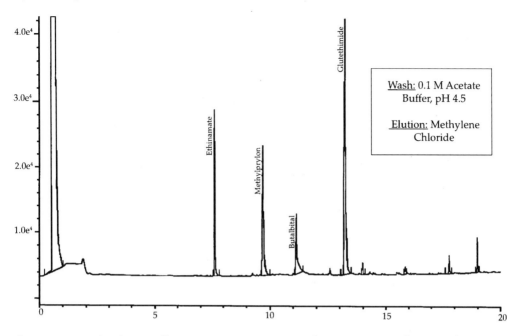

Fig. 15. pH and solvent effects in separation B. Loading pH = 4.5; elution solvent = methylene chloride.

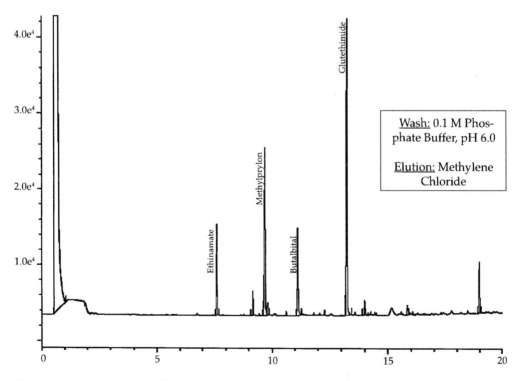

Fig. 16. pH and solvent effects in separation C. Loading pH = 6.0; elution solvent = 50:50 hexane-ethyl acetate.

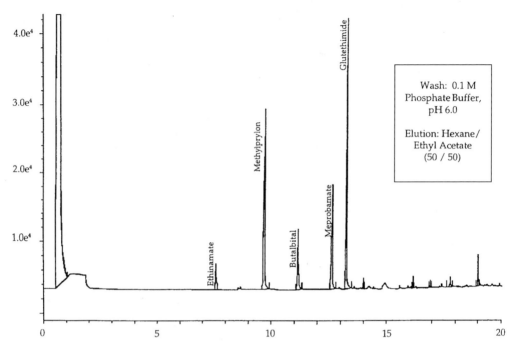

Fig. 17. pH and solvent effects in separation D. Loading pH = 6.0; elution solvent = methylene chloride.

Our challenge now is to determine whether or not recovery can be improved on any of the drugs. The results of our second attempt can be seen in Fig. 15. All conditions were held the same except that the elution solvent was changed to methylene chloride. The recovery of glutethimide remained the same and ethinamate recovery dropped off slightly. A significant loss of recovery is seen for methylprylon, and butalbital, and meprobamate disappeared altogether. These are not the results we had hoped for and are probably a result of lower solvent strength and/or solubility of the sample in the elution solvent.

In the next attempt the elution solvent was left as it was in the previous attempt and the pH of the sample application was changed to 6.0. Figure 16 shows the outcome. We have still not recovered the meprobamate. Recoveries of the butalbital and the methylprylon have declined slightly and the recovery of the ethinamate deteriorated. It appears that results are poorer.

In the next attempt, the application pH remained at 6.0 but the elution solvent was changed back to methylene chloride. Figure 17 shows the results, which are an improvement in general recovery. The meprobamate has been recovered but now the ethinamate has almost disappeared.

You can begin to see the effect of elution solvent polarity and solubility in these types of examples. In this case we were fortunate and chose the optimum set of conditions on the first try, but this will not occur in most cases. However, if you proceed methodically, changing one variable at a time, you will eventually find the best conditions for optimizing your extraction. Remember, there will always be trade-offs. Hopefully, they won't prevent you from attaining your goal of a quick, efficient, clean extraction.

The results show that the conditions used in Fig. 14 were the optimal ones for the drugs in this mix. This series demonstrates that the analyst may have to sacrifice the recovery of one compound to optimize recovery of others. It is hoped that the analyst will be able to find conditions that will be optimal for all drugs desired in a screen, but this will not always be the case.

6.5 THE USE OF SELECTIVE ELUTION

This example illustrates how selective we can become if the compounds of interest have different physical characteristics. Various lipid classes have different solubility characteristics that can be used to purify or separate these compounds (1).

The following classes of lipids can be separated from adipose tissues or serum in excellent yields and purity:

- Fatty acids
- Phospholipids
- Cholesterol esters
- Cholesterol
- Triglycerides
- Diglycerides
- Monoglycerides

Figure 18 illustrates the basic structures of these lipid classes. Figure 19 demonstrates a separation scheme for lipid compounds reported in the literature.

The authors of this book thought that this approach demonstrated enough significant principles and a unique way of applying them that a detailed review (Section 6.5.1) was worthwhile. If you work with any of these classes of compounds, there is something valuable to be learned from this example. Section 6.5.1 demonstrates a separation scheme for lipid compounds reported in the literature. This method, when developed, required three separate 500-mg columns. See if you can use what you have learned so far to do it on two columns. Table 1 shows the lipid recoveries obtained using this method.

6.5.1 The Separation of Lipids from Serum and Tissues by Selective Elution on 500-mg CLEAN-UP Extraction Columns (CUNAX503)

1. **Prepare sample.**
   Tissues
   a. Homogenize sample using 1 g of wet tissue to 1 mL of chloroform.
   b. Centrifuge to separate particulates.
   c. Retain supernatant for application onto conditioned SPE column in Step 2.
   Serum or plasma
   a. Plasma or serum: Make a chloroform extract of the samples.
      Dilution 1:1, serum to chloroform.
   b. Mix/vortex.
   c. Centrifuge to separate particulates.
   d. Retain supernatant for application onto conditioned SPE column in Step 2.

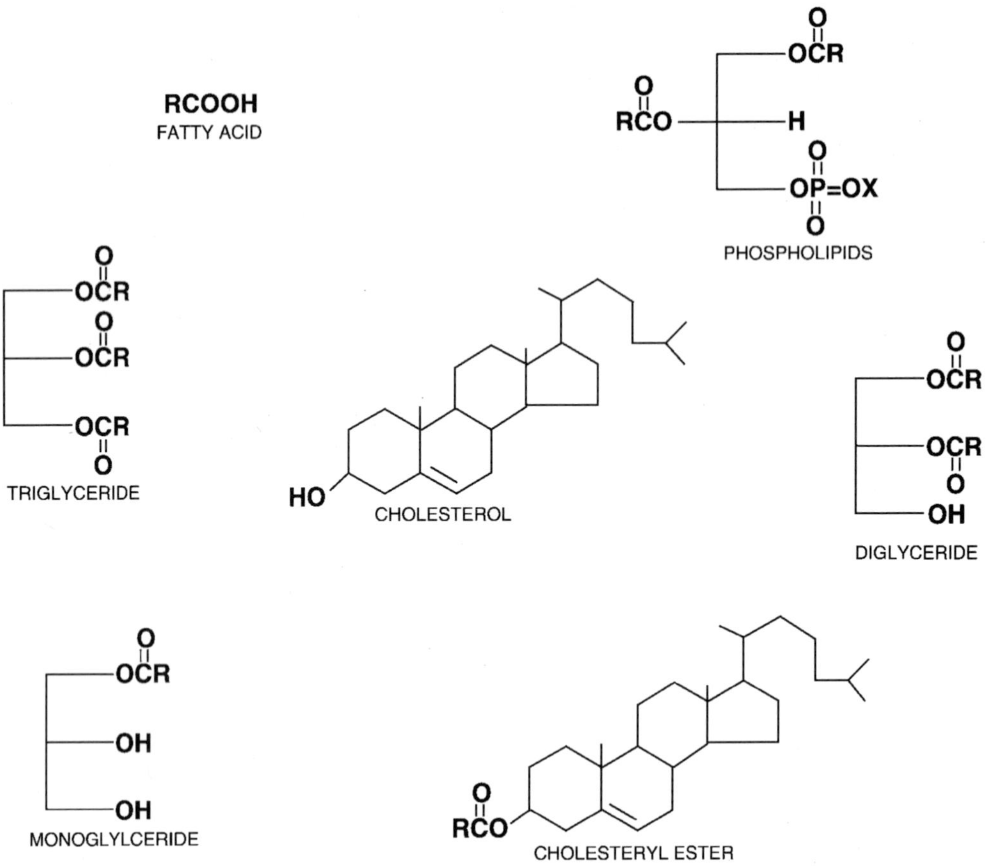

Fig. 18. Base structures of tissue and plasma lipids.

2. **Condition CLEAN-UP extraction column.**
   1 × 3 mL of CH3OH; aspirate.
   1 × 3 mL of ethyl acetate; aspirate.
   1 × 3 mL of CH$_2$Cl$_2$; aspirate.
   3 × 3 mL of hexane; aspirate.
3. **Apply sample.**
   Load at 1 mL/min.
4. **Wash column.**
   1 × 1 mL CHCl$_3$
   All lipid classes will be retained at this point.
5. **Elute cholesterol esters, triglycerides, cholesterol, diglycerides, and monoglycerides.**
   1 × 4 mL CHCl$_3$–IPA (2:1).
   Elute at 1–2 mL/min.
   Dry down eluate.
   Reconstitute in 1 mL hexane for further extraction.
   Phospholipids and fatty acids are still on the column.
6. **Elute fatty acids from the column used in Step 5.**
   1 × 4 mL acetic acid-diethylene (2:98).
   Analyze by method of your choice.

Step 1: Initial Isolation of Lipids

> The SPE column is an amine functional SPE column.
> Precondition the column with three column volumes of hexane.
> Add the sample extracts after the sample preparation step above.

Fatty acids, phospholipids, cholesterol esters, triglycerides, cholesterol, diglycerides, and monoglycerides are retained on the SPE column.

Step 2: To the SPE column from **step 1** add solvent A-2:1 chloroform in isopropanol

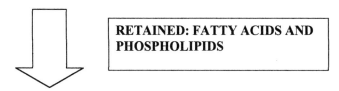

RETAINED: FATTY ACIDS AND PHOSPHOLIPIDS

ELUTED OFF THE COLUMN:
Cholesterol Esters
Triglycerides
Cholesterol
Diglycerides
Monoglycerides

Step 3: To the SPE column from **Step 2** add solvent B-2% acetic acid in diethyl ether.

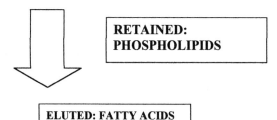

RETAINED: PHOSPHOLIPIDS

ELUTED: FATTY ACIDS

Step 4: To the SPE column from **step 3** add solvent C-methanol.

ELUTED PHOSPHOLIPIDS

Fig. 19. Lipid separation scheme (continued on pp. 126 and 127.)

7. **Elute phospholipids.**
   1 × 4 mL of MeOH.
   Analyze by method of your choice.
8. **Condition a second new CLEAN-UP extraction column**
   1 × 3 mL of CH₃OH; aspirate.
   1 × 3 mL of ethylacetate; aspirate.
   1 × 3 mL of CH₂Cl₂, aspirate.
   3 × 3 mL of hexane; aspirate.
9. **Apply sample.**
   Load reconstituted eluant from Step 5.
   Load at 1 mL/min.

Using Step 1 again:
Step 1: Initial Isolation of Lipids

Perform the isolation of Fatty Acids and Phospholipids first, then use the additional isolation step 5.

Cholesterol esters, triglycerides, cholesterol, diglycerides, and monoglycerides are retained on the SPE column.

Step 2: To the SPE column from **step 1** add solvent D-Hexane

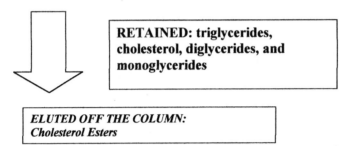

RETAINED: triglycerides, cholesterol, diglycerides, and monoglycerides

ELUTED OFF THE COLUMN:
Cholesterol Esters

Step 3: To the SPE column from **step 2**
add an additional preconditioned amine SPE columns,
to catch the eluants from the first SPE column.
Add solvent E - 1% diethyl ether, 10% methylene chloride in hexane
to the SPE column.

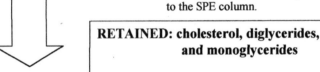

RETAINED: cholesterol, diglycerides, and monoglycerides

ELUTEd: Triglycerides

Step 4: To the SPE column from **step 3** add solvent F 5% ethyl acetate in hexane.

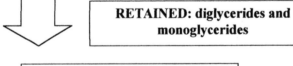

RETAINED: diglycerides and monoglycerides

ELUTED: Cholesterol

Fig. 19. (*continued*)

10. **Elute cholesterol esters.**
    1 × 4 mL hexane.
    Analyze by method of your choice.
11. **Condition a third new CLEAN-UP extraction column**.
    1 × 3 mL of CH_3OH; aspirate.
    1 × 3 mL of ethyl acetate; aspirate.
    1 × 3 mL of $CH2Cl_2$; aspirate.
    3 × 3 mL of hexane; aspirate.

Step 5: To the SPE column from **step 4** add solvent G- 15% ethyl acetate in hexane.

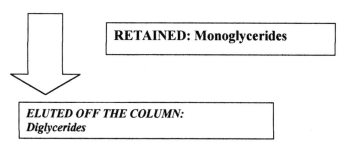

RETAINED: Monoglycerides

ELUTED OFF THE COLUMN:
Diglycerides

Step 6: To the SPE Column from **Step 5** add solvent H – 2:1 chloroform- methanol.

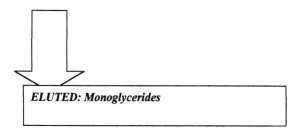

ELUTED: Monoglycerides

Fig. 19. (*continued*)

12. **Attach the two columns.**
    Using an adapter, connect the column from step 11 to the bottom of the column used in step 10*.
13. **Elute triglycerides.**
    To the top of the 2 connected columns:
    1 × 1 mL of diethyl ether-methylene chloride-hexane (1:10:89).
    Analyze by method of your choice.
14. **Elute cholesterol.**
    Separate top and bottom column.
    To top column†:
    1 × 16 mL of ethylacetate-hexane (5:95).
    To bottom column:
    1 × 4 mL of ethyl acetate-hexane (5:95).
    (Combine eluants analyze by method of your choice.)
15. **Elute diglycerides.**
    To the top column from step 14.
    1 × 8 mL of ethyl acetate-hexane (15:85).
    Analyze by method of your choice.
16. **Elute monoglycerides.**
    To the top of column from step 15.
    1 × 4 mL of chloroform-methanol (2:1).
    Analyze by method of your choice.

Table 1
Lipid Recoveries

Analyte	Recovery	SD	% Contamination
Fatty Acids	98.9 %	4.7%	1.16%
Phospholipids	98.4%	5.3%	2.03%
Cholesterol Esters	96.7%	4.9%	Trace
Triglycerides	96.7%	2.5%	Trace
Cholesterol	100.0%	4.1%	1.13%
Diglycerides	101.4%	7.8%	1.96%
Monoglycerides	97.3%	5.3%	1.15%

*The second column is necessary to collect excess cholesterol that breaks through either because it overloads the column or, more likely, because the cholesterol is chromatographing down the column.

†The top column will contain diglycerides, monoglycerides, and 90% of the cholesterol; the bottom column will contain approximately 10% of the cholesterol, which migrated off the top column and is collected on the bottom column.

6.5.2 Mechanisms Behind Selective Elution

The initial gross liquid-liquid extraction of lipids from serum was accomplished with chloroform. The extract was applied to the first extraction column. The first elution system eluted the uncharged compounds while the free fatty acids and phospholipids (charged compounds) were retained. The pH was lowered to elute the free fatty acids. The sorbent strength was increased to bring off the phospholipids.

The uncharged compounds eluted from the first column were then applied to the second and third columns and the sorbent strength was gradually increased to separate the compounds by classes.

The sorbent system used to elute the triglycerides cause the cholesterol to migrate down the column. This is not a desired or recommended effect but the researcher compensated by adding the additional column to collect the migrating compound. Perhaps this effect could be eliminated by adjusting the solvent combination.

Although this part of the technique may not be pure SPE by definition, the results are certainly indisputable (Table 1).

REFERENCE

[1]Kaluzny, M., Duncan, L., Merritt, M., and Epps, D. Rapid separation of lipid classes in high yield and purity using bonded phase columns.
Second Annual Symposium on "Sample Preparation and Isolation Using Bonded Silicas, Philadelphia, 1985.

Chapter 7

Separation of Analytes from Their Matrices

7.1 INTRODUCTION

Solid phase extraction has shown great versatility in the separation of many analytes from different matrices. The most common matrices are biological fluids such as whole blood and urine; however, many different separations from unusual matrices have been accomplished. This chapter reviews a wide range of procedures that illustrate the separation of analytes from their matrices. General rules for matrix preparation are given in Table 1.

7.1.1 Is It a Gas, Liquid, or Solid?

The state of the material can change the method of preparation sample. For example, most separations use the liquid form of a sample. This allows for the filtering effects of the silica backbone. Dissolving the material in a solvent can achieve a degree of separation by the solubility of the analyte versus its matrix. Drugs in tissues may be analyzed by homogenization or by mixing of the tissue sample with the sorbent material and the passing of solvents through the sorbent. Gases can be easily passed through the silica surface for absorption.

7.1.2 Aqueous, Organic, or Nonpolar?

One simple rule of thumb in dissolving materials into the matrix or other liquid is that like dissolves like. Polar materials are soluble in polar solvents (water, alcohol). Nonpolar materials can be dissolved in nonpolar solvents (hexane, methylene chloride).

From: *Forensic Science and Medicine:*
Forensic and Clinical Applications of Solid Phase Extraction
Edited by: M. J. Telepchak, T. F. August, and G. Chaney © Humana Press Inc., Totowa, NJ

Table 1
General Rules for Matrix Preparation

a. Dissolve solids or powders.

A homogenized form of the sample must be used.

Any solid should be dissolved into its liquid form. Example: when a drug has an affinity
for lipids (e.g., red blood cells), the sample should be homogenized before separation.

b. Filter or centrifuge suspended solids.

The most common form of this is the sample preparation of tissues.

The cells are first disrupted by osmotic pressure or enzymatic digestion.

The cell residues can be centrifuged to separate cellular fluid from the tissue cells.

c. Gross extraction

In cases where the analyte is a minor constituent of the mixture, a simple liquid-liquid
extraction can remove most of the major contaminants.

d. Dilution

In some cases, dilution of the sample can aid in isolating the analyte.

e. Precipitating proteins

One common extraction strategy is to precipitate the proteins in a blood or plasma sample
by the addition of a solvent (e.g., methanol or acetonitrile), strong salt solution (zinc
chloride), or a strong acid solution (perchloric, formic, or trichloroacetic acid).

f. Deconjugation

A common route of biotransformation is the formation of conjugates whereby the drug
combines with a neutral sugar to form a glucuronide. Hydrolysis with strong acids
and bases or enzyme hydrolysis with β-glucuronidase will remove this attachment.

Acid hydrolysis offers the advantage of speed, works with minimal expense, but may
cause chemical breakdown of the primary analyte or create many more contaminants
than you began with. Acid or base hydrolysis can be achieved in an autoclave in 15–20 min.

Enzyme hydrolysis works especially well if stability is a problem; however, it takes a
longer period of time to work completely. Enzyme hydrolysis can take from 3 to 6 h or
longer to work.

7.1.3 Do We Need to Prepare Our Samples?

In some cases, no sample preparation is needed because the matrix is so dissimi-
lar to the analyte that physical separation would work. For example, iron salts in a
rock however, sample can be separated by a magnet without any elaborate separation
procedures. In most cases, isolation of the analyte from its matrix is required.

7.2 URINE

Urine is the yellow, amber, or clear fluid produced by the kidneys for the removal of metabolic waste and other substances from the body. It is formed continu-
ously and stored in the urinary bladder. An average healthy person produces 1–2 L of
urine daily.

7.2.1 Composition

The composition of urine is 95% water. The remaining 5% is composed of sugars, amino acids, creatinine, urea, and other products of metabolism. The physical and
chemical composition of urine is highly variable, changes considerably with the nature

and composition of the diet and amount of endogenous metabolites, and depends on other factors such as body weight, emotional status, rate of metabolism, and so forth. At the moment of voiding, the urine is usually clear (transparent). On standing the urine may become cloudy, turbid, or develop a flocculent precipitant as a result of the mucus present from the urinary tract or lipid deposition.

7.2.2 Characteristics

Urine is the most widely used matrix; many drugs also form conjugates that are excreted in the urine requiring some form of deconjugation (acid hydrolysis or enzyme β-glucuronidase hydrolysis).

Urine has variable composition with a high degree of variability in the amount of salt and other byproducts of metabolism. Pigments and proteins may also be present. Drugs are seen in a delayed form; in most cases the disappearance of the drug from the blood results in its appearance in the urine.

7.2.3 General Sample Preparation

In most cases, dilution and buffering are the only sample preparation steps. If solids exist, centrifugation or filtering may be needed.

7.2.4 Acid Hydrolysis of Urine

1. To 5 mL of urine add internal standard and 500 μL of concentrated hydrochloric acid. Mix/vortex.
   a. Autoclave
2. Autoclave for 20 min at 121°C. Cool.
3. Centrifuge for 10 min at 670g and discard pellet.
4. Add 1000 μL of 7.4 M NH$_4$OH. Mix/vortex.
5. Adjust the sample pH to 6.0 ± 0.5 with 1–3 mL of phosphoric acid.
   b. Boiling water bath
   Use the same procedure as in (a) but place the sample into a boiling water bath for 20 min instead of an autoclave.
   c. Block Heater
   Use the same procedure as in (a) but place the sample into a block heater at 90°C for 30 min instead of an autoclave.

Note: Acid hydrolysis is used for basic conjugates. Some drugs have acid conjugates that need a basic hydrolysis (e.g., THC conjugates). Sodium or potassium hydroxide is used in place of hydrochloric acid to hydrolyze the conjugates.

7.2.5 Enzymatic Hydrolysis of Urine

1. To 5 mL of urine, add internal standard and 2 mL of β-glucuronidase.
   β-Glucuronidase solution is made at a concentration of 5000 Fishman units (FU) per milliter of 1.0 M acetate buffer, pH 5.0.
   It is recommended that β-glucuronidase obtained from *Patella vulgate* or limpets be used. In some cases other enzyme sources may be recommended (such as type IX–A– *E. coli* used for THC metabolites).
2. Hydrolyze at 65°C for 3 h. Cool the sample.
3. Centrifuge for 10 min at 670g and discard the solid pellet.
4. Adjust the sample pH to 6.0 ± 0.5 with approx 700 μL of 1.0 M NaOH.

Note: Depending on the analyte, the time for hydrolysis can vary from 1–3 to 24 h.

7.3 BLOOD

Blood is the fluid that circulates in the arteries, veins, and capillaries in humans and many animals. Blood is essential for life and plays a role in every major body function. In humans, blood is a complex mixture in which a number of living cells are suspended. The average volume of blood in a 70-kg adult is approximately 5 L. Blood travels in a continuous cycle throughout the body by the pumping action of the heart. The blood serves many functions:

1. Cellular respiration and the exchange of oxygen in hemoglobin;
2. Distribution of nutrients, food, hormones, and drugs;
3. Transportation of cells for immunity and cellular defenses;
4. Maintenance of the precise pH environment for cell function.

SPE has been used widely for the isolation and separation of drugs, hormones, endogenous products of metabolism, and other substances from the blood matrix.

7.3.1 Composition

Blood is a complex suspension of various components. The fluid portion of whole blood is called plasma. Whole blood is made up of 55% plasma fractions and a 45% cellular portion.

Plasma can be harvested by centrifugation of anticoagulated whole blood. The cellular portion consists of red blood cells, white blood cells, and platelets. Serum is a clear liquid exudate from clotted blood.

7.3.2 Plasma Proteins

The total protein content of plasma is 7.0–7.5 g/100 mL of plasma. This is the major part of solids in plasma. The separation of individual proteins from plasma is accomplished by the use of various solvents, electrolytes, or both to remove different protein fractions in accordance with their solubility.

7.3.3 Characteristics of Whole Blood

Whole blood has a high protein content from hemoglobin. Blood-cell materials are present and some drugs may be transported within the cell. Most drugs form conjugates; glucuronides and sulfates are the primary conjugates in humans.

7.3.4 Blood Sample Preparation

1. **Osmotic breakdown**
   a. To 1 mL of whole blood, plasma, or serum, add internal standard and 4 mL of distilled water.
   b. Mix/vortex and let stand for 5 min.
   c. Centrifuge at 670g for 10 min and discard the pellet.
   d. Adjust the pH of the supernatant accordingly by the addition of a buffer solution.
2. **Protein precipitation (using polar solvents such as methanol or acetonitrile)**
   a. Use 2 parts solvent to 1 part plasma serum.
   b. Mix and let stand for 5–10 min.

c. Vortex the sample and centrifuge the precipitate.

d. Collect the supernatant and buffer before extraction.

Notes: The organic solvent should be diluted with aqueous buffers to reduce the solvent strength and ensure the appropriate ionization state.
Acetonitrile is considered the most effective solvent for disrupting protein binding.
Lower ratios of organic solvents (10–30%) may also work.

3. **Acid treatment**
   a. Strong acids such as formic, perchloric, or trichloroacetic acid can disrupt the proteins and their structures.
   b. Add 50 μL of 0.1–1.0 *M* perchloric or formic acid to 1 mL of serum or plasma.
   c. Use a dilution of 10% trichloroacetic acid.
   d. Mix the sample and let stand for 5–10 min.
   e. Vortex the sample and centrifuge ($670g$ for 5–10 min) to drop out the precipitate.
   f. Analyze the supernatant.

4. **Inorganic salts**
   Ammonia sulfate or zinc sulfate (10–20%) can be used to precipitate proteins (1:1 dilution).

5. **Sonication**
   a. Sonicate the biological fluid for 15 min at room temperature.
   b. Add an appropriate pH buffer, mix, and vortex.
   c. Centrifuge at $670g$ for 15 min.
   d. Discard the pellet and analyze the supernatant.

7.4 HAIR

The use of hair as a matrix for the screening of drugs has been widely published. Hair offers multiple advantages as a matrix:

- Hair collection can be done in a simple and noninvasive manner. This eliminates the "invasion of privacy" issues found with the collection of urine and blood.
- Hair samples can document a longer period of time for drug exposure.
- Hair is more difficult to adulterate.
- Hair is remarkably stable, allowing for retesting years later. For example, cocaine was detected in hair samples of Chilean mummies >2000 yr old.

Hair also presents some major problems:

- The testing must be able to detect drugs at picogram-per-milliliter levels.
- The uptake of drugs into the hair may vary depending on the hair color. For example, blond hair has a lesser chance of the deposition of drugs than black hair.
- A number of environmental factors, such as the use of hair products, may affect the integrity of the hair shaft, thus affecting the uptake of drugs into the hair.

Hair continues to be used in drug testing despite its shortcomings.

7.4.1 Hair Sample Preparation

The preparation of hair samples is performed easily in most cases by the following steps:

1. Samples are usually identified as to the portion of hair collected and the length reported from the tip.

2. A sample aliquot (20–50 mg) s placed into a culture tube and is washed with an initial amount of methanol to remove external contamination. The sample is rinsed in 2 mL of methanol, incubated for 10 min by swirling, and the methanol is then decanted off.

3. Two milliliters of fresh methanol or (0.1 mL sodium hydroxide) are added to the tube and are heated 2 h at 70–75°C.

4. After the digestion of the sample and the heating period, the supernatant is decanted to a clean test tube and the solvent is evaporated at 40°C to dryness.

5. The dried sample can be reconstituted with buffer and the SPE extraction can be performed.

Note: Acid or base may also be used in addition to methanol to digest the samples.

7.5 SWEAT

Sweat is the secretion of exocrine glands in the transdermal layer of moist skin surfaces. The presence of various drugs in sweat often makes it an ideal matrix for monitoring drug intake, especially in screening for drugs of abuse. Many drugs have been identified in sweat, including ethanol, amphetamines, cocaine, heroin, morphine, methadone, methamphetamine, and phencyclidine.

7.5.1 Collection Device

A sweat patch may consist of an adhesive layer on a thin transparent film of surgical dressing to which an absorbent pad is attached. The dressing allows for the exchange of gases and water vapor to escape but prevents the escape of the nonvolatile components of sweat. Over a period of several days the compounds in the sweat saturate the pad and concentrate.

7.5.2 Sample Preparation

Sweat patches are removed after use, stored by placing the unit onto an index card, and kept frozen at 30°C until preparation. Sample preparation consists of thawing to room temperature, removal of the absorbent pad from the collection device, and extraction of the pad with the extraction solution. The extraction solution is a mixture of 0.1% Triton X-100 (surfactant) in an appropriate buffer. After agitation and mixing, the extraction solutions are collected, buffered, and subjected to SPE extraction.

7.6 SALIVA

Saliva has been proposed as an alternative biological specimen for screening for drugs of abuse and various other analytes (e.g., HIV, cotinine) for the life insurance industry. It is readily available, noninvasive, and is easily prepared for analysis. Its disadvantages are a limited quantity of sample, low levels of detection, and a short surveillance time (drug detection window).

7.6.1 Composition

Saliva is a fluid from the human oral cavity that is secreted as a combination of three glandular fluids. The parotid gland secretes serous fluid, the sublingual gland secretes mucus, and the submandibular gland secretes both serous and mucus fluids. A minor source of saliva is mucosal transudate, which is the fluid from passive trans-

Table 2
Potential Analytes for Saliva Testing

17-Hydroxyprogesterone	DHEA-binding glycoprotein	Methaqualone
Acetaminophen	Diazepam	Nortriptyline
Amitriptyline	Digoxin	Phenobarbital
Amobarbital	Epidermal growth factor	Phenytoin
Androstenedione	Estradiol	Primidione
CA19-9	Ethanol	Progesterone
Caffeine	GH release factor	Secobarbital
Carbamazepine	Inhibiting factor	Sex hormones
Cholesterol	HIV antibodies	Binding globulins
Cocaine	IgA	Testosterone
Corticosterol-binding globulin	Insulin-like growth factor I	Theophylline
Cortisol	Insulin-like growth factor II	Transforming growth factor
	Lithium	alpha

port of fluid through crevicular spaces (i.e., cheek and gum). Saliva is an excellent matrix for drugs of abuse, hormones, proteins, and infectious agents. Currently, saliva can be best described as a qualitative index and not a quantitative tool.

7.6.2 Analytes

Table 2 lists potential analytes for saliva testing.

7.6.3 Collection Procedure

Currently a number of saliva collection devices are on the market (Saliva Diagnostics [Vancouver, BC], STC Technologies [Bethlehem, PA], Starstadt [Princeton, NJ], etc.). These devices allow for the collection of an adequate sample volume in a simple manner. For a sample to be considered valid an immunological test is performed on the sample. In most cases an IgG level is taken, and if the results are >0.5 ng/mL the sample is considered valid.

7.6.4 Sample Preparation

Saliva is usually prepared by dilution with buffer and direct application of the sample onto a conditioned sample column.

7.7 MECONIUM

Substance abuse is a major social problem in the United States. Drug abuse during pregnancy is a serious social issue and a grave concern to the obstetrician and pediatrician. Fetal drug exposure can lead to a high incidence of perinatal complications such as stillbirths, abruptio placentae, fetal stress, and increased newborn mortality and morbidity. Newborn complications include prematurity, low birth weight, asphyxia, pneumonia, congenital malformations, cerebral infarcts, and drug withdrawal. The screening of neonates born to suspected abusers is essential to the prompt intervention and follow-up care.

The use of meconium as an alternative specimen in neonatal drug screening has been widely used. It has a number of distinct advantages over blood and urine:

- Meconium is easily obtained. It is often difficult to obtain an adequate sample of blood and urine.
- Meconium measures drug exposure over a longer period of time than other specimens.
- Blood or urine can be negative if the mother abstains a few days before delivery.
- Organ tissue often is difficult to obtain and process.

7.7.1 Meconium Sample Preparation

Meconium is prepared for SPE by the following procedure:

1. Samples are kept in the frozen state until analysis.
2. A thawed sample is weighed. The usual sample size is between 0.1 and 1 gram.
3. Two milliters of alcohol are added.
4. The sample is mixed using a clean wooden applicator and vortex mixed to yield a suspension.
5. The suspension is centrifuged (670g for 5 min) and the supernatant is decanted.
6. To the supernatant add the internal standard buffer to the appropiate pH and vortex to completely mix.

The sample is ready to be added to a conditioned SPE column.

7.8 TISSUE

Tissues have been long used as the matrix of choice for forensic applications, especially in autopsy cases where the blood has been degraded or hemolyzed to the extent that the extraction efficiency may be affected. In addition, recent studies have shown that postmortem drug levels are site-dependent (1–3) with heart blood giving higher levels than femoral blood.

Incorrect interpretation of these results can cause questions as to the validity of the analytical result. Tissue analyses are often necessary to interpret postmortem blood samples correctly. The major problem in doing tissue extractions is the inability of tissue homogenates to pass through the tightly packed bonded SPE columns. This situation has been alleviated by the use of bonded packing materials that have larger particle sizes (XtrackT SPE columns).

Homogenization followed by enzyme digestion and/or protein precipitation and centrifugation of samples has been used for kidney, liver, and intestinal tissues. Brain tissue has a high lipid content and may require digestion with lipase before extraction (4).

Some sample preparation methods follow.

7.8.1 Tissue Sample Preparation Procedures

7.8.1.1 Brain Tissue for Cocaine and Metabolites (5)

1. Sample approximately 1 g of brain tissue.
2. Add 0.2 M Tris buffer, pH 6.3, and internal standard (bupivicaine).
3. Homogenize for 5 s.
4. Centrifuge to separate the supernatant from the cellular materials.
5. Apply the supernatant to a large particle size SPE tube (i.e., XtrackT®).

7.8.1.2 Brain Tissue-Alternative Procedure (6)

1. To 1 g of brain tissue add 5 mL of 0.1 *M* perchloric acid.
2. Homogenize the sample for a few seconds.
3. Centrifuge to remove cellular materials.
4. Apply the supernatant to a preconditioned SPE column.

7.8.1.3 Enzymatic Digestion of Liver Tissue (7)

Depending on which drug is needed, a number of procedures may be used.

1. Liver (1 g) is minced with 3 mL of water in a homogenizer.
2. To 0.4 g liver homogenate (0.4 mL) add internal standard and buffer solution.
3. Centrifuge: Remove pellet and apply the supernatant to the SPE tube.

XtrackT is a registered trademark of United Chemical Technologies, Inc.

ENZYME-DIGESTED SAMPLE

To the homogenate prepared above, different kinds of enzymes may be added to break up tissue samples. Adjustment of the pH may be required after enzyme digestion.

ENZYMES

- Protease Subtilisin Carlsberg at pH 10.5
- β-Glucuronidase at pH 7.4

PROCEDURE

To the sample homogenate above, adjust the pH to the operating pH of the enzyme.
Add the enzyme to the sample.
Incubate for the specified period of time.
Adjust the pH and apply the sample to the SPE column.

OTHER TISSUES INTESTINE (8)

To 3 grams of tissue 10 mL of water was used.
The sample was homogenized for a few seconds.
The tissue homogenate was extracted with chloroform.
The chloroform layer was separated and evaporated to dryness.
The dried residue was reconstituted in methanol and applied to the SPE column.

MUSCLE

Chlortetracycline in swine muscle (9).
Pulverized frozen tissue using a mortar and pestle.
Added glycine in acid and homogenized the entire mixture.
Centrifuge the sample and pour off the supernatant.
Apply the supernatant to the SPE column.

BONE

Vancomycin in bone (10).
A weighed bone sample is cut up and pulverized in a blender with dry ice.
Water is added.
The sample is sonicated for 20 min.
After separation by centrifugation the supernatant is applied to a prepared SPE column.

7.9 OCULAR FLUIDS

7.9.1 Introduction

The need for a reliable tool to determine drug levels at the time of death has pushed investigation into the determination of drugs in alternative matrices, such as the eye.

7.9.2 Physiology

The human eye consists of three distinct chambers:

- **Anterior Chamber**
  This chamber is filled with aqueous humor.
  This chamber is primarily located anterior to the iris and lens of the eye.
  The fluid in this chamber is primarily water containing between 0.1% and 0.6% protein and serves the function of continually washing the surface of the eye.
  Drugs given topically cross through Schlemmís channels and concentrate in this chamber of the eye.
- **Posterior Chamber**
  This chamber produces aqueous humor.
  This chamber is located posterior to the anterior chamber.
  This chamber forms the blood aqueous barrier of the eye.
- **Vitreous Chamber**
  This chamber has a network of collagen and hyaluric acid fibrils and is the large chamber that forms a major part of the eye.
  Vitreous humor is the fluid that is located inside the vitreous chamber of the eye. It has a volume of 4 mL. The composition of this fluid is 98–99% water and 0.2% protein. The exchange of drugs is controlled by the blood-ocular barrier located within the vitreous chamber.
- The leakage of fluid in the blood-ocular barrier can be seen in a number of clinical situations such as inflammation, age, and diabetes.

7.9.2.1 Advantages of Vitreous Humor

Vitreous fluids have low protein content and are easily prepared.
Vitreous humor is readily available and easily obtained. Vitreous humor can be used as an alternative where blood is not available.

7.9.2.2 Issues of Vitreous Humor Drug Levels

Drug concentrations vary considerably from blood levels.

The validity of kinetic conditions of healthy subjects cannot be extended to the kinetics of intoxication cases. Further research is needed to extend the value of this determination.

7.9.3 General Sample Preparation

Take 0.5–1.0 mL of vitreous or aqueous humor and add 2 mL of 0.1 *M* phosphate buffer, pH 6.0. Add this sample onto a conditioned SPE column.

7.10 AMNIOTIC FLUID

7.10.1 Introduction

The use of drugs by expectant mothers has necessitated the development of methods for matrices that will identify prenatal drug exposure. For example, it has been estimated that 50 million Americans have used cocaine at least once and approximately 8 million use it in a regular basis (1).

Roughly one-third of the 8 million users are women with 10% using cocaine at least once during their pregnancy (2). During the past 10 years every major urban medical center has reported an increased incidence of positive drug findings during neonatal testing (3). Detection of the drug is usually performed by urine specimens obtained from the mother; however, metabolite determination is limited by its short half-life and the variability in the elimination of this drug. Meconium was proposed as a better indicator of drugs in the maternal-fetal circulation; however, this hypothesis is currently not supported. The use of amniotic fluid for this purpose has been proposed.

7.10.2 Physiology

The amniotic fluid is the solution that circulates from the mother to the fetus. This solution is normally obtained after parturition. Amniotic fluid is a viscous, whitish-colored solution.

7.10.3 SPE Procedure—Sample Preparation

One milliliter of amniotic fluid is diluted with 3 mL of 0.025 *M* phosphate buffer, pH 4.0, and applied to the SPE column.

7.10.3.1 SPE Method

Column: Due to the viscosity of the sample, a larger particle size SPE column was used in this procedure. The CLEAN SCREEN® large particle size solid phase extraction columns (XRDAH515) were obtained from United Chemical Technologies, Inc. (Bristol, PA). *See* Table 3.

7.11 NAILS

7.11.1 Intoduction

Forensic applications have pushed the use of alternative matrices as the determinant of prior drug use. Nails are a useful matrix, especially when a historical aspect of drug use is needed. The only limitation for this procedure is that the amount of drug seen is often very low. More research is needed to make this matrix a useful tool.

Table 3
SPE of Cocaine in Amniotic Fluid

Conditioning	2 mL elution solvent (see below)
	1 mL methanol
	3 mL water
	3 mL 0.025 *M* phosphate buffer, pH 4.0.
Sample Addition	Add the diluted amniotic fluid sample at 1–2 mL/min.
Column Wash	2 mL water
	Dry under vacuum (>15 mm Hg) for at least 2 min.
	6 mL methanol
	Dry under vacuum (>15 mm Hg) for at least 2 min.
Column Elution	8 mL of freshly prepared elution solvent
	methylene chloride/isopropanol/ammonium hydroxide (78:20:2 v/v/v)
	Evaporate to dryness at 40°C using a gentle stream of nitrogen.
Derivatization	Add 30 μL of MTBSTFA to the dried sample cap and react at 90°C for 60 min.
	Analytes were detected by GC-MSD in SIM mode.
Results	The results of this study indicated that amniotic fluid is a useful indicator of cocaine exposure to the fetus.
Source	Winecker, R., Goldberger, Bruce A., Tebbett, I., Behnke, M., Eyler, F. D., et al. Detection of cocaine and its metabolites in amniotic fluid and umbilical cord tissue. *J. Anal. Toxicol.* 21:97–101, 1997.

Listed below is the preparation of nail samples for the detection of cocaine, benzoylecgonine, norcocaine, cocaethylene, morphine, 6-monoacetyl morphine, codeine, and hydrocodone.

7.11.2 Nail Sample Preparation

Approximately 3–5 mm of the unatttached anterior portion of the nail was clipped. Approximately 100 mg of nail is used per sample. Each sample was immediately washed with 3 mL of methanol repeated twice.

The washed nails are dried in an oven at 60°C for 2 h.

The washed nails are cut into smaller pieces, reweighed and placed into 3 mL of phosphate buffer, 0.1 *M*, pH 5.0. The samples are placed into an ultrasonic bath for 1 hour and soaked in the phosphate buffer for 72 h.

7.11.3 SPE Method

COLUMN—The CLEAN SCREEN solid phase extraction columns (ZSDAU020) were obtained from United Chemical Technologies, Inc. (Bristol, PA). *See* Table 4.

7.12 CURRENCY

7.12.1 Introduction

The exchange of illicit cocaine for money by drug dealers has provided an unusual demonstration of how selective and sensitive methods can be developed for detecting the passive contamination of our currency.

Table 4
SPE of Basic Drugs in Nails

Conditioning	3 mL methanol
	2 mL water
	1.5 mL 0.1 M phosphate buffer (pH 6.0).
Sample Addition	Add the solubilized nail sample (in pH 5.0 phosphate buffer) at 1–2 mL/min.
Column Wash	2 mL water
	1.5 mL 0.1 M hydrochloric acid
	2 mL methanol
	Dry under vacuum ($\geq$15 mm Hg) for at least 10 min.
Column Elution	3 mL of freshly prepared elution solvent methylene chloride–isopropanol–ammonia (78:20:2 v/v/v)
	Analytes were detected by GC-MSD in SIM mode.
Source	Engelhart, D., Lavins, E., and Sutheimer, C. Detection of drugs of abuse in nails. *J. Anal. Toxicol.* 22 314–318, 1998.

7.12.2 Study Populations

Ten single dollar bills from various cities were examined for the presence of cocaine. Individual bills were purified with methanol and extracted with solid phase extraction. The SPE extracts were analyzed by GC-MS. Cocaine was identified and qualified by full-scan spectroscopy and quantified by SIM.

7.12.3 Sample Isolation

A single bill was extracted with 10 ml of methanol
3 mL of 2 M sodium acetate buffer, pH 4.0, were added to the methanol.
Samples were filtered through a fritted filter onto the SPE column.

7.12.4 Results

The results for this study indicated that cocaine was present in 79% of the currency samples, in 54% of the samples in amounts of more than 1 microgram per bill.

Source: Oyler, J., Darwin, D., and Cone, E. Cocaine contamination of United States paper currency. J. Anal. Toxicol. 20:213–16, 1996.

7.13 SEBUM

7.13.1 Introduction

Sebum is an oily substance produced in the sebaceous glands and composed of wax esters of fatty acids. Most sebaceous glands are associated with hair follicles and have ducts that open to the hair shaft. The rate of sebum secretion is highly variable and is dependent on body region, number of follicles, and individual variables. Sebum secretion rate is also dependent on skin temperature.

Sebum is collected by noninvasive techniques including application of lipid-absorbent tape (Sebutape—Cu Derm Corp., Dallas, TX) or other absorbent film to the skin surface and the use of cigarette rolling paper against the skin.

7.13.2 Sample Preparation

1. Sebum was collected from the foreheads of the subjects.
2. Sebutape patches were weighed before and after application.
3. Before application the subject's forehead was cleansed with isopropyl alcohol and allowed to dry for 1 min.
4. Sebum was collected for a period of 1–2 hours.
5. Patches were removed, and placed into a test tube; the internal standard solution and 3 mL of hexane were added. The patches were immersed in the extraction solution for 3 hours at room temperature.
6. The organic extraction solution was placed into a 6-mL tube and 3 mL of a buffer solution was added to the patches, mixed, and added into the organic extraction solution.
7. The combined extracts were mixed and centrifuged and the organic (hexane) solution was discarded.
8. SPE was performed on the combined extracts.

Source: Joseph, R., Oyler J, Wstadik A, Ohuoha C, and Cone E. Drug testing with alternative matrices I. Pharmacological effects and dispsition of cocaine and codeine in plasma, sebum and stratum corneum. *J. Anal. Toxicol.* Abstract from 1997 SOFT Annual Meeting, October 1997.

Selected Readings

Cirmele, V., Kintz, P., and Mangin, P. Determination of cronic flunitrazepam abuse by hair analysis using GC–MS–NCI. J. Analyt. Toxicol. 20:596–598, 1996.

Cone, E. J., Yousefnejad, D., Darwin, W. D., Maguire, T. Testing human hair for drugs of abuse. II: Identification of unique cocaine metabolites in hair of drug abusers and evaluation of decontamination procedures. J. Analyt. Toxicol. 15:250–255, 1991.

Goldberger, B., Darraj, A., Caplan, Y., and Cone, E. J. Detection of methadone, methadone metabolites and other illicit drugs of abuse in the hair of methadone treated subjects. J. Analyt. Toxicol. 23:526–530, 1998.

Hold, K., Wilkins, D., Crouch, D., Rollins, D., and Maes, R. Detection of stanozolol in hair by negative ion chemical ionization mass spectroscopy. J. Analyt. Toxicol. 20:345–349, 1996.

Kikura, M., Pragst, F., Hunger, J., Thor, S. Distinction between amphetamine-like OTC drug use and illegal amphetamines/methamphetamine use by hair analysis. SOFT/TIAFT Meeting (Abstract), 1995.

Kintz, P., Jamey, C., Cirmele, V., Brenneisen, R., and Ludes, B. Evaluation of acetylcodeine as a specific marker of illicit heroin in human hair. J. Analyt. Toxicol. 22:425–429, 1998.

Kintz, P., Cirmele, V., Sengler, C., Mangin, P. Testing human hair and urine for anhydroecgonine methyl ester, a pyrolysis product of cocaine. J. Analyt. Toxicol. 19:479–486, 1995.

Moore, C., Deitermann, D., and Lewis, D. The analysis of neonatal hair for drugs of abuse—a case study. Clin. Chem. 42:205–209, 1996.

Negrusz, A., Moore, C., and Perry, J. (1998) Detection of doxepin and its metabolite desmethyldoxepin in hair following drug therapy. J. Analyt. Toxicol. 22:531–535, 1998.

Rothe, M., Pragst, F., Hunger, J., and Thor, S. Determination of carbamazepine and metabolites in the hair of epileptics. SOFT/TIAFT Meeting (Abstract), 1995.

Slawson, M., Wilkins, D., and Rollins, D. The incorporation of drugs into the hair: Relationship of hair color and melanin concentration to phencyclidine incorporation. J. Analyt. Toxicol. 22:406–413, 1998.

Wang, W. L., and Cone, E. J. Testing human hair for drugs of abuse IV. Environmental cocaine contamination and washing effect. Forensic Sci. Int. 70:39–51, 1995.

Suggested Readings

Brown, D. J. The pharmacokinetics of alcohol excretion in human perspiration. Meth. Find. Exp. Clin. Pharmacol. 7:539–544, 1985.

Cook, C. E. Phencyclidine disposition after intravenous and oral doses. Clin. Pharmacol. Exp. Ther. 31:625–634, 1985.

Gorodetzky, C. W., Kulberg, M. P. Validity of screening methods for drugs of abuse in biological fluids.II.Heroin in plasma and saliva. Clin. Pharmacol. Exp. Ther. 15:579–587, 1974.

Henderson, G. L., Wilson, B. K. Excretion of methadone and metabolites in human sweat. Res. Commun. Chem. Pathol. Pharmacol. 5:18 1–8, 1973.

Ishiyma, I. The significance of drug analysis of sweat in respect to rapid screening for drug abuse. Z. Rechtsmed. 82:251–256, 1979.

Smith, F. P., Liu, R. H. Detection of cocaine metabolite in perspiration stains, menstrual bloodstains and hair. J. Forensic. Sci. 31:1269–1273, 1986.

Suzuki, S., Inoue, T., Hori, H., and Inayama, S. Analysis of methamphetamine in hair, nail, sweat and saliva by mass fragmentography. J. Analyt. Toxicol. 13:176–178, 1989.

Vree, T. B., Muskens, A. T., and Van Rossum, M. Excretion of amphetamines in human sweat. Arch. Int. Pharmacodyn. Ther. 199:311–317, 1972.

Suggested Readings: General

Schramm, W., Smith, R. H., Craig, P. A., and Kidwell, D. A. Drugs of abuse in saliva: A review. J. Analyt. Toxicol. 16:1–9, 1992.

Cone, E. J., and Huestis, M. A. Urinary excretion of commonly abused drugs following unconventional means of administration. Forensic Sci. Rev. 1:121–139, 1989.

Idowu, O. R., and Caddy, B. A review of the use of saliva in the forensic detection of drugs and other chemicals. J. Forensic. Sci. Soc. 22:123–135, 1982.

Alcohol/Ethanol

Schwartz, R. H., O'Donnell, R. M., Thorne, M. M., Getson, P. R., and Hicks, J. M. Evaluation of a colorimetric dipstick test to detect alcohol in saliva: A pilot study. Ann. Emerg. Med. 18:1001–1003, 1989.

Jones, A. W. Inter- and intra-individual variations in the saliva/blood alcohol ratio during ethanol metabolism in man. Clin. Chem. 25:1394–1398, 1989.

Amphetamines

Wan, S. H., Matin, V., Azarnoff, D. L. Kinetics, salivary excretion of amphetamine isomers and effect of urinary pH. Clin. Pharmacol. Ther. 23:585–590, 1978.

Suzuki, S. T., Inoue, T., Hori, V., Inayama, S. Analysis of methamphetamine in hair, nail, sweat and saliva by mass fragmentography. J. Analyt. Toxicol. 13:176–178, 1989.

Barbiturates

Inaba, T., and Kalow, W. Salivary excretion of amobarbital in man. Clin. Pharmacol. Ther. 18:558–562, 1975.

Dilli, S., Pillai, R. Analysis of trace amounts of barbiturates in saliva. J. Chromatogr. 190:113–118, 1980.

Peat, M. A., Chem, C., Finkle, B. S. Determination of methaqualone and its major metabolite in plasma and saliva after a single oral dose. J. Analyt. Toxicol. 4:114–118, 1980.

Benzodiazepines

Tjaden, U. R., Meeles, M. T. H. A., Thys, C. P., Van Der Kaay, and M. Determination of some benzodiazepines and metabolites in serum, urine and saliva by high performance liquid chromatography. J. Chromatogr. 181:227–241, 1980.

Hallstrom, C., Piraino, G. J., and Ruch, E. Diazepam concentrations in parotid saliva, mixed saliva and plasma. J. Clin. Pharmacol. Ther. 24:720–725, 1978.

Hart, B. J., Wilting, J., De Gier, J. J. Stability of benzodiazepines in saliva. Exp. Clin. Pharmacol. 10:21–26.

Cocaine

Peel, H. W., Perrigo, B. H., Mikhael, N. Z. Determination of drugs in the saliva of impaired drivers. J. Forensic Sci. 29:185–189, 1984.

Cone, E. J., Kumor, K., Thompson, L. K., and Scherer, M. Correlation of saliva cocaine levels with plasma levels and with pharmacologic effects after intravenous cocaine administration in human subjects. J. Analyt. Toxicol. 12:200–206, 1988.

Jenkins, A. J., Oyler, J. M., and Cone, E. J. Comparison of heroin and cocaine concentrations in saliva with concentrations in blood and plasma. J. Analyt. Toxicol. 19:359–374, 1995.

Kato, K., Hillsgrove, M., Gorelick, L., Darwin, W. D., Cone, E. J. Cocaine and metabolite excretion in saliva under stimulated and non-stimulated conditions. J. Analyt. Toxicol. 17:338–341, 1993.

LSD

Twitchett, P. J., Fletcher, S. M., Sullivan, A. T., and Moffat, A. C. Analysis of LSD in human body fluids by high performance liquid chromatography, fluorescence spectroscopy and radioimmunoassay. J. Chromatogr. 150:73–84, 1978.

Francom, P., Andrenyak, D., Lim, H. K., Bridges Foltz, R., Jones, R. T. Determination of LSD in urine by capillary column gas chromatography and electron impact mass spectroscopy. J. Analyt. Toxicol. 12:1–8, 1988.

Nicotine

Curvall, M., Elwin, E., Kazami-Vala, E., Warholm, C., and Enzell, C. R. The pharmacokinetics of cotinine in plasma and saliva from non-smoking healthy volunteers. Eur. J. Clin. Pharmacol. 38:281–287, 1990.

Jarvis, M. Comparison of tests used to distinguish smokers from non-smokers. Am. J. Public Health 77:1435–1438, 1987.

Etzel, R. A review of the use of saliva cotinine as a marker of tobacco smoke exposure. Prev. Med. 19:190–197, 1987.

Opiates

Cone E, Welch P, Mitchell J, Paul B (1991) Forensic drug testing for opiates: I. Detection of 6-acetylmorphine in urine as an indicator of recent heroin exposure; drug and assay considerations and detection times. J. Analyt. Toxicol. 15:1–7, 1991.

Gorodetzky, C., and Kullberg, M. Validity of screening methods for drugs of abuse in biological fluids. II. Heroin in plasma and saliva. Clin. Pharmacol. Ther. 15:579–587, 1974.

Cone, E. Testing human hair for drugs of abuse I. Individual dose and time profiles of morphine and codeine in plasma, saliva and urine compared to drug induced effects on pupils and behavior. J. Analyt. Toxicol. 14:1–7, 1990.

Kang, G., and Abbott, F. Analysis of methadone and metabolites in biological fluids with gas chromatography mass spectroscopy. J. Chromatogr. 231:311–319, 1982.

Phencyclidine

Bailey, D., and Guba, J. Measurement of phencyclidine in saliva. J. Analyt. Toxicol. 311–313, 1980.

Cook, C. Phencyclidine disposition after intraveneous and oral doses. Clin. Pharmacol. Ther. 31:625–634, 1991.

Tetrahydrocannabinoids

Thompson, L., and Cone, E. Determination of delta-9-tetrahydrocannabinol in human blood and saliva by high performance liquid chromatography with amperometric detection. J. Chromatogr. 421:91–97, 1987.

Huestis, M., Dickerson, S., and Cone, E. Can saliva THC levels be correlated to behavior? AAFS Abstract 92-2, Colorado Springs, 1992.

Suggested Readings: Drugs of Abuse

Moore, C., and Negrusz, A. Drugs of abuse in meconium. Forensic Sci. Rev. 7:103–118, 1995.

Cocaine

Lewis, D., Moore, C., and Leikin, J. Cocaethylene in meconium samples. Clin. Toxicol. 32:697–703.

Lombardero, N. Measurement of cocaine and metabolites in urine, meconium and dipers by gas chromatography-mass spectroscopy. Ann. Clin. Lab. Sci. 23:385–394, 1993.

Oyler, J., Darwin, D., Preston, K., Suess, P., and Cone, E. Cocaine disposition in meconium from newborns of cocaine abusing mothers and urine of adult drug users. J. Analyt. Toxicol. 20:453–462, 1996.

Shulman, S. Meconium testing for cocaine metabolite: Prevalence, perceptions and pitfalls. Am. J. Obstet. Gynecol. 168:1449–1456, 1985.

Opiates

Moore, C., Deitermann, D., Lewis, D., and Leikin, J. The detection of hydrocodone in meconium. Two case studies. J. Analyt. Toxicol. 19:514–518, 1995.

Tetrahydrocannabinoids

Schwartz, R., and Hawks, R. Laboratory detection of marijuana use. JAMA 254:788–792, 1985.

REFERENCES

[1]Rorig, T., and Prouty, R. A nortriptyline death with unusually high tissue concentrations. J. Anal. Toxicol. 13:303–305, 1989.

[2]Rorig, T., and Prouty, R. Fluoxethine overdosage: A case report. J. Anal. Toxicol. 13:305–307, 1989.

[3]Rorig, T., Rundle, D. and Leifer, W. Fatality from metoprolol overdosage. J. Anal. Toxicol. 11:231–232, 1987.

[4]Corasinti, M., Strongoli, M., and Nascito, G. Determination of paraquat in rat brain using ion pair solid phase extraction and reversed phase HPLC with UV detection. J. Chromatog. 527:189–195, 1990.

[5]Moore, C., Browne, S., Tebbett, I., and Negruz, A. Determination of cocaine and its metabolites in brain tissue using high flow solid phase extraction columns and high performance liquid chromatography. Forensic Sci. Intl. 53:215–219, 1992.

[6]Smith, P., and Heath, D. Paraquat lung: A reapprasal. Thorax 29:643–653, 1974.

[7]Cordonnier, J., Van den Heede, J., and Heyndrickx, A. A rapid isolation of acidic and basic drugs from human tissue. Intl. Analyst 1:28–34, 1987.

[8]Demedts, P. Application of the combined use of fused silica capillary columns and npd for the toxicological determination of codeine and ethylmorphine in human overdosage. J. Anal. Toxicol. 7:113–115, 1983.

[9]Branchflower, W., Mc Cracken, R. and Rice, D. Determination of chlorotetracycline residue in tissues using high performance liquid chromatography with fluorescent detection. The Analyst 114:421–423, 1989.

[10]Greene, S., Abdalla, T., Morgan, S., and Bryan, C. L. High pressure liquid chromatographic analysis of vancomycin in plasma, bone, atrial appendage tissue and pericardial fluid. J. Chromatogr. 417:121–28, 1987.

[11]Bermejo, A. Morphine determination by gc-ms in human vitreous humor and comparison to radioimmunoassay. J. Anal. Toxicol. 16:372–374, 1992.

[12]Logan, B., and Stafford, D. High performance liquid chromatography with column switching for the determination of cocaine and benzoylecgonine concentrations in vitreous humor. J. Forens. Sci. 35:1303–1309, 1990.

[13]Midgley, J. Analysis of acidic metabolites of biogenic amines in bovine retina, vitreous and aqueous humor by gas chromatography-negative ion chemical ionization mass spectroscopy. J. Neurochem. 55:842–848, 1990.

[14]Burkett, G., Yasin Salih, Y., Palow D. Patterns of cocaine binging- effects on pregnancy. Am. J. Obstet. Gynecol. 171:372–379, 1994.

[15]Fox C. Cocaine use in pregnancy. J. Am. Board. Fam. Pract. 7:225–228, 1994.

[16]Dusick, A. M., Covert, R. F., Schreiber, M. D., Yee, G. T. Risk of intercranial hemorrhage and other adverse outcomes after cocaine exposure in a cohort of 323 very low birth weight infants. J. Pediat. 122:438–445, 1993.

Cocaine

[17]Jariwala, L., and Shaw, R. Clinical, pathological and toxicological findings of licit and illicit drugs in stillborns, newborns and infants. Calif Assoc. Toxicol. Newsletter Winter 22–25, 1990.

[18]Roe, D., Little, B., Bawdon, R., and Gilstrap, L. Metabolism of cocaine by the human placenta: implications for fetal exposure. Am J Obstet Gynocol 163:715–718, 1990.

[19]Ferko, A., Barberi, E., DiGregorio, G., and Ruch, E. Determination of cocaine and its metabolites in parotid saliva, plasma, urine and amniotic fluid in pregnant and non-pregnant rats. Res Comm Subst Abuse 12:1–17, 1991.

[20]Sandberg, J., and Olsen, G. Microassay for the simultaneous determination of cocaine, norcocaine, benzoylecgonine, and benzoylnorecgonine by high performance liquid chromatography. J Chromatogr 525:113–121, 1990.

Amphetamines

[21]Crimele, V., Kintz, P., and Mangin, P. Detection of amphetamines in fingernails; an alternative to hair analysis. Arch. Toxicol. 70:68–69, 1984.

[22]Suzuki, O., Hattori, H., and Asano, M. Nails as useful materials for the detection of methamphetamine and amphetamine abuse. Forensic Sci Int 24:9–16, 1984.

Cocaine and Benzoylecgonine

[23]Miller, M., Martz, R., and Donnelly, B. Drugs in keratin samples from hair, fingernails, and toenails. Second International Meeting on Clinical and Forensic Aspects of Hair Analysis, Genoa, Italy, June 6–8, 1994.

Fenfluramine and Phentermine

[24]Lewis, D., Moore, C., and Leikin, J. Detection of fenfluramine and phentermine in hair and nails. Abstract—SOFT Meeting, Albuquerque, NM, Oct. 4–6, 1998.

Chapter 8

Solid Phase Extraction Troubleshooting

Extraction problems that can arise with solid phase extraction are not unlike those that occur with any type of chemical extraction process, including recovery and contamination problems. Since SPE usually requires columnar flow processes, liquid flow problems are possible and more unique to this methodology. On the positive side, SPE offers many advantages over traditional liquid extractions–including reduced sample and solvent volumes, prevention of emulsions, greater partition efficiency (improved recovery, selectivity, and precision), fewer steps, and shorter analysis time– and is amenable to automation. Nonetheless, problems can and do occur; this chapter addresses the most commonly encountered SPE problems and offers suggestions for their resolution. Possible method problems are categorized as:

- Flow problems
- Contamination problems
- Recovery problems
- Nonextraction problems

8.1 FLOW PROBLEMS

Vacuum, pressure, gravity, or capillary forces can facilitate the physical flow of liquids through an SPE column. Regulation of flow rates is a critical aspect of extraction efficacy, particularly at sample application and elution steps. Flows that are too slow add unnecessary time to the analysis and may facilitate entrapment of unwanted matrix components in terminal pores of the sorbent (see Chapter 2, Figure 12). Flows that are too fast can adversely affect recovery of target analytes, especially when ion-™exchange mechanisms are employed. It is important to realize, however, that SPE flow characteristics are rather crude in comparison to HPLC, owing to greater variation in

From: *Forensic Science and Medicine:*
Forensic and Clinical Applications of Solid Phase Extraction
Edited by: M. J. Telepchak, T. F. August, and G. Chaney © Humana Press Inc., Totowa, NJ

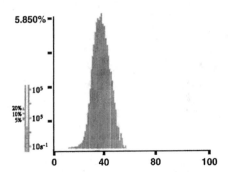

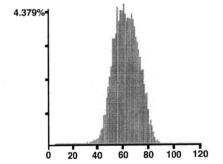
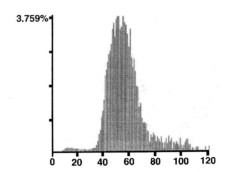

Fig. 1. Particle size distribution.

particle shape and size and a nonpressurized (open) flow system. For this reason, some inconsistency in flow from column to column is expected and normal. These slight flow variations are not likely to cause notable variance in assay performance. SPE flow problems are characteristic of one or more of the following:

- Matrix viscosity or particulates
- Insufficient or variant flow source
- Manufacturing defects–silica "fines," defective frits, assembly variations

Manufacturing processes can create flow problems dependent on the competence to monitor sorbent particle and pore size. Histograms of particle size distribution can show evidence of "fines," or particles that are significantly smaller in size than the average particle size for given batch of sorbent (Figure 1).

If the particle distribution is too wide (resulting in higher number of fines), then restricted or irregular flows may result (Figure 2). Fines that are actually smaller than the frit pore diameter can escape the columns and contaminate eluates. The appear-

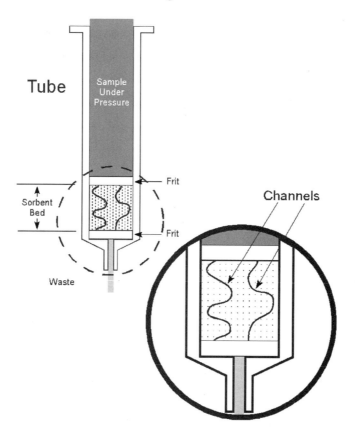

Fig. 2. Sorbent bed channeling.

ance of a white crystalline residue in elution tubes after drydown may indicate excessive fines in the column.

Another manufacturing source of flow problems is defective frits. Frits hold the sorbent in place in the column (at top and bottom of the sorbent bed). The pore sizes of frits are selectable and should be considered in any analysis based on both the sample matrix and the size of the molecules being extracted. If the frit pore diameter is not uniform or is an inappropriate size, restricted flow can occur. Also, frits that are cut from sheets of polyethylene can have rough or unevenly cut edges that allow liquids to channel down the sides of the column rather than through the sorbent bed. This occurrence can also allow sorbent itself to leak out during shipping or handling, thus reducing the expected column capacity for the analysis. The type of frit used can also affect flow properties. Polyethylene frits are characteristically hydrophobic and therefore are naturally resistant to aqueous phases. Glass-weave frits are available that are hydrophilic and subsequently less resistant to aqueous samples (a disadvantage is cost, however).

A third possibility of manufacturing contribution to flow problems is in the column assembly process. Columns that are packed too tightly will produce more restrictive flows; conversely, if columns are not packed tightly enough, flows can be too fast, resulting in recovery and selectivity problems. Procedures for assembly of SPE cartridges do vary. Machine or automated packing processes are more uniform, but as with any instrumentation, variations can occur from day to day. Many SPE columns, particularly specialty phases, are frequently hand-packed. Operator variation is not uncommon. Quality assurance departments rely on spot-checking assembled cartridges at various intervals; not all manufacturers routinely check flow parameters.

Flow problems may also occur from insufficient force to initiate and maintain flow necessary for the particular matrix or column configuration. Insufficient or poorly regulated vacuum is a typical cause of flow problems. Reasons for insufficient vacuum can be the source itself; sink-type aspirator sources do not usually have sufficient vacuum force to pull and hold a seal on most vacuum chambers. Electrical vacuum pumps can also lack sufficient torr force, depending on tube length (from source to chamber), the size of the vacuum chamber, the number of samples being processed, and the matrix viscosity. Conversely, too much vacuum can collapse tubing and also impede flow. Be sure tubing has sufficient wall strength to sustain its shape under vacuum. Bad seals or warped heads on the manifold can allow leaks to occur and result in low vacuum. If a vacuum source is weak, vapor locks can occur, whereby the vacuum force applied cannot disrupt the surface tension of the liquid in the column. In such cases, a "bump" in vacuum (or pressure) is required to disrupt the liquid surface and initiate flow. A pipet bulb serves as an excellent tool for creating a brief positive pressure to initiate flow. Other tools to evaluate source flow problems are a vacuum or pressure gauge, and "dummy" SPE cartridges without sorbent to determine if the frit pore diameter is too small to allow flow of the sample matrix.

Flow problems are more often a factor of the matrix being analyzed. Extremely viscous samples, or samples with a high amount of particulates, can clog both frits and sorbent pores. There are generally two ways to alter flow characteristics of "difficult" samples: either change the matrix or change the column. If the matrix is viscous, or contains particulates, fibrin, mucus, proteins, or other cellular components, you can alter the matrix by diluting, filtering, centrifuging, and sonicating the sample, or by precipitating proteins. You can also alter column characteristics by going to a larger sorbent particle and/or pore size, increasing the sorbent surface area (larger diameter column), decreasing the sorbent bed depth, or increasing the frit pore diameter or the frit type (hydrophobicity).

Often the easiest solution to matrix flow problems is to dilute the sample. Dilution of dense or viscous samples with water or an appropriate buffer will very often reduce the resistance to flow. However, there can be several disadvantages to dilution of samples. First, the diluent may itself compete for binding sites on the sorbent, resulting in decreased sorbent capacity and possible "breakthrough" of target analytes. High ionic strength diluents can affect both hydrophobic and ionic binding mechanisms. Next, increased sample volume can also produce migration (band broadening) of bound analytes through the sorbent bed. The result can be breakthrough during sample application or subsequent washes, or inefficient elution of target analytes. Weakly bound analytes are particularly susceptible to these phenomena. Finally, high volumes of aqueous liquids applied to hydrophobic phases may desolvate the phase and reduce binding capacity. Addition of a small amount of polar organic solvent

(<10% v/v) such as methanol to the sample mix can help maintain proper solvation of the phase.

Filtration is another common means to remedy sample matrix problems. A particularly useful tool is silanized glass wool. After column conditioning, a small pinch of glass wool is pushed into the SPE cartridge using forceps or an applicator stick; the wool should rest loosely, just on top of the column frit. Apply the sample to the column, and then remove the glass wool prior to column washes. Samples that are otherwise completely resistant to flow without some manipulation will usually pass through the wool and the column without problem. Also, the surface area of the glass wool is relatively small, so sample loss is minimal. Other means of filtering are available, including syringe-type filter cartridges, standard filter paper, gauze, and so on. Any means is acceptable provided that your target compounds are not bound to any filter surfaces, or are bound to macromolecules that would be filtered.

Centrifugation is useful, especially for macroparticulates and cellular components.

Sonication can disrupt fibrin and mucosal constituents, as well as proteins and cellular components, dependent on sonic frequency and duration. This technique can be very useful, but may be somewhat time-consuming, and usually requires centrifugation as well.

Precipitation of proteins can be accomplished by addition of organic solvents or acids to the sample. Protein removal generally leaves a very clean matrix, but care must be taken that compounds of interest are not highly bound to proteins. Acid precipitation will usually require further matrix adjustment to provide proper pH and ionic strength for sample application to the SPE column. Organic precipitation usually does an adequate job of protein removal, and the sample can simply be diluted back to an aqueous character with a buffer. Acetonitrile and dilute acetone (10%) are very good solvents for protein precipitation in biological samples (1:1 ratio). A "standing" time of 10–15 min is recommended, followed by centrifugation. If the sample is to be analyzed on a hydrophobic phase, dilution of the organic supernatant to an 80–90% aqueous sample is required for proper retention on the sorbent.

If manipulation of the matrix is not desirable, then there are options to alter the column characteristics. The first is to try a larger particle/pore size. Most standard SPE products offer a 40–60 µm particle size with a 60 Å pore diameter. Special phases are available that offer an average 150-µm particle with a 200 Å pore size. These high-flow sorbents are ideal for extremely viscous sample types. A word of caution is that flows can be too fast, resulting in decrease or irregular recoveries.

Another factor to consider in the column is the frit pore diameter. Figure 3 shows a variety of frits in different diameters and thickness. The most common source of matrix flow problems is clogged frits. For standard 40–60 µm particle sorbents, the frits are typically 20 µm. Particulates or proteins will often clog the top frit before the sample ever reaches the sorbent. If larger frits are needed based on the matrix, then you will also affect to use larger particle size sorbents. The type of frit used will also impact flow characteristics; polyethylene frits are hydrophobic in nature and therefore naturally resistant to aqueous liquids. Hydrophilic frits are available that are less resistant to the flow of aqueous samples. These are usually in the form of glass-weave design and can be expensive.

Porous Polyethylene

10 Micron porosity (¹/₁₆" thickness)

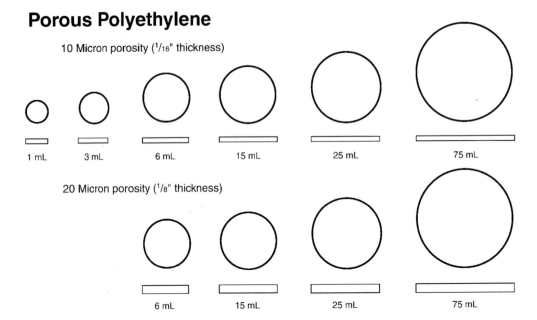

| 1 mL | 3 mL | 6 mL | 15 mL | 25 mL | 75 mL |

20 Micron porosity (¹/₈" thickness)

| 6 mL | 15 mL | 25 mL | 75 mL |

Porous Stainless Steel

15 Micron porosity (¹/₁₆" thickness)

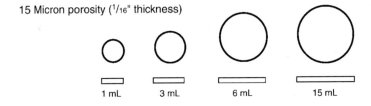

| 1 mL | 3 mL | 6 mL | 15 mL |

Fig. 3. Porous frits.

Changing the surface area will also affect the flow characteristics of SPE columns. Spreading the sample over a larger surface by using a wider-diameter cartridge will sometimes improve flow. Conversely, a narrower column may improve deficiencies in the flow source and facilitate better flow. Changing the depth of the sorbent bed may also impart different flow dynamics. Similar to HPLC, the packing diameter and length relates to the amount of backpressure present in the system. A guide is to use the least amount of sorbent that provides sufficient capacity for your target compounds and matrix, packed in a cartridge that is suitable for your sample volume. Tapered or wide-mouth cartridge types allow use of larger sample volumes while maintaining small sorbent volumes. Positive pressure sources, in which the sample is pushed through from the top of the cartridge rather than pulled from the bottom, can provide more precise flow control and appear less prone to flow difficulties. Positive pressure manifolds are on the market, and most automated SPE systems utilize positive pressure. Figure 4 shows a variety of tube sizes available in SPE.

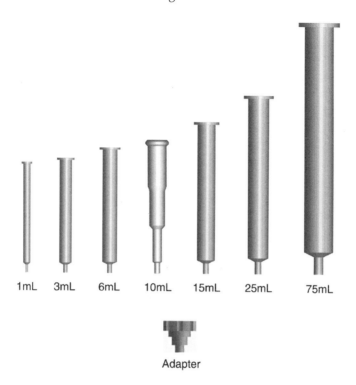

1mL 3mL 6mL 10mL 15mL 25mL 75mL

Adapter

Fig. 4. Tube sizes.

8.2 Contamination Problems

The evolution of SPE has provided devices and methodology for more sensitive analyses, and thus the requirement for increased selectivity and purity of extracts. Contamination from SPE products is becoming a less frequent problem owing to improved manufacturing processes. The likelihood of encountering SPE contaminants is generally dependent on the concentration range of target analytes and the mode of detection employed. Quality manufactured SPE devices should not contribute measurable contaminants above low nanogram (ppb) levels. Below nanogram levels, contribution is possible and may require prewashing of the column using a strong wash or washes. Assuming the strongest eluotropic solution to be used is the elution solvent, this solvent is recommended for the prewash at 10–20 times the bed volume (3–4 mL for a 200-mg column). Acids used for sample washes may also leach surface phthalate esters from cartridge wall or frits, so prewashes with these solutions may further reduce contaminants. The final prewash should always be the elution solvent, followed by routine conditioning steps. Prewashes, as well as conditioning, also serve to remove fines and dust that can be created by physical abrasion of sorbent particles during shipping and storage.

The most common contamination sources directly attributable to SPE devices are plasticizers/phthalates from the polypropylene cartridge or polyethylene frits, and various polymer residuals and phthalates from the sorbent. Figure 5 displays SPE column components, and Table 1 details predictable contaminants and their sources.

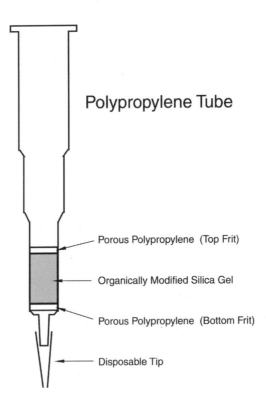

Fig. 5. Extraction tube components.

An easy method to assess whether contamination is coming from the SPE column is to pass a routine volume of elution solvent through the column, and collect and analyze per your procedure; process and analyze an equal volume of the same elution solvent that is not passed through a column. If the contaminant shows in only the column sample, then the SPE device contribution is evident. If the contaminant appears in both or neither of the samples, then reagent or other source(s) is causal. While contaminant contribution from SPE columns can occur, a much greater likelihood of contamination or interference exists from other sources. If you encounter a contamination problem, suspect everything! Table 2 shows a checklist of non-SPE-related contamination sources. You need to systematically isolate and eliminate these sources when tracking down a contamination.

Impurity or interfering peaks are seen in many assays, especially when the highest sensitivity is required or multiple purification steps are needed in the analysis (i.e., chemical derivatization). In many cases the origin of the impurity may not interfere with the primary analysis owing to the chromatographic separation.

The following examples show how impurities can be present and affect the results of our analyses.

<u>Example 1: Contaminants Present</u>

Figure 6 illustrates the separation of codeine and morphine using, trimethylsilyl (TMS) derivatives. Chromatogram A represents the separation of aqueous standards

Table 1
Possible Contaminants of Components of SPE Cartridges

Compound	Column components		
	Polypropylene housing	Polyethylene frit	C18 Bonded porous silica
C8 Alkene		–	X
C9 Alkene	–	–	X
C10–C16 Alkenes	X	–	X
C17–C28 Alkenes	X	X	
C8–C28 Alkanes	–	–	X
Naphthalene	–	–	X
Biphenyl	X	–	–
Acenaphthene	X	–	–
2,6-di-tert-Butyl-*p*-cresol	X	–	–
2,6-di-tert-Butyl-*p*-quinone	X	–	–
Phenol	X	–	–
Methyl octadecanoate	X	–	–
Dimethyloctadecylsilanol	–	–	X
Decamethylpentasiloxane	–	–	X
Dodecamethylhexasiloxane	-	–	X
Tetradecamethylheptasiloxane	–	–	X
Diethyl phthalate	–	–	X
Dibutyl phthalate	X	X	X
bis (2-Ethylhexyl) phthalate	X	X	X
bis (2-Ethylhexyl) adipate	X	–	–

directly derivatized in a test tube. Chromatogram B represents the actual extraction by SPE of the same standards as in chromatogram A.

In chromatogram B, peak 3 represents an unknown contaminant peak occurring after the morphine peak. The source of this contaminant has not been identified. In this case the peak is well separated from the peaks of interest.

Figure 7 illustrates an unknown peak seen in the separation of tetrahydrocannabinoids (THCs) when derivatized with *bis*-silytrifluoroacetamide (BSTFA) with 1% trimethylchlorsilane (TMCS). Many of our contaminants possess similar functional groups to the analytes of interest that may derivatize and be seen in our final analysis. The chromatographic process separates these peaks from the analytes of interest.

The interferent peak seen in Figure 7 has been identified as a plasticizer from the polyethylene frits in the SPE tube. Columns and frits have compounds that impart flexibility to the plastic. The plasticizers in these components cause interferant peaks especially seen in THC analysis owing to the low detection limits needed for this analysis. In most cases we can reduce the potential for interferents by conditioning the SPE column first with the strongest solvent being used (elution solvent) before conditioning our column.

Table 2
Non-SPE-Related Contaminant Sources

Gas chromatograph
- Column bleed
- Syringes
- Septum
- Liners, glass wool, or deactivated silica guard column
- Dirty detector
- Contaminated gases

Liquid chromatograph
- Guard columns (old)
- Column contamination
- HPLC filters

Robot parts
- O-Rings

Extraction manifolds
- Luer lock connectors (if not using a Clean-Thru configuration)

Miscellaneous sources
- Syringes
- Solvents
- Pipet tips
- Derivatization reagent–improper storage (air, moisture, etc).
- Injection vials
- Sample storage containers
- Vial septum
- Plasma bags–di-2-ethyl hexyl phthalate
- Test tube caps
- Sample contaminants
- Evaporator needles

Polymers from slow-release drug formulations
- Triethyl citrate
- Tributyl citrate
- Acetyl triethyl citrate
- Dibutyl sebacate
- Diethyl phthalate
- Dibutyl phthalate
- Triacetin

Impure standards
Impure derivatizing agents

SAMPLE NAME: 300 MG/ML STD

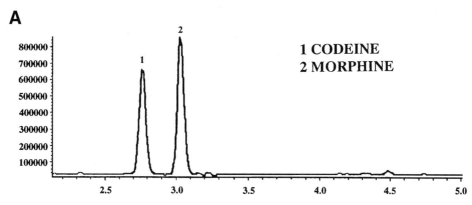

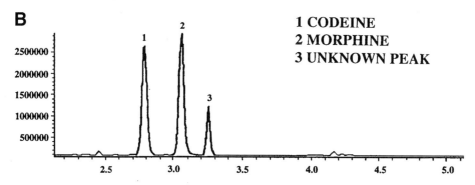

Fig. 6. (A) Neat standards of morphine and codeine TMS. **(B)** Morphine and codeine TMS after solid phase extraction.

Example 2: Contaminant Interference–Isotopic Ratio

Figure 8 shows multiple plasticizer peaks with one peak appearing as a shoulder on the chromatogram of the combined ions. Inspection of the single ion tracings indicates that these peaks are separated; however, the abundance of one of the isotope ions is significant. The analyst must make sure that the isotopic ratios are calculated on the correct peak or the confirmation criteria may not be met.

The sources of many interferents are usually not from the components of the SPE columns.

For example:

- Endogenous interferents from the matrix may be present. This may become problematic, as the concentration of endogenous interferents varies with each sample and patient.
- Solvents and buffers may contain impurities that may interfere with our analysis. In some cases, the use of an old or impure derivatization reagent can give us interferent peaks that may compromise the analysis. In all cases, the use of fresh reagents will minimize these problems.

Table 3 lists possible sources of contaminants.

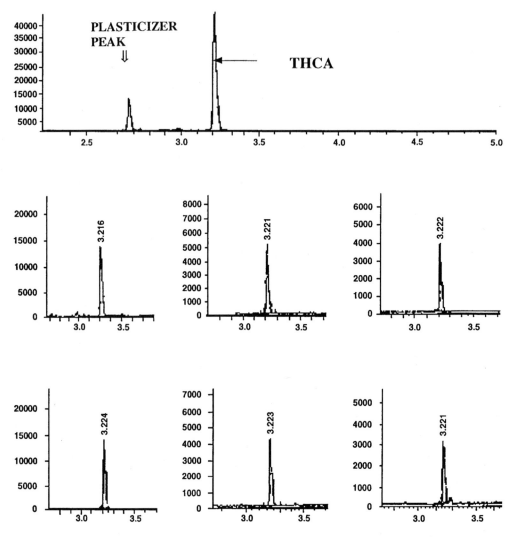

Fig. 7. THC analysis (TMS derivatives) SIM and individuals ions.

8.3 RECOVERY PROBLEMS

The issues in this section may seem like a review of earlier material; however, rereading them in the light of troubleshooting and the different slant on the presentation will help you understand how to troubleshoot problems relating to the issues.

An often-touted advantage of SPE is improved recovery and reproducibility over conventional liquid extractions. Recoveries do not meet expectations, however. Like any analytical process, careful and systematic approaches to problem solving in SPE will usually reward a successful and robust method. The principal difference between SPE and liquid-liquid extractions is that SPE involves columnar flow kinetics vs homogenous mixing to achieve partition of target compounds from the matrix. As flow parameters can directly affect method performance, appropriate attention to flow is essential. (Please note the word "appropriate," not paranoid; in some instances, there

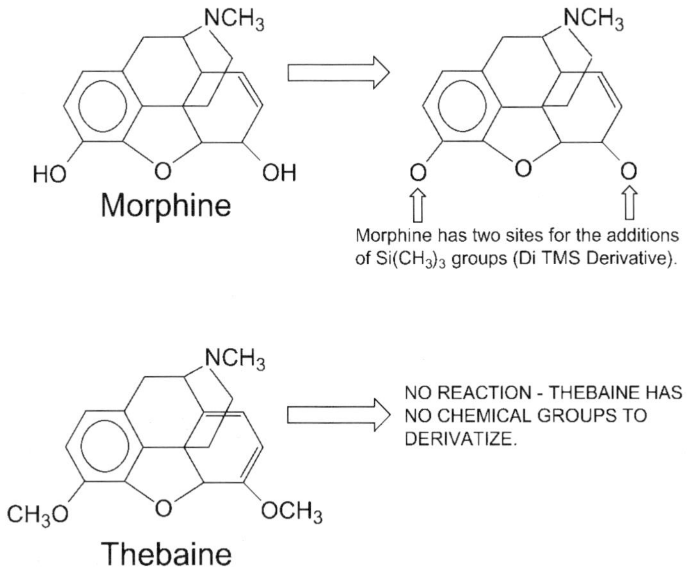

Fig. 8. THC analysis (TMS derivatives) SIM and individual ions showing plasticizer peak.

Table 3
Contaminant Checklist

The following should be considered as possible contaminant sources:
- Reagents, solvents, water, internal standards
- Reusable glassware, caps (soap)
- Disposable plastics–tubes, pipet tips
- Reagent lines, tubing–plastics, Teflon, bacteria (reagent bottles and automated systems); perform scheduled cleaning with dilute bleach
- Equipment–manifolds (lids, luers), pipettors/dilutors, valves, syringes, evaporators (tips, tubing, hardware)
- Sample containers–polycarbonate bottles, plasma bags, clot tubes
- Instrumentation–inlets, injectors (liners, guard columns, inlet seals, septa, ferrules, silanizing reagent, glass, glass wool, O-rings, syringes, wash bottles), gases/mobile phase, column degradation, column overload, detectors
- Matrix interferences–drug delivery polymers, or nonoptimized method

Other factors to consider are the pattern and frequency of the interference:
- Does it appear in all samples, or is it random?
- Does it occur in every batch or sporadically?

Analysis of a water blank can help rule out matrix effects or contribution.
- Analyst bias is possible if the problem does not occur in every batch. (Multiple analysts may not be following the same protocol or technique. **Do not assume–verify.**)
- Walk through all steps of the procedure and look for likely sources of contamination:

Old reagents–near or past expiration, or "bottom of the barrel"

New reagents–improper strength, source, preparation new/different supplier of reagents or supplies

Dirty equipment

Recent maintenance or other changes to equipment

has been an overemphasis on flows, making SPE more difficult than necessary. In addition to flow, the sorbent surfaces must be made physically and chemically receptive to the bonding kinetics of desired elements in the sample. Finally, numerous chemical factors must be considered to optimize methods, with the sorbent being an additional variable not present in liquid-liquid extractions. Keep in mind that there is an optimal balance between sensitivity (recovery) and selectivity or cleanliness of the end product. Recovery is a relative asset to overall extraction performance. In an optimized method, recovery is a balance between sensitivity and selectivity. Chromatographic signal-to-noise ratio (S/N) and resolution of interfering substances are paramount to absolute recovery. If acceptable limits of detection are achieved (with no interfering compounds) at only 30% recovery, then a higher recovery may not be necessary. In fact, a higher target analyte recovery may also increase interferences and noise. Evaluate the performance of the method on the optimal recovery needed to sustain the required S/N, not on an absolute percent recovery.

Most SPE procedures have five fundamental steps:

1. ***Conditioning:*** Solvates the SPE column and normalizes column environment to the sample; removes microparticulates and interferents
2. ***Sample application:*** Diffusion of sample through sorbent bed for binding of target compounds to sorbent functional groups; exclusion of macromolecules for initial cleanup
3. ***Wash:*** Remove excess sample matrix and unretained compounds
4. ***Dry:*** Remove aqueous or immiscible solvents to prepare sorbent for elution solvent
5. ***Elution:*** Disrupt functional binding mechanisms and selectively release compounds for collection and analysis

Each of the preceding steps can have an impact on method recovery and reproducibility. Each requires optimization specific to the compounds and matrix being analyzed. Chemical and flow processes must be considered. Variables include the matrix, the target analyte(s), the sorbent, and the solvents employed. Before discussing in detail the five fundamental steps of SPE, let us review the bonding mechanisms.

8.3.1 SPE Bonding Mechanisms

Hydrophobic bonding, also called reversed phase or nonpolar bonding, occurs via attraction of like hydrocarbon groups. This is also referred to as van der Waals forces or dispersion forces. The bond strength is relatively weak at 1–5 kcal/mol, with increasing strength as the number of hydrocarbon atoms increases. Hydrophobic phases are alkyl chains and/or rings, with a wide range of chain lengths from C2 to C18 common. Capacity of reversed phase sorbents is dependent on the alkyl chain configuration and the total carbon loading (%) on the silica substrate. Bonding is similar to classical liquid-liquid extraction dynamics, and is both polarity- and solvent-strength-dependent. A polar and low ionic strength sample matrix favors retention. Effective bonding also requires that the target analytes be in a neutral state. Ionization state can have a profound impact on both recovery and cleanliness of reversed phase extractions. Reversed phase mechanisms are very common in drug extraction applications.

Polar bonding, also called hydrophilic or normal phase bonding, occurs by hydrogen bonding and/or dipole interactions. Compounds that are hydrogen donors–

such as hydroxyls, carboxylic acids, and amines–are characteristic of polar bonding. Bond energy is moderately strong at 3–10 kcal/mol. Organic sample matrices favor retention on polar sorbents. While polar bonding as a primary mechanism of extraction is less common in drug analysis, it is important to realize that some polar bonding is likely to occur when using silica-based sorbents, including reverse phase. This is due to the presence of silanols on silica surfaces (*see* Chapter 2, Figures 4 and 2, silanol groups) These Si–OH groups are very active and readily bond with analytes containing polar functional groups. At pH above 4.0, the silanols are charged (–) and form ion pairs with available compounds (pi-pi and dipole-dipole interactions). At pH below 3.0, silanols are neutral and readily form H-bonds with hydrogen donor species in the sample (most polar analytes). The bond strengths can be quite strong and require a strong polar solvent to disrupt the bonds for elution. These secondary polar interactions are common, especially when extracting acids or amines with active hydrogen sites.

Ion-exchange bonding mechanisms are electrostatic interactions between oppositely charged sorbents and analytes. Bonding is reversible by changing pH conditions or by introducing competing ions with greater sorbent affinity than the compounds of interest (displacement). Bonding energy can be very strong (50–250 kcal/mol), which makes this an ideal mechanism for superior extraction cleanup provided the bonding is selective for target analytes. Strong bonds allow use of strong washes (aqueous acids and buffers, polar organics, and mixtures of organics) to remove matrix contaminants without loss of target analytes. This translates to cleaner extracts (high S/N) and typically higher absolute recoveries. Capacity of ion-exchange sorbents can be measured directly as milliequivalents/gram.

Bonds can be cation-exchange, in which a negatively charged sorbent (anionic) binds with positively charged analytes (cations, charged bases). Base compounds must be 2 pH units below their pK_a for full ionization (2 units above pK_a to be non-ionized). Bonds can also be anion-exchange, in which positively charged sorbents (cationic) bind with negatively charged analytes (anions, charged acids). Acidic compounds must be 2 pH units above their pK_a for full ionization (2 units below pK_a to be non-ionized).

Various functional acids or amines are bonded to silica or resins as ion exchangers; a summary of ion-exchange sorbents is shown in Table 1 in Chapter 10.

Mixed-mode SPE columns are prevalent in drug extractions because they offer multiple binding mechanisms for improved sensitivity and excellent sample cleanup. A mixed-mode sorbent employs two or more binding mechanisms in the same column. Most common in drug extractions are reversed phase with ion exchangers. When using mixed-mode extractions, the elution solvent must be able to reverse or disrupt all bonding mechanisms simultaneously, so pH, polarity, and solubility must all be considered. Mixed-mode sorbents can be manufactured by blending sorbents of each functional type, or they can be true copolymers whereby different functional silanes are polymerized to the substrate. Each has advantages and limitations. Blended phases can offer greater capacity flexibility by altering the blend to change carbon loading or milliequivalent levels of ion exchangers. Copolymers have limits on carbon-loading and ion-exchange capacity by the nature of available bonding sites on the substrate; however, copolymers typically yield greater lot-to-lot reproducibility, as no physical blending of phases is required.

8.3.2 The Five Fundamental Steps of SPE

8.3.2.1 Conditioning

Conditioning of solid phase sorbents serves several functions. Solid phase columns are shipped dry for reasons of stability and packaging. To facilitate activation of sorbent functional groups, a suitable wetting agent must be applied. The purpose is to expand the functional binding sites away from the solid surface, exposing them to the diffusive flow of the sample and reagents. Characteristics of a good wetting or solvation solvent are:

- Miscible with aqueous matrices (sample and buffers)
- Diffuses easily into sorbent pores (low surface tension)
- High mass transfer of HCl bonds with sorbent alkyl chains (expands chains)
- Universal elution of polar and nonpolar contaminants on sorbent (also fines)

Methanol is frequently used in reversed phase procedures because it meets all these conditions.

The conditioning or solvation process facilitates extension of functional carbon chains, creating a receptive stationary phase on the silica or resin backbone. Insufficient solvation can occur if too little solvent is applied, or more often if the solvent is swept too quickly through the sorbent bed. Excessive flow creates insufficient contact for adequate H–C interaction to occur. In addition, excessive flow rate and/or redrying of the sorbent may result in channeling of the sorbent bed (Fig. 2). If excessive vacuum or pressure is applied to SPE columns, liquids will take the path of least resistance and channels or tunnels will form in the sorbent bed. Channeling is detrimental to efficient extraction and recovery because it reduces the available surface area for sample contact. In essence, sorbent capacity is significantly reduced, because only a portion of the sorbent is successfully solvated. Recovery is further reduced because successive liquid steps will also flow faster through the channels, thus reducing contact time for effective mass transfer.

While channeling is most undesirable, it is sometimes overemphasized to a point of procedural paranoia. Channeling is not likely to occur in properly packed columns provided moderate care is taken during conditioning steps. Generally, flow rates between 0.5 and 3.0 mL/min are acceptable to allow sufficient solvent-sorbent contact for solvation, without causing channeling. It is not necessary to keep solvent continually on the sorbent provided low flow rates are maintained. Drying of sorbent beds requires elevated flows for at least 5–10 min; judicious attention to conditioning steps will prevent channeling and ensure effective solvation of the sorbent. If you have walked away from the manifold and feel too much time has passed between conditioning steps, simply start over to resolvate. However, if channels have formed due to high flows or excessive drying, then reconditioning will not correct the problem.

Disk-type columns have evolved in part to overcome channeling problems. Because of reduced bed depths and rigid supports, channeling does not occur even at higher flow rates. This makes disks ideal for larger sample volumes by allowing higher flows and reducing the time to draw the sample through the column. Environmental applications have used disk sorbents for processing liter volumes of water. Disk cartridges are finding their way into pharmaceutical and drug testing because they also offer the advantages of using less solvents for processing. Capacity can be an issue and should be evaluated based on analyte concentration and matrix considerations. Disk problems have also been found when dealing with particularly dirty matrices.

A second purpose of column conditioning is to chemically prepare the sorbent environment to allow optimal contact and binding of the sample. Proper pH and ionic strength are important parameters to facilitate mass transfer between the matrix and the sorbent. Reversed phase sorbents are effective for extraction of compounds from aqueous matrices because they favor retention of "like" hydrocarbon moieties, but repel the polar matrix itself. Organic matrices do not allow effective bonding of analyte constituents because the matrix competitively impedes mass transfer of analytes. High ionic strength buffers do likewise. Polar sorbent extractions are just the opposite in that they favor organic matrices because polar solvents will disrupt H and pi bonds, the primary polar bonding mechanisms. Column pH conditions are usually driven by the desired ionization state of target analytes. Un-ionized compounds favor retention in reversed phase systems. In most cases, the pH of the sample and that of the sorbent should be equivalent for optimal binding.

A final function of conditioning is to remove dust, fines, and residual polymer impurities from the sorbent. Physical abrasion of silica particles in shipping and storage will create microparticulates. It can also create additional silanol binding sites. Methanol (or another polar organic) will wash away most impurities and, to a small degree, block silanols.

8.3.2.2 Sample Application

It is useful to again consider the similarities of SPE and HPLC. In both cases a partitioning occurs between mobile and stationary phases. Of course the efficiency and resolution of HPLC are much greater than that of SPE because of a much higher number of theoretical plates. SPE overcomes fewer theoretical plates by using start-stop flow processes vs continuous flow as in HPLC (SPE is sometimes referred to as digital chromatography). For optimal performance, each SPE step must either promote full retention or full elution of the target compounds, or secondarily, provide sample cleanup. The success of these processes is dependent on both chemical and physical aspects of the extraction. When the analyte remains predominantly bound to the matrix because of incomplete partitioning into the stationary phase, then breakthrough occurs. Breakthrough is the ineffective retention of target analytes on the solid phase sorbent, resulting in low analyte recovery. During sample application the most common cause of breakthrough is flow rates that exceed the sorbent affinity for binding of target compounds. This results from inadequate mass transfer of the analyte to sorbent binding sites. Other considerations for breakthrough include:

- Improper conditioning
- Improper loading solvent (ionic strength, organic strength)
- Flow rate–insufficient diffusion and mass transfer (residence time)
- Volume overload–weakly retained analytes migrate with the matrix
- Mass overload–capacity is insufficient (analyte or matrix)
- Incorrect sorbent for the target analyte

Conditioning and matrix factors have been discussed previously. Flow rate, as in conditioning steps, is again critical to ensure adequate contact of sample through pores of the sorbent. Excessive flow rates can result in breakthrough and/or band broadening. It is desirable to concentrate the target compound in a very narrow band at or near the top of the sorbent bed. Well-optimized methods will demonstrate this bonding pattern. When analytes are weakly retained, they will migrate with the mobile phase, either escaping the sorbent or spreading through the bed. The disadvantage is that subsequent washes may further migrate the compounds, causing additional break-through. In such cases, even slight chemical variations (such as changes in reagents) or operator variances in flow control will yield reproducibility problems. Sample flow is even more critical in ion-exchange procedures, as the binding kinetics are slower than reversed or normal phase mechanisms. Conversely, flows that are too slow can allow matrix components to trap inside terminal pores, potentially resulting in increased interferences and lower recovery. Recommended flow rates for sample application are about 1–2 mL/min.

Breakthrough due to sample volume or mass overload can be avoided by decreasing the sample size, if possible, or by increasing the sorbent volume. Most often, mass overload due to insufficient sorbent capacity is due to matrix competition for binding sites. A final cause of analyte breakthrough is an incorrect selection of the solid phase column for the compound of interest and/or the sample matrix.

A troubleshooting procedure to determine sources of breakthrough is discussed later.

8.3.2.3 Column Wash

Column washes are typically a series of solvent applications, usually in increas-ing order of polarity or eluting strength, for purpose of removing unwanted matrix components without disruption of isolate bonds. Water, buffers, weak acids, organic solvents, and organic mixtures are common wash solvents. Wash selection is based on the polarity and solubility characteristics of the matrix and the target compounds. It is recommended to use the strongest and the greatest volume of wash solvents that do not cause desired isolates to migrate or elute. This provides maximum cleanup of interferences without loss of recovery. Flow rates in wash steps should remain in the 1–3 mL/min range, but variation is usually less critical to recovery than in other steps. Table 4 lists recommended safe wash (and elution) volumes.

8.3.2.4 Column Drying

Drying of the column bed after wash steps facilitates removal of aqueous components that could contaminate the extract, and prepares the sorbent for phase change when eluting with organics that are immiscible with the wash solvents. Dry times vary dependent on the vacuum or pressure source and the column configuration. Typically 3–5 min at elevated vacuum or pressure is sufficient. It is possible to gauge dryness by touching the cartridge around the sorbent bed; if it feels noticeably cooler than ambient temperature, then drying is not complete. In some instances aqueous droplets may adhere to the walls of the cartridge. These can be removed with a twisted tissue or cotton tip applicator.

It is also possible to overdry the sorbent in some reversed phase applications. Hydrophobic bonding depends on accessibility of alkyl chains for H–C interactions. Release of these bonds also requires that the elution solvent have the same accessibil-ity to the retained compound to effect disruption of bonding. If sorbents are dried to the point of desolvation, the analytes are entrapped by physical restriction to the liber-

Table 4
Safe Wash and Elution Volumes

	Margin of Safety for Assay Reproducibility			
	Typical wash parameters		Typical assay parameters	
Sorbent mass (mg)	Safe wash volume (mL)	Assay wash volume (mL)	Safe elution volume (mL)	Assay elution volume (mL)
100	2.5	1.5	0.5	0.75
200	5.0	3.0	1.0	1.5
500	7.5	4.5	2.5	4.0
1000	25.0	15.0	5.0	8.0

Specifics of analyte and matrix interactions with sorbent will determine optimum conditions.

ating elution solvent. This has been reported in barbiturates and THC analysis using reversed phase methodology on mixed-mode columns.

8.3.2.5 Sample Elution

In the sample application and wash steps it was desirable to keep isolates fully retained in a narrow band on the sorbent. For elution, it is desirable to completely, yet selectively, elute all the isolate in as minimal a volume as possible. Using minimal elution volume ideally provides greater selectivity and less solvent to concentrate for analysis (guidelines for safe elution volumes are listed in Table 4). The elution solvent strength should be the weakest solvent that completely disrupts all binding mechanisms of the analyte as needed (hydrophobic, polar, and/or ion exchange).

Once again, flow rates become a very critical factor in analyte recovery. For the same reasons already discussed, appropriate flows are essential to allow kinetic transfer of analyte from the stationary phase to the mobile phase (elution solvent). This is the one step in which slower is better. Gravity flow is desirable if possible. Sometimes a short bump of vacuum or pressure will initiate the flow, and then gravity flow will continue.

Attention to correct pH, polarity, and solubility will yield both optimal recovery and selectivity for the method. If ion-exchange mechanisms are used, the elution solvent must have sufficient pH strength to reverse the electrostatic bonds. Cation exchange is frequently used for the extraction of basic (alkaline) drugs. Base drugs are ionized by pH adjustment 2 units below their pK_a, resulting in high-energy electrostatic bonds to the charged acidic sorbent. Elution solvents often utilize ammonium hydroxide to reverse the ionic state of the drugs with subsequent release from ionic bonds. It is critical that the pH of the elution solvent be at least 2 units above the analyte pK_a to fully protonate the compound. Ammonium hydroxide quickly becomes weak pH decreases when exposed to air, so the elution solvent must be prepared shortly before its use. Stock source of ammonium hydroxide can also weaken, so it is recommended to purchase small bottles. Problems of improper pH are the most common difficulty with ion-exchange procedures.

Recovery problems can be very frustrating to solve by trial and error. A more systematic approach is to view the problem as "Where did it go?"

There are limited possibilities:

- Analyte was unretained at the sample application and lost with the matrix (breakthrough).
- Analyte was unretained during wash steps and lost with washes (breakthrough).
- Analyte was retained in the elution step and remains bound to the sorbent.

Another nonextraction possibility is that the analyte was bound to a sample container or preextractant and never reached the extraction column (active sites on glass or plastic, protein precipitate). Examples of drugs with absorption problems include tetrahydrocannabinoids and tricyclic antidepressants.

If your measured recovery is only 50%, then the other 50% of the compound has to be somewhere. To determine the fate of the target analyte, it is useful to perform a mass balance. A mass balance is a quantitative accounting for all of a known concentration of analyte applied to the SPE column. It is accomplished by the individual collection and analysis of every liquid fraction to exit the column. Aqueous fractions can be passed through a nonselective sorbent (such as a C18) for minimal cleanup, and then eluted (no washes) using the same elution solvent as the primary method. This assumes that the elution solvent is correct for the analyte (pH, polarity, and solubility). While these eluates will not necessarily be very clean, they should provide an indication whether analyte is present or not. By analyzing each mobile phase that has passed through the column, it should be possible to detect whether or not breakthrough is occurring and, if it is, then where. If no analyte is detected in these fractions, then it directs the search back to the sorbent and/or the elution solvent. A series of elution profiles can be conducted by spiking standards onto columns and trying various elution solvents to determine which best eluted the pure compound. Tip: If you identify an eluting solvent that gives very little or no elution of target analytes, then you may have an excellent wash solution. A similar approach can be applied to different sorbent types to determine which did or did not retain the compound.

In addition, be sure that your analyte is not significantly bound to plasma proteins, and that it does not have affinity for active sites on glassware or plastics (including sample containers).

8.4 NONEXTRACTION PROBLEMS

Frequently when troubleshooting extraction problems, many other potential causes of low recovery or contamination are overlooked. An effective analytical approach is to work backward. In chromatographic analyses that means to look at the detection factors first:

- Are the analytes of interest (at the required concentration) detectable by the selected instrumentation?
- Are correct ions selected for SIM/GC-MS?
- Are exact or nominal masses selected? (Affects sensitivity.)
- Are GC conditions correct? (Column phase, temperatures.)

You should be able to adequately detect neat standards of your analyte before assuming that the extraction is the problem. Working backward:

- Are derivatives correctly employed?
- Are the derivatives correct/ideal for the compound functional groups?
- Are the derivatives stable in existing conditions? (Temperature, humidity, analysis time.)

Is the reconstitution solvent appropriate for the compound? (Solubility, reactivity, polarity.)

For example, some sympathomimetic amines are less soluble in ethyl acetate than they are if the ethyl acetate is combined with a small amount of isopropanol (80:20). The polar amines prefer the increased polarity of the mixture, and are subsequently better dissolved.

Next are evaporation considerations:

- Are the target compounds heat-labile?

Evaporative loss can be minimized by decreasing temperature and/or adding a keeper solvent. These are compounds with relatively high boiling points that can absorb heat energy and prevent lower-boiling compounds from evaporative loss.

Properly developed and validated SPE methods are extremely robust. Problems that do arise can be systematically identified and eliminated. It is useful to keep a few columns from the original lot that was validated; SPE columns are very stable, and having an original column on hand can help determine whether a problem is related to a new column lot or to other sources. If you can eliminate the column as a problem source, then you can focus on reagents, instrumentation, or technique. It is also recommended to check out at least two or three lot numbers of columns during validation to ensure reproducibility. Last, do not overlook technical support available from column manufacturers. Sample preparation is their expertise, and they can provide technical assistance as well as extensive method references.

REFERENCES

Majors, R. E. A Review of modern solid-phase extraction, current trends and developments in sample preparation. LC-GC Supplement, 1998.

Majors, R. E. Trends in sample preparation. LC-GC 14:9, 1996.

Majors, R. E. Liquid extraction techniques for sample preparation. LC-GC. 14:11, 1996.

Bouvier, E. S. P., Majors, R. E., eds. SPE method development and troubleshooting. LC/GC 13:11, 1995.

Bouvier, E. S. P., Martin, D. M., Iraneta, P. C., Capparella, M., Cheng, Y., and Phillips, D. J. A novel polymeric reversed-phase sorbent solid-phase extraction. LC-GC. 15:2, 1997.

Bouvier, E., Martin, D., Iraneta, P., Capparella, M., Phillips, D., Cheng, Y., Bean, L. A new water-wettable solid phase extraction sorbent for the analysis of drugs in biological fluids phillips. Waters Column. VI:3.

Sample preparation and isolation using bonded silicas, proceedings of the second annual international symposium. Analyt. Int., 1985, Philadelphia, PA.

J & W Scientific. AccuBond® SPE reference guide. (B029-0001).

Alltech Assoicates. Factors that determine the capacity of an SPE packing bed, technical tips.

Zief, M., Kiser, R. Solid-phase extraction for sample preparation. J. T. Baker Corp., 1988.

Foery, R. F., Artis, M., Ramakrishnan, K. S., and Rutter, R. Absorption characteristics of plastic containers for urinary delta 9-THCA. Soc. of For. Toxicol., 1995.

United Chemical Technologies. The science of solid phase extraction workshop presented at the International Association of Forensic Toxicologists, Melbourne, Australia, 2003.

Burke M, Optimization of SPE for drugs of abuse. Int. Sorbent Tech, Tucson, AZ.

Klink, F. E. Solid phase extraction technology and techniques for the pharmaceutical laboratory, ACS, short course, 2000.

Chapter 9

Drug Methods for the Toxicology Lab

The following chapters will outline specific analytical methods that have been published or have been developed in the laboratory that highlight the use of solid phase extraction. Each section has been referenced to provide the technical information necessary to perform these methods and to investigate different derivatization methodologies, separation conditions, and other issues encountered in performing these assays. Most methods will include a brief description of the primary drugs, metabolites, and cross-reactive drugs. Various methods for separation and derivatization will also be presented, with additional references.

9.1 AMPHETAMINE AND METHAMPHETAMINE BY GC-MS

Amphetamine and methamphetamine are potent central nervous system stimulants that are categorized as phenylethylamine derivatives. The chemical structures of these compounds can be seen in Figure 1. "Over the counter "decongestants (or sympathomimetics) that contain phenylpropanolamine or pseudoephedrine give false positive readings for the immunological screening tests; however, they are not confirmed because of the use of derivatization procedures that give different retention times and ion ratios. The metabolism of methamphetamine and amphetamine is seen in Figure 2.

9.1.1 Amphetamines in Urine: Manual Method with a Dual-Derivatization 200-mg CLEAN SCREEN Extraction Column (1,2) (ZSDAU020 or CSDAU020)

1. **Prepare sample.**
   a. To 2 mL of urine add internal standard(s)* and 1 mL of 0.1 *M* phosphate buffer, pH 6.0.
   b. Mix/vortex.
   c. Sample pH should be 6.0 ± 0.5. Adjust pH accordingly with 0.1 *M* monobasic or dibasic sodium phosphate.

From: *Forensic Science and Medicine:*
Forensic and Clinical Applications of Solid Phase Extraction
Edited by: M. J. Telepchak, T. F. August, and G. Chaney © Humana Press Inc., Totowa, NJ

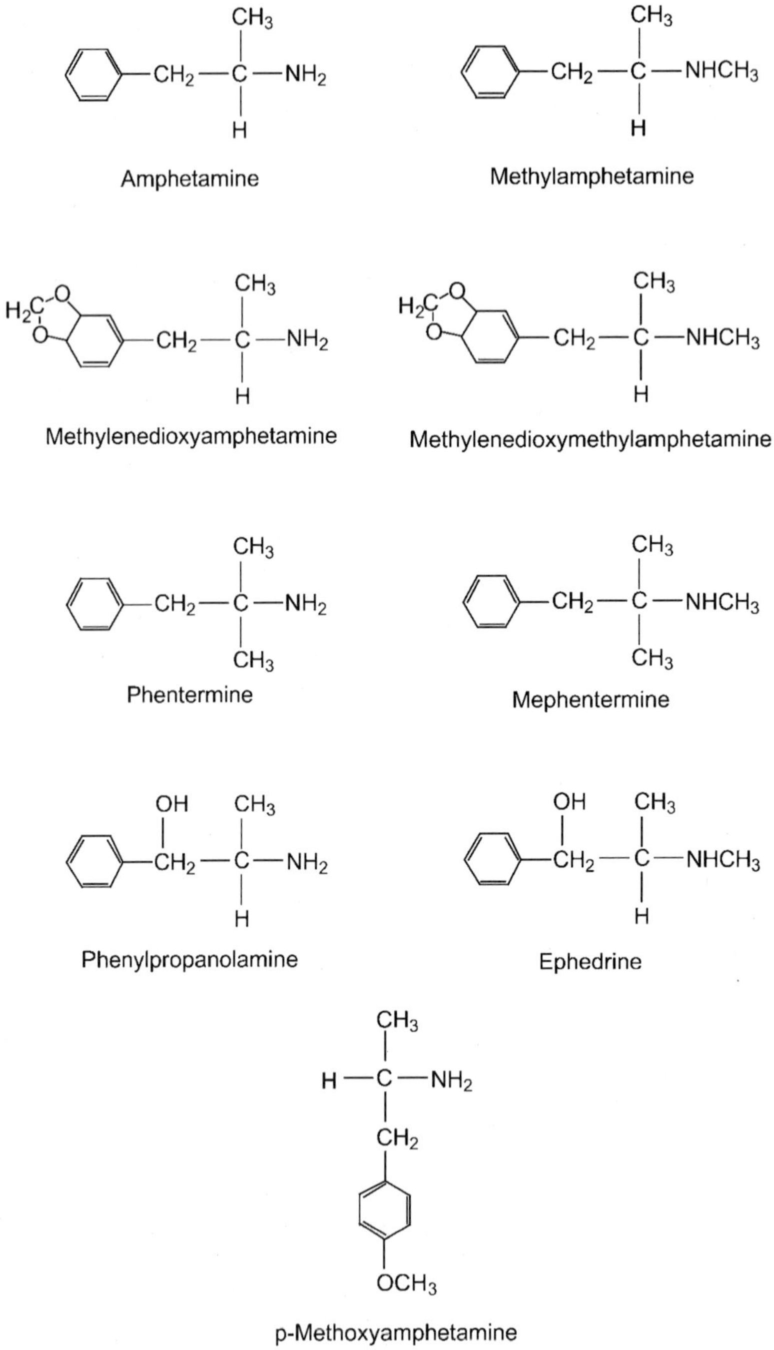

Fig. 1. Chemical structures of amphetamines.

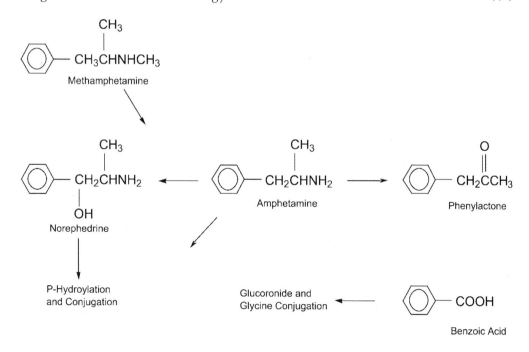

Fig. 2. Human metabolism of methanphetamine and amphetamine.

2. **Condition CLEAN SCREEN extraction column.**
   1×3 mL of CH_3OH; aspirate.
   1×3 mL of DI H_2O; aspirate.
   1×1 mL of 0.1 M phosphate buffer, pH 6.0; aspirate.
   Note: Aspirate at ≤3 in. Hg to prevent sorbent drying.
3. **Apply sample.**
   Load at 1–2 mL/min.
4. **Wash column.**
   1×3 mL of DI H_2O; aspirate.
   1×1 mL of 1.0 M acetic acid; aspirate.
   1×3 mL of CH_3OH; aspirate.
       Dry column (5 min at ≥10 in. Hg).
5. **Elute amphetamines.**
   1×3 mL of CH_2Cl_2–IPA–NH_4OH (78:20:2); collect eluate at 1–2 mL/min.
   Note: a. Prepare elution solvent daily.
          b. Add isopropanol to the ammonia solution mix, then add methylene chloride.
          c. The apparent pH of this solution should be approx 11.0.
6. **Evaporate eluate.**
   Evaporate to dryness at ≤40°C under a gentle stream of nitrogen.
7. **Dual derivatization.**
   a. Reconstitute the sample with 50 μL of ethyl acetate and 50 μL of N-Methyl-
      trimethyltrifluoroacetamide.
   b. Overlayer with nitrogen gas and cap each tube tightly.
   c. Allow to react for 10 min on the multiblock heater at 70°C.
   d. Remove the samples and allow to cool.

Table 1

Analyte	Primary ion[†]	Secondary ion	Tertiary ion
Amphetamine	240	118	91
D$_5$-Amphetamine*	244	123	91
Methamphetamine	254	210	118
D$_5$-Methamphetamine*	258	213	118

*Suitable internal standards include D$_5$-amphetamine and D$_5$-methamphetamine.
[†]Quantification ion.

   e. Add 25 µL of MBHFBA (make sure that this derivatization reagent is dissolved before use).
   f. Cap tightly and place onto the multiblock heater at 70°C for an additional 5 min.
8. **Quantitate.**
   a. Inject 1–2 µL onto the GC-MS (see GC-MS conditions).
   b. Monitor the following MSTFA derivative ions (GC-MS):

9.1.2 Amphetamines from Human Urine: Automated Method with a 200-mg CLEAN SCREEN Extraction Column (2,3) (CSDAU203 or CCDAU203)

1. **Prepare sample.**
   a. To 2 mL of urine add internal standard(s)* and 1 mL of 0.1 *M* phosphate buffer, pH 6.0.
   b. Mix/vortex.
   c. Sample pH should be 6.0 ± 0.5.
   d. Adjust pH accordingly with 0.1 *M* monobasic or dibasic sodium phosphate.
2. **Place sample onto the RapidTrace module.**
   Follow the procedure listed on the page 152.
3. **Remove samples from the RapidTrace module.**
4. **Evaporate eluate.**
   Evaporate to dryness at ≤40°C under a gentle stream of nitrogen.
5. **Dual derivatization.**
   a. Reconstitute the sample with 50 µL of ethyl acetate and 50 µL of MSTFA.
   b. Overlayer with nitrogen gas and cap each tube tightly.
   c. Allow to react for 10 min on the multiblock heater at 70°C.
   d. Remove the samples and allow to cool.
   e. Add 25 µL of MBHFBA (make sure that this derivatization reagent is dissolved before use).
   f. Cap tightly and place onto the multiblock heater at 70°C for an additional 5 min.
6. **Quantitate.**
   a. Inject 1–2 µL onto the GC-MS (see Section 9.1.2.2).
   b. Monitor the following ions (GC-MS):

9.1.2.1 Settings on Rapid Trace

9.1.2.2 GC-MS Conditions for the Analysis of Amphetamines

1. **GC Column**
   a. An RTx 5, DB-5 or, HP-5 capillary column may be used for this analysis.
   b. Column specifications are 30 m long × 0.25 mm inner diameter and 0.25 µm film thickness.

Table 2

Analyte	Primary ion[†]	Secondary ion	Tertiary ion
Amphetamine	240	118	91
D_5-Amphetamine*	244	123	91
Methamphetamine	254	210	118
D_5-Methamphetamine*	258	213	118

*Suitable internal standards include D_5-amphetamine and D_5-methamphetamine.
[†]Quantification ion.

Table 3

Step	Source	Destination	mL	mL/min	Liq. Chk
1. Condition	MeOH	Aq.	3.0	18	No
2. Condition	H_2O	Aq.	3.0	18	No
3. Condition	PO_4	Aq.	1.0	18	No
4. Load	Sample	Bio.	3.1	1.0	No
5. Purge—cannula	H_2O	Cannula	6.0	30	No
6. Rinse	H_2O	Bio.	3.0	12	No
7. Rinse	Aceta	Aq.	1.0	12	No
8. Rinse	MeOH	Aq.	3.0	12	No
9. Dry	Time = 5 min				
10. Collect	Elut	Fractl	4.0	1.0	No
12. Purge—cannula	MeOH	Cannula	4.0	30	No
13. Purge—cannula	H_2O	Cannula	4.0	30	No

Load cannula depth = 1   Mix volume = 0.5
Mix cannula depth = 0   Mix volume = 0.5
Mix cycles = 2   Reagent mix cycles = 2

Table 4

Reagent setup

No.	Reagent	Abbreviation	Sip speed
1.	H_2O	H_2O	30
2.	Methanol	MeOH	30
3.	Phosphate buffer pH 6.0	PO_4	30
4.	HCl 0.1 *M*	HCl	30
5.	Elution	Elut	15
6.	0.1 *M* Acetic acid	Aceta	30
7.	Hexane	Hex	30
8.	—		30
9.	Mixing vessel	Mixer	15
10.	Sample	Sample	15

Column air push volume 2
Column air push volume speed multiplier = 2

Table 5

No.	Waste	Abbreviation
1.	Waste aqueous	Aq.
2.	Waste organic	Org.
3.	Biohazard	Bio.

2. Oven Conditions
   a. Starting temperature = 100°C hold for 1.0 min
   b. Increase at a rate of 25°C/min
   c. Final temperature = 250°C
   d. Hold for 5 min
3. Analytical Conditions
   a. EM V at autotune value
   b. Dwell time = 50 ms
   c. Solvent delay = 6.2 min
   d. Purge-off time = 0.4 min
   e. Transfer line temperature = 250°C
   f. Injection temperature = 250°C
   g. Equilibration time = 0.5 min
   h. Start time = 2.8 min

9.1.2.3 Procedural Notes

INTERFERENCES

No interferences were noted using the GC-MS confirmation procedure as listed. A prepared standard of phentermine, phenylpropanolamine, caffeine, pseudoephedrine, dextromethorphan, methylenedioxyamphetamine (MDA), methylenedioxymethamphetamine (MDMA), and phenethylamine did not interfere with the procedure. Normal controls run with the procedure did not affect the GC-MS determination of amphetamine and methamphetamine. The analyses in this control include benzoylecgonine, secobarbital, diazepam, cannabinoids, methadone, methaqualone, morphine, codeine, phencyclidine, and propoxyphene.

LIMIT OF DETECTION AND CONFIRMATION CUTOFF

The initial limit of detection (LOD) was determined to be 5.0 ng/mL for amphetamine and methamphetamine. The limit of quantification (LOQ) for amphetamine and methamphetamine was found to be 150 ng/mL. The LOQ of this procedure is lower than the 500 ng/mL confirmational cutoff, assuring the ability to distinguish this analyte below the cutoff value.

LINEARITY

The linearity of this method is as follows:
Amphetamine   150–3000 ng/mL
Methamphetamine   150–1500 ng/mL

Table 6

Analyte	Primary ion[†]	Secondary ion	Tertiary ion
Amphetamine	190	91	118
D$_5$-Amphetamine*	194	91	123
Methamphetamine	204	118	160
D$_5$-Methamphetamine*	208	118	163

*Suggested internal standards for GC-MS: D$_5$-amphetamine and D$_5$-methamphetamine.
[†]Quantitation ion.

9.1.3 Other Derivatization Methods

9.1.3.1 Fluoracylate with PFAA (1)

Pentafluoropropionic acid anhydride (PFAA or PFPA) is one compound of a class of acid anhydrides that are used to derivatize amine groups. The excess reagent must be removed before GC-MS analysis to prevent the injection of acidic reactant and reaction byproducts onto the GC column (2).

1. **Sample preparation.**
   To the evaporated sample or standard tube:
   a. Add 50 µL of PFPA (PFAA).
   b. Overlay with nitrogen gas and cap.
   c. React for 20 min at 70°C.
   d. Evaporate to dryness at ≤40°C.
   e. Reconstitute with 100 µL of ethyl acetate.
2. **Quantitate.**
   a. Inject 1–2 µL onto the GC-MS.
   b. Monitor the following ions (GC-MS):

9.1.3.2 Keeper Solvents

The use of a "keeper" solvent such as dimethyl formamide (DMF) has been used to cut down on the loss of these compounds due to their volatile nature. An amount (30–50 µL) of high-purity DMF is added to the elution solvent before evaporation. The use of 0.1 *M* HCl in methanol has also been used to form the hydrochloride salts of the amphetamine analytes.

9.1.3.3 4-CB (4-Carboxyhexylfluorobutyryl Chloride) Derivatives (3)

4-CB is a commonly used derivatization reagent for amphetamines; however, methamphetamine ions can result from the presence of ephedrine or pseudoephedrine. This effect may become exaggerated when a new injection insert liner is used. The presence of this artifact has caused NIDA to allow a positive methamphetamine (>500 ng/mL) only when in addition amphetamine is present in excess of 200 ng/mL (4).

1. **Sample Preparation.**
   To the evaporated sample or standard tube:
   a. Add 200 µL of 4-carboxyhexylfluorobutyryl chloride in 1-chlorobutane (1:100 v/v).
   b. Overlay with nitrogen gas and cap.
   c. React for 15 min at 50°C.

Table 7

Analyte	Retention time (min)	Primary ion[†] ion	Secondary	Tertiary ion
Amphetamine	8.28	294	266	248
D_5-Amphetamine*	8.28	297	269	250
Phentermine	8.41	308	280	261
MDA	8.41	135	162	308
Methamphetamine	8.90	308	280	262
D_5-Methamphetamine*	8.90	312	284	266
Phenylpropanolamine	9.58	295	295	338
Ephedrine	9.71	308	280	398
Pseudoephedrine	11.21	308	280	398
MDMA	11.37	162	308	280

*Suggested internal standards for GC-MS: D_5-amphetamine and D_5-methamphetamine.
†Quantitation ion.

     d. Add 300 μL anhydrous ethanol.
     e. Overlay with nitrogen gas and cap.
     f. React for 15 minutes at 50°C.
     g. Evaporate to dryness at ≤45°C.
     h. Reconstitute with 100 μL of ethyl acetate.

2. GC conditions:
     a. Column: HP-5 12.5 *M* × 0.2 mm i.d. x 033 μm film thickness.
     b. Oven program: 60°C; hold 1 min to 225°C at 20°C/min with a hold time of 0.75 min, then 70°C/min to 260°C; hold for 2 min (total time = 12.5 min).
     c. Injector temp = 210°C.
     d. Transfer line = 285°C.
     e. Solvent delay = 4 min.
     f. Electron multiplier = Autotune value.
     g. Purge-off time = 0.75 min.

3. Quantitate.
     a. Inject 1–2 μL onto the GC-MS.
     b. Monitor the following ions (GC-MS):

9.1.3.4 HFBA (Heptafluorobutyric Acid Anhydride) Derivatives (5)

Heptafluorobutyric acid anhydrides are acylation reagents that derivatize the amine function on the amphetamine molecule.

1. Sample preparation.
To the evaporated sample or standard tube:
     a. Add 50 uL of heptafluorobutyric acid anhydride.
     b. Overlay with nitrogen gas and cap.
     c. React for 15 min at 75°C.
     d. Evaporate to dryness at ≤50°C.
     e. Reconstitute with 100 μL of ethyl acetate.

Table 8

Compound	Rentition time (min)	Primary ion[†]	Secondary ion	Tertiary ion
Amphetamine	6.32	330	240	159
D_5-Amphetamine*	6.32	243	121	92
Phentermine	6.4	254	91	210
Phenylpropanolamine	6.77	240	169	330
Propylhexidrine	6.89	254	210	162
Methamphetamine	7.04	344	254	210
D_5-Methamphetamine*	7.04	258	213	119
Ephedrine	7.19	254	210	344
Pseudoephedrine	7.52	254	210	344
MDMA	9.06	162	254	210

*Suggested internal standards for GC-MS: D_5-amphetamine and D_5-methamphetamine.
[†]Quantitation ion.

Table 9

Mass Spectral Characteristics of Substituted Fluorine Derivatives of Amphetamine, Methamphetamine and MDMA (6)

Compound	Derivative	Base peak	Secondary peak (%)	Tertiary peak (%)
Amphetamine	Trifluoro (1)	140	118 (90%)	91 (44%)
	Pentafluoro (2)	190	118 (68%)	91 (34%)
	Heptafluoro (3)	240	118 (61%)	91 (35%)
	Perfluoro (4)	440	516 (1.1%)	118 (42%)
Methamphetamine	Trifluoro (1)	154	110 (35%)	118 (30%)
	Pentafluoro (2)	204	160 (33%)	118 (22%)
	Heptafluoro (3)	254	210 (22%)	118 (11%)
	Perfluoro (4)	454	530 (0.2%)	410 (32%)
MDMA	Trifluoro (1)	154	162 (72%)	135 (54%)
	Pentafluoro (2)	204	162 (46%)	160 (46%)
	Heptafluoro (3)	254	210 (36%)	162 (47%)
	Perfluoro (4)	454	410 (34%)	162 (46%)

Reaction conditions:

1. Trifluoroacetic acid anhydride (TFAA) — 40°C—15 min
2. Pentafluoropropionic acid anhydride (PFAA or PFPA) — 75°C—15 min
3. Heptafluorobutyric acid anhydride (HFBA or HFAA) — 60°C—40 min
4. Perfluorooctanoyl chloride (PFO) — 60°C—30 min

2. GC conditions.
   a. Column: HP-5 12.5 m × 0.2 mm i.d. × 0.33 μm film thickness.
   b. Oven program: 60°C; hold 1min to 225°C at 20°C/min with a hold time of 0.75, then 70°C/min to 260°C; hold for 2 min (total time = 12.5 min).
   c. Injector temp = 210°C.
   d. Transfer line = 285°C.
   e. Solvent delay = 4 min.
   f. Electron multiplier = autotune value
   g. Purge-off time = 0.75 min.
3. Quantitate.
   a. Inject 1–2 μL onto the GC-MS.
   b. Monitor the following ions (GC-MS):

9.1.4 Periodate Degradation of Interfering Ephedrine (7)

The ingestion of over-the-counter sympathomimetic agents provides a significant degree of cross- reactivity and chromatographic difficulties when injected with amphetamines or methamphetamines. Ephedrine, pseudoephedrine, and phenylpropanolamine can often be oxidized to noninterfering substances by the addition of periodic acid in an alkaline environment. The following procedures have been used to eliminate the cross-reactivity of these interferents.

9.1.4.1 Procedure 1

   a. For every milliliter of sample add 250 μL of 1.6 *M* periodic acid solution.
   b. Add also 300 μL of 1.6 *M* potassium hydroxide solution.
   c. Vortex (a white precipitate should form).
   d. Add 2 mL of phosphate buffer, 0.1 *M* pH 6.0.
   e. Vortex and centrifuge.
   f. Transfer the supernatant to the SPE column for separation.
   Solutions: 1.6 *M* Periodic acid solution
   a. To 200 mL of distilled water add 91.2 g of periodic acid.
   b. Dilute to 250 mL with distilled water.
   c. Store at room temperature in glass—prepare fresh daily.
      1.6 M Potassium hydroxide
   a. Dissolve 22.44 g of potassium hydroxide in 250 mL of distilled water.
   b. Mix (**Caution:** This solution may become hot while mixing).
   c. Store at room temperature in glass.

9.1.4.2. Procedure 2 (8)

   a. Bring all urine samples, calibrators, controls, and standards to room temperature.
   b. Transfer 2 mL of each sample to a 13 x 100 mm test tube and add internal standard.
   c. Add 1 mL of 1.0 *N* sodium hydroxide and 0.5 mL of saturated sodium periodate solution.
   d. Mix and incubate at room temperature for at least 10 min.
   e. Add 1 mL of 1.0 *N* HCl.
   f. Add 1 mL of 0.1 *M* phosphate buffer, pH 6.0.
   g. Adjust the pH of each sample to pH 6.0 ± 0.5 with 1.0 *N* NaOH or HCl as indicated by pH paper.
   h. Apply the prepared solution to the SPE column for isolation.

Table 10
Ions of Amphetamine Pro-Drugs

(a) Clobenzorex® (Underivatized) (10)

Drug	Primary ion	Secondary ion	Tertiary ions	Other ions
Clobenzorex	125	364	118	91
4-Hydroxy Metabolite (1)	125	330	364	118

The 4 hydroxy-metabolite is determined at approximately the same levels as the amphetamine produced by the metabolic interconversion of this drug. This metabolite has a longer half-life than the parent drug and is useful as an indicator of Clobenzorex ingestion.

(b) Fenproporex (Underivatized) (11)

Drug	Primary ion	Secondary ion	Tertiary ions	Other ions
Fenproporex	293	240	118	91

Solutions: Saturated sodium periodate solution
a. Add 10 g of sodium periodate to 100 mL of distilled water.
b. Shake and add additional sodium periodate until excess crystals are seen.
c. Store at room temperature in glass—prepare fresh daily.

9.1.5 New Issues in the Determination of Amphetamine and Methamphetamine

9.1.5.1 Amphetamine or Methamphetamine Pro-Drugs

Drugs that are metabolized to amphetamine or methamphetamine (precursor drugs) are potentially significant concerns in the screening and interpretation of amphetamine-positive drug screening results. Fenproporex® (3-[1-(methyl-2-phenylethyl) amino] propane-nitrile) and Clobenzorex® (2-chlorobenzylamphetamine) are examples of anorectic drugs that are available in Mexico and other countries. These drugs metabolize to significant amounts of amphetamines in humans (9,10). Currently 14 drugs on the market are known to metabolize to amphetamine or methamphetamine in the human body (11). There is very little information on the metabolic profiles of these compounds, making the distinction between abuse and legal medicinal use very difficult.

9.1.5.2 Designer Drugs

Other clandestine drugs such as MDMA (Ecstasy), MDEA (Eve), and MBDB and its metabolite BDB have been used as recreational drugs that have significant toxicological impact. For example, MDMA has a chemical structure similar to that of methamphetamine and the hallucinogen mescaline, so this agent can have both stimulant and psychedelic effects. These new designer drugs are highly addictive, have neurotoxin potential, and are listed as Schedule 1 agents in the US Drug Enforcement Code, as they have no legitimate medical purpose.

Methods for the isolation of MDA and MDMA have been published using the amphetamine SPE method and use different mass spectral ions for SIM determination. A review of some of these methods is given below.

Table 11
Ions of Designer Drugs

Drug	Primary ion*	Secondary ion	Tertiary ions
3,4-Methylenedioxy- methamphetamine (MDMA)	254	210	162, 135, 389
3,4- Methylenedioxy- amphetamine (MDA)	240	162	135, 375
4-Hydroxy-3-methoxy- methamphetamine (HMMA-Di HFBA)	360	254	210, 587
4-Hydroxy-3-methoxy- amphetamine (HMA-Di HFBA)	360	240	163, 573
3,4 Dihydroxy- methamphetamine (HHMA-Tri-HFBA)	515	254	210, 542, 769
3,4 Dihydroxy- amphetamine (HHA-Tri-HFBA)	515	240	210, 542, 755

*Quantitation ion.

9.1.5.3 Chiral Isomers

A discussion about the various optical isomers of these compounds is beyond the scope of this book; however, the importance of chirality in these compounds gives both significant differences in the pharmacodynamics and pharmacokinetics, and has forensic significance. For example, pharmacodynamic differences can be seen in the actions of thalidomide in that only one isomer is responsible for birth defects. Another example is the *D* form of propoxyphene (Darvon®), which is an analgesic, and the *L* form (Novrad®) which is an antitussive.

Pharmacokinetic differences are seen with different isomers having different protein binding and renal clearance values. Differences of a forensic nature can separate plant drugs from chemically synthesized agents (e.g., cocaine), identify legitimate vs clandestine manufactured drugs, and help determine the use of drugs that commonly metabolize to amphetamines.

9.1.5.4 Derivatization Procedure for HFBA Derivatives, MDA, MDMA, and MDEA

Sample preparation
To the eluted sample using the amphetamine SPE procedure:
1. Add 0.1 mL of 1% HCl in Methanol.
2. Dry sample down at 50–60°C.
3. Add 35 μL of HFBA (heptafluorobutyric acid anhydride) and 100 μL of ethyl acetate.
4. Incubate at 70°C for 15 min.

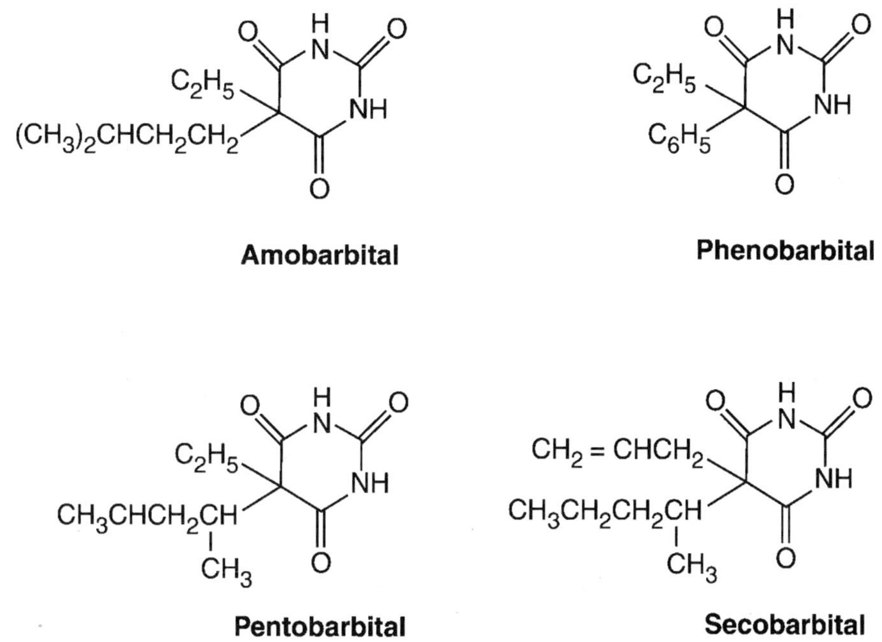

Fig. 3. Chemical structures for barbituric acids.

5. Dry down using a stream of nitrogen with no heating.
6. Reconstitute the dry sample with 100 µL of ethyl acetate.
7. Inject 1–2 µL onto the GC-MS system.

9.2 BARBITURATES IN URINE (1)

Barbiturates are central nervous system depressants and have been useful pharmacological agents since the 1940s (Figure 3). Barbiturates are potential drugs of abuse due to their hypnotic and sedating effects, so the screening of urines for barbiturates is widely practiced. This section reports on a method for the confirmation and quantitation of barbiturates in human urine by GC-MSD with selective ion monitoring (SIM). Sample preparation was automated by the use of CLEAN SCREEN DAU-SPE columns on the Zymark RapidTrace Workstation. We validated this method for five commonly prescribed barbiturates (amobarbital, butabarbital, pentobarbital, phenobarbital, and secobarbital).

Experimental Standards

All analytical standards—amobarbital, butabarbital, hexobarbital, phenobarbital, pentobarbital, and secobarbital—were acquired from Alltech Applied Science (State College, PA).

Instrumentation

A Hewlett Packard Model 5890 gas chromatograph and a Model 5971A mass spectroscopy system were used with a Model 7673 autosampler. Data were collected on HP DOS Chemstation (Rev 2.0) software on a PC equipped with Windows 3.1. A

DB-5® (30 m, 0.25 mm i.d. with 0.25 μm film) capillary column was used for the separation of our compounds. This column has a 5% phenyl and 95% dimethylsiloxane stationary phase equivalent to a DB-5 or HP-5 capillary column.

Analytical Conditions
The GC-MSD oven temperature program was as follows:

Initial temperature 60°C; hold for 1 min; increase to 300°C at a rate of 20°C/min; hold for 2 min.

The injector temperature was set at 250°C. Ultrapure helium was used as the carrier gas at a 30 mL/min flow rate.

The mass selective detector operated in the selective ion monitoring mode with the photomultiplier voltage set by the autotune program.

The GC-MSD interface temperature was 280°C.

Selected ions (see Table 22) were monitored at a dwell time of 25 ms.

Results
Chromatography

Each analyte is completely separated from each other and is baseline resolved (Figure 4).

Linearity

All analytes gave linear curves from 50–2000 ng/mL. The coefficient of correlation for all analytes was greater than 0.995.

Recovery

The recovery of all analytes ranges from 85%–120%.

DB-5 is a registered trademark of J & W Scientific (Folsom, CA).

Assay Variability

The validation of each assay was accomplished by the running of five replicate injections of seven calibration levels (50, 100, 250, 500, 1000, 1500, and 2000 ng/mL) put in a random sequence for 3 analytical days. All dilutions of the stock solutions were prepared fresh for each analytical day.

Each analyte gave precise and consistent results with a less than 6.5% relative standard derivatization (RSD) for both the interday and intraday variability.

Stability

There were no stability problems encountered in both urine samples stored in the refrigerator over a period of 1 wk and prepared samples stored on the autosampler tray for >60 h at room temperature.

Sensitivity

This assay has adequate sensitivity and selectivity. It was developed on a 2-mL urine sample with a 50-ng/mL lower limit of detection. In normal analytical circumstances, concentrations in the range of 2000–10,000 ng/mL are observed.

Summary

A rapid, reliable, and robust method for the quantification of five barbiturates is presented. The results for the interday and intraday variability indicated that all analytes using the automated SPE preparation gave reliable and precise results. This method could easily be modified to analyze other barbiturates, such as aprobarbital, barbital, butalbital, mephobarbital, and other barbiturates.

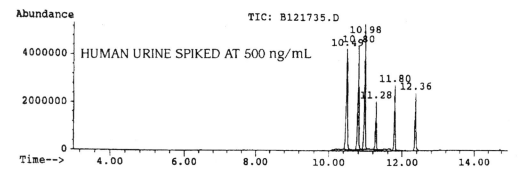

Fig. 4. Barbiturate analysis chromatograms.

Table 12

Drug	Primary ion[+]	Secondary ion	Tertiary ion
Amobarbital	156	141	157
Butabarbita	156	141	157
Hexobarbital*	221	157	236
Pentobarbital	156	141	197
Phenobarbital	204	232	117
Secobarbital	168	167	195

*Suggested internal standard for GC-MS: hexobarbital or a deuterated barbiturate analog.
[+]Quantitation ion.

9.2.1 Barbiturates in Urine: Manual Method (2)

For GC or GC-MS Confirmations Using a 200-mg CLEAN SCREEN Extraction Column (ZSDAU020 or CSDAU0203)

1. **Prepare sample.**
   a. To 2 mL of urine add internal standard(s)* and 1 mL of 0.1 M phosphate buffer, pH 6.0.
   b. Mix/vortex.
   c. Sample pH should be 6.0 + 0.5. Adjust pH accordingly with 0.1 M monobasic or dibasic sodium phosphate.
2. **Condition extraction column.**
   1 × 3 mL of CH_3OH; aspirate.
   1 × 3 mL of DI H_2O; aspirate.
   1 × 1 mL 0.1 M phosphate buffer, pH 6.0; aspirate.
   Note: Aspirate at <3 in. Hg to prevent sorbent drying.
3. **Apply sample.**
   Load at 1–2 mL/min.
4. **Wash column.**
   1 × 3 mL of DI H_2O; aspirate.
   1 × 1 mL of 0.1 M acetic acid; aspirate.

Table 13

Drug	Primary ion[†]	Secondary ion	Tertiary ion
Amobarbital	156	141	157
Butabarbital	156	141	157
Butalbital	168	167	181
Hexobarbital*	221	157	236
Pentobarbital	156	141	197
Phenobarbital	204	232	117
Secobarbital	168	167	195
Thiopental	172	157	173

*Suggested internal standard for GC-MS: hexobarbital or a deuterated barbiturate analog.
†Quantitation ion.

Dry column (5 min at >10 in. Hg).
1 × 2 mL of hexane; aspirate.
5. Elute barbiturates.
1 × 3 mL hexane–ethyl acetate (50:50).
6. Dry eluate
a. Evaporate to dryness at ≤40°C.
b. Reconstitute with 100 µL ethyl acetate.
7. Quantitate
a. Inject 1–2 µL onto the chromatograph.
b. Monitor the following ions (GC-MS):

9.2.2. Barbiturates in Urine: Automated Method (3)

For GC or GC/MS Confirmations Using 200-mg CLEAN SCREEN Extraction Column (CSDAU203 or CCDAU203)

1. Prepare sample.
a. To 2 mL of urine add internal standard(s)* and 1 mL of 0.1 *M* phosphate buffer, pH 6.0.
b. Mix/vortex.
c. Sample pH should be 6.0 ± 0.5. Adjust pH accordingly with 0.1 *M* monobasic or dibasic sodium phosphate.
2. Place samples onto the Zymark RapidTrace.
3. Run the RapidTrace procedure.
See Section 9.2.2.1 for details.
4. Remove sample and dry eluate.
a. Evaporate to dryness at ≤40°C using a TurbVap® or equivalent evaporator.
b. Reconstitute with 100 µL of ethyl acetate.
5. Quantitate.
a. Inject 1–2 µL onto chromatograph.
b. Monitor the following ions (GC-MS):

Table 14

Step	Source	Destination	mL	mL/s	Liq. Chk
1. Condition	MeOH	Aq.	2.0	18	No
2. Condition	H$_2$O	Aq.	2.0	18	No
3. Condition	PO$_4$	Aq.	2.0	18	No
4. Load	Sample	Bio.	3.1	1.0	No
5. Purge—cannula	H$_2$O	Cannula	6.0	30	No
6. Rinse	H$_2$O	Bio.	4.5	12	No
7. Rinse	Aceta	Bio.	2.0	12	No
8. Dry	Time = 3 min				
9. Rinse	Hex	Org.	3.0	12	No
10. Dry	Time = 2.0 min				
11. Collect	Elut	Fractl	4.0	1.2	No
12. Purge—cannula	MeOH	Cannula	4.0	30	No
13. Purge—cannula	H$_2$O	Cannula	4.0	30	No

Load cannula depth = 1   Column air push volume = 2
Mix cannula depth = 0   Column air push volume
speed   multiplier = 2
Mix cycles = 2
Mix volumes = .5
Mix speed = .6
Reagent mix cycles = 2

Table 15

Reagent setup

No.	Reagent	Abbreviation	Sip speed
1.	H$_2$O	H$_2$O	30
2.	Methanol	MeOH	30
3.	Phosphate buffer pH 6.0	PO$_4$	30
4.	1 *M* HCl	HCl	30
5.	Elution solvent*	Elut	15
6.	Acetic acid 0.1 *M*	Aceta	30
7.	Hexane	Hex	30
8.	—		30
9.	Mixing vessel	Mixer	30
10.	Sample	Sample	15

Table 16

No.	Waste	Abbreviation
1.	Aqueous	Aq.
2.	Organic	Org.
3.	Biohazard	Bio.

*The elution solvent for this assay is hexane-ethyl acetate (50:50). Make the elution solvent fresh daily.

Table 17

Drug	Primary ion[†]	Secondary ion	Tertiary ion
Amobarbital	156	141	157
Butabarbital	156	141	157
Butalbital	168	167	181
Hexobarbital*	221	157	236
Pentobarbital	156	141	197
Phenobarbital	204	232	117
Secobarbital	168	167	195
Thiopental	172	157	173

*Suggested internal standard for GC-MS: hexobarbital or a deuterated barbiturate analog.
†Quantitation ion.

9.2.2.1 RapidTrace Settings for Barbiturates

9.2.3 Barbiturates in Urine Manual Procedure (4)

For GC or GC-MS Confirmations Using CLEAN SCREEN Reduced Solvent Volume Extraction Columns (CSDAU083)

1. **Prepare sample.**
   a. To 1 mL of urine add internal standard(s)* and 1 mL of 0.1 M phosphate buffer, pH 6.0.
   b. Mix/vortex.
   c. Sample pH should be 6.0 ± 0.5. Adjust pH accordingly with 0.1 M monobasic or dibasic sodium phosphate.
2. **Condition extraction column.**
   1 × 0.5 mL of CH_3OH; aspirate.
   1 × 0.5 mL of DI H_2O; aspirate.
   1 × 0.25 mL of 0.1 M phosphate buffer, pH 6.0; aspirate.
   Note: Aspirate at ≤3 in. Hg to prevent sorbent drying.
3. **Apply sample.**
   Load at 1–2 mL/min.
4. **Wash column.**
   1 × 0.5 mL of DI H2O; aspirate.
   1 × 0.5 mL of 0.1 M acetic acid; aspirate.
   Dry column (5 min at ≥10 in. Hg).
   1 × 0.1 mL of hexane; aspirate.
5. **Elute barbiturates.**
   2 × 0.75 mL hexane-ethyl acetate (50:50).
6. **Dry eluate.**
   a. Evaporate to dryness at ≤40°C.
   b. Reconstitute with 100 µL of ethyl acetate.
7. **Quantitate.**
   a. Inject 1–2 µL onto chromatograph.
   b. Monitor the following ions (GC-MS):

Table 18

Drug	Primary ion[†]	Secondary ion	Tertiary ion
Amobarbital	156	141	157
Butabarbital	156	141	157
Butalbital	168	167	181
Hexobarbital*	221	157	236
Pentobarbital	156	141	197
Phenobarbital	204	232	117
Secobarbital	168	167	195
Thiopental	172	157	173

*Suggested internal standard for GC-MS: Hexobarbital or deuterated barbiturate analog.
[†]Quantitation ion.

9.2.4 Barbiturates in Urine Automated Procedure

For GC or GC-MS Confirmations Using CLEAN SCREEN Reduced Solvent Volume (4) Extraction column (CSDAU083)

1. **Prepare sample**
   a. To 1 mL of urine add internal standard(s)* and 0.5 mL of 0.1 M phosphate buffer, pH 6.0.
   b. Mix/vortex.
   c. Sample pH should be 6.0 ± 0.5. Adjust pH accordingly with 0.1 M monobasic or dibasic sodium phosphate.
2. **Place sample onto the Zymark RapidTrace.**
3. **Run the RapidTrace Procedure.**
   See Section 9.2.4.1 for details.
4. **Remove samples and dry eluate.**
   a. Evaporate to dryness at ≤40°C using a TurboVap or equivalent evaporator.
   b. Reconstitute with 100 µL of ethyl acetate.
5. **Quantitate.**
   a. Inject 1–2 µL onto chromatograph.
   b. Monitor the following ions (GC-MS):

9.2.4.1 RapidTrace Settings for Analysis of Barbiturates Using a Reduced Solvent Volume Column

9.2.5 Chemical Derivatives of Barbiturates

Chemical derivatization has been commonly performed to improve on the peak shape of barbiturates. The most common reaction performed on barbiturates is alkylation by the use of trimethylanilinium hydroxide. This gives very stable derivatives that chromatograph well.

Table 19

Step	Source	Destination	mL	mL/s	Liq. Chk
1. Condition	MeOH	Org.	0.5	6	No
2. Condition	H$_2$O	Aq.	0.5	6	No
3. Condition	PO$_4$	Aq.	0.5	6	No
4. Load	Sample	Bio.	1.7	1.2	No
5. Purge—cannula	H$_2$O	Cannula	6.0	30	No
6. Rinse	H$_2$O	Bio.	0.5	8	No
7. Rinse	Ac4.5	Bio.	0.5	8	No
8. Dry	Time = 3 min				
9. Rinse	Hex	Org.	0.1	8	No
10. Dry	Time = 2.0 min				
11. Collect	Hex/EtAc	Fractl	1.5	2	No
12. Purge—cannula	MeOH	Cannula	4.0	30	No
13. Purge—cannula	H$_2$O	Cannula	4.0	30	No

Load cannula depth = 1   Column air push volume = 2
Mix cannula depth = 0   Column air push volume speed multiplier = 2
Mix cycles = 2   Mix speed = .6
Mix volume = .5   Reagent mix cycles = 2

Table 20

Reagent setup

No.	Reagent	Abbreviation	Sip speed
1.	H$_2$O	H$_2$O	30
2.	Methanol	MEOH	30
3.	Phosphate pH 6	PO$_4$	30
4.	Acetate, pH 4.5	Ac4.5	30
5.	Elution solvent	Elut	15
6.	0.1 M acetic acid	Aceta	30
7.	Hexane	Hex	30
8.	Hexane-EtAc 50:50	Hex: EtAC	30
9.	Mixing vessel	Mixer	30
10.	Sample	Sample	15

Table 21

No.	Waste	Abbreviation
1.	Aqueous	Aq.
2.	Organic	Org.
3.	Biohazard	Bio.

Table 22
Selected Properties of Barbiturates

Compound	RT[a]	pK$_a$	Ions Major (amu)	Ions Minor I (amu)	Ions Minor 2 (amu)	Comments
Amobarbital	10.8	8.0	156	141	157	Short-acting
Butabarbital	10.5	7.9	141	156	157	Hypnotic
Hexabarbital	11.8	8.3	221	157	236	Internal STD
Pentobarbital	10.9	8.0	156	141	197	Short-acting
Phenobarbital	12.4	7.5	204	232	117	Anticonvulsant
Secobarbital	11.3	8.0	168	167	195	Short-acting

Other barbiturates

Compound	Est RT[a]	pK$_a$	Ions			Comments
Aprobarbital	9.8	7.8	167	141	124	
Barbital	8.9	7.8	156	141	98	
Butalbital[c]	10.5[b]	7.9	168	167	124	
Butethal	10.5	8.1	141	156	98	
Mephobarbital[d]	12.9	7.7	218	117	146	
Metharbital[d]	8.9	8.2	170	155	112	
Probarbital	9.7	8.0	156	141	169	
Talbutal	10.9	7.8	167	168	195	
Thiamylal[e]	12.1	7.3	184	185	212	
Thiopental[e]	11.S	7.5	172	157	173	

[a]Actual retention time on this analytical system.
[b]Calculated retention time based on historical data.
[c]Used for migraines.
[d]Anticonvulsant.
[e]Ultrashort anesthetic induction agent.

The reagent is MethElute®* or 0.2 *M* trimethylanilinium hydroxide (TMPAH) in methanol and is available from various sources.

Procedure

1. The eluted sample is evaporated to dryness at 40°C with a stream of dry nitrogen.
2. 100 μL of ethyl acetate and 25 μL of TMPAH are added to the dried sample.
3. Mix and vortex the sample.
4. Place onto a heater block at 75μC for 20 min.
5. Remove the tube from heat.
6. Allow to cool to room temperature and inject 1–2 μL onto the GC-MS system.

The GC separation conditions are the same as the nonderivatized barbiturate assay; however, monitor the following ions:

Table 23

Retention time	Compound	Primary ion[b]	Second ion (% base)	Third ion (% base)
6.2 min	Butalbital	196	195 (60%)	209 (14%)
6.5 min	Amobarbital	169	184 (86%)	226 (8%)
6.6 min	Pentobarbital	169	184 (90%)	225 (7%)
6.8 min	Secobarbital	196	195 (70%)	181 (37%)
7.7 min	Hexobarbital[a]	235	169 (26%)	171 (16%)
7.8 min	Phenobarbital	232	175 (18%)	117 (11%)

[a]Internal standard peak.
[b]Quantitation ion.
Methelute® is a registered trademark of Pierce (Rockford, IL).

Table 24
Pharmacokinetic Parameters of Benzodiazepines

Generic Name	Trade Name	Dose (mg)	Duration	Half-life	Blood	Urine
Alprazolam	Xanax®	0.25–1 mg	0.5–7 hr	12–15 hr	30 h	72 h
Chlordiazepoxide	Librium®	5, 10 , 25 mg	1–8 hr	5–30 hr	24+ h	days
Clonazepam	Rivotril®	0.5, 2.0 mg	1–12 hr	19–60 hr	96 h	168 h
Diazepam	Valium®	2, 5, 10 mg	0.3–7 hr	20–100 hr	72 h	days
Flunitrazepam[a]	Rohypnol®	1, 2 mg	0.5–12 hr	9–25 hr	18 h	72 h
Flurazepam	Dalmane®	15, 30 mg	1–6 hr	20–100 hr	140 h	days
Lorazepam	Ativan®	0.5, 1, 2 mg	0.5–7 hr	12–15 hr	36 h	72–96 h
Temazepam	Restoril®	15, 30 mg	1–8 hr	9–12 hr	72 h	48 h
Triazolam	Halcion®	0.125 mg	0.5–6 hr	1.5–4 hr	6 h	48 h

[a]Not legally distributed in the United States.

9.3 BENZODIAZEPINES

Benzodiazepines are agents that are frequently prescribed for the symptomatic treatment of anxiety and sleep disorders. They were introduced in the 1960s and have replaced barbiturates for many indications. They are safe agents, having a large therapeutic index and a relatively low incidence of pharmacological addiction. Table 24 lists some of the pharmacokinetic parameters of these agents.

Table 25 summarizes some of the analytical challenges in benzodiazepine analysis.

9.3.1 Benzodiazepines in Urine for GC or GC-MS Confirmations Using 200 mg CLEAN SCREEN Extraction Column (ZSDAU020 or ZCDAU020)

1. Prepare sample—β-glucuronidase hydrolysis.
   a. To 5 mL of urine add internal standard(s)* and 2 mL of β-glucuronidase solution.
   b. β-glucuronidase solution contains 5000 FU/mL Patella vulgata in 0.1 *M* acetate buffer, pH =5.0.

Table 25
Benzodiazepine Assay Challenges

A. Poor/ limited solubility in water
   Solubility issues are the key to variable analytical recovery.
B. Analytical concentrations
   Due to the low doses of these agents, nanogram -per-milliliter concentrations must be
      detected.
C. Metabolism
   The metabolism of many of these agents can yield similar metabolic products.
D. Glucuronides
   Glucuronide formation is a major metabolic route for these compounds.
   All samples must be hydrolyzed or deconjugated before analysis.
E. Chemical derivatization
   In most cases chemical derivatization with silylation reagents must be done to improve on
      the detection and confirmation of these compounds.
F. Chemical diversity
   The wide range of chemical diversity, such as pK_a, makes it difficult to achieve maximum
      extraction efficiency across the entire range of benzodiazepines in a single extraction.

A number of SPE procedures have been developed for these agents.

   c. Mix/vortex.
   d. Hydrolize for 3 h at 65°C.
   d. Centrifuge for 10 min at 670g and discard pellet.
   e. Cool before proceeding.
2. **Condition CLEAN SCREEN extraction column.**
   1 × 3 mL of CH_3OH; aspirate.
   1 × 3 mL of DI H_2O; aspirate.
   1 × 1 mL of 0.1 M phosphate buffer, pH 6.0.
   Note: Aspirate at ≤3 in. Hg to prevent sorbent drying.
3. **Apply sample.**
   Load at 1 mL/min.
4. **Wash column.**
   1 × 2 mL of DI H_2O; aspirate.
   1 × 2 mL of 20% acetonitrile in 0.1 M phosphate buffer, pH 6.0; aspirate.
   Dry column (5 min at ≥10 in. Hg).
   1 × 2 mL of hexane; aspirate.
5. **Elute benzodiazepines.**
   1 × 3 mL of ethyl acetate; collect eluate at 1–2 mL/min.
6. **Dry eluate.**
   Evaporate to dryness at ≤40°C.
7. **Derivatize.**
   a. Add 50 μL of ethyl acetate and 50 μL of bissilytrifluoroacetamide (BSTFA) with
   1% trimethylcholrosilane (TMCS)
   b. Overlayer with N_2 and cap. Mix/vortex.
   c. React 20 min at 70°C. Remove from heat source to cool.
   Note: Do not evaporate BSTFA solution.

Table 26

Generic name	Trade name	Primary ion[b]	Secondary ion	Tertiary ion
Alprazolam	Xanax®	308	279	204
α-Hydroxyalprazolam-TMS		381	396	383
Chlordiazepoxide	Librium®	282	283	284
Clonazepam	Rivotril®	387	352	306
Diazepam	Valium®	256	283	221
Nordiazepam-TMS		341	342	343
Flurazepam	Dalmane®			
Desalkylflurazepam-TMS		359	341	245
Hydroxyethylflurazepam		288	287	289
Lorazepam-TMS	Ativan®	429	430	347
Oxazepam-TMS[a]	Serax®	86	109	307
Prazepam[a]		269	241	324
Temazepam-TMS	Restoril®	343	283	257
Triazolam	Halcion®	313	314	342
α-Hydroxytriazolam-TMS		415	417	430

[a]Suggested internal standard for GC-MS: prazepam, D5-oxazepam.
[b]Quantitation ion.
Note: Flurazepam does not extract under these conditions; however, metabolites such as desalkyflurazepam and hydroxyethylflurazepam will extract with high recovery.
Source: UCT Internal Publication.

9.3.2 Benzodiazepines in Serum or Plasma for HPLC Analysis: 200-mg CLEAN SCREEN Extraction Column (ZSDAU020 or ZCDAU020)

1. Prepare sample.
   a. To 1 mL of serum add internal standard and add 1.0 mL of 0.1 *M* phosphate buffer, pH 6.0.
   b. Mix/vortex.
   c. Sample pH should be 6.0 ± 0.5. Adjust pH accordingly with 0.1 *M* monobasic or dibasic sodium phosphate.
2. Condition CLEAN SCREEN extraction column.
   1 × 3 mL of CH₃OH; aspirate.
   1 × 3 mL of DI H₂O; aspirate.
   1 × 1 mL of 0.1 *M* phosphate buffer, pH 6.0
   Note: Aspirate at ≤3 in. Hg to prevent sorbent drying.
3. Apply sample.
   Load at 1 mL/min.
4. Wash column.
   1 × 2 mL of DI H₂O; aspirate.
   1 × 2 mL of 20% acetonitrile in 0.1 *M* phosphate buffer, pH 6.0; aspirate.
   Dry column (5 min at ≥10 in. Hg).
   1 × 2 mL of hexane; aspirate.

5. **Elute benzodiazepines.**

1 × 3 mL of ethyl acetate; collect eluate at 1–2 mL/min.

6. **Dry eluate.**

Evaporate to dryness at ≤40°C.

7. **Reconstitute.**

Reconstitute in mobile phase.

8. **Quantitate.**

Inject sample onto HPLC.

Source: UCT internal publications.

8. **Quantitate.**

a. Inject 1–2 µL of sample onto chromatograph.

9.3.3 Serum Benzodiazepines by HPLC 100-mg CLEAN-UP C2 Extraction Column (CEC02111)

I. **Reagents:**

1. **Saturated sodium borate buffer, pH 9.5.**

a. Dissolve 10 g of sodium borate in 950 mL of DI H_2O.

b. Adjust pH to 9.5 with 10 *N* sodium hydroxide. Add DI water to bring total volume to 1000 mL.

2. **0.01 *M* Potassium phosphate buffer, pH 6.0.**

a. Dissolve 1.36 g of monobasic potassium phosphate in 950 mL of DI H_2O.

b. Adjust pH to 6.0 with 1 *N* sodium hydroxide. Add DI water to bring total volume to 1000 mL.

3. **Mobile phase:**

18.5% Acetonitrile

26.5% Methanol

55.0% Potassium phosphate buffer, pH 6.0 (0.01 *M*)

II. **Extraction method:**

1. **Prepare sample.**

Add 200 µL of sodium borate buffer to 0.5 mL of serum. Vortex.

2. **Conditioning steps.**

2 × 1 mL of methanol.

2 × 1 mL of DI H_2O.

Do not let column dry out.

(vacuum settings should be 3–5 in. Hg)

3. **Apply sample to column.**

a. Add buffered sample to top of column.

b. Pull through at a flow of 1–2 mL/min.

4. **Wash column.**

1 × 1 mL of DI H_2O.

Dry column 2–3 min under vacuum (15–20 in. Hg).

5. **Elute benzodiazepines.**

2 × 0.5 mL of methanol.

6. **Inject sample.**

a. Dry eluate under nitrogen and minimal heat.

b. Reconstitute with 100 µL of mobile phase.

c. Inject 15–20 µL onto HPLC.

Source: UCT internal publication.

9.3.4 Flunitrazepam

Flunitrazepam (Figure 5) is marketed worldwide by Roche Pharmaceuticals under the trade name Rohypnol®. It is a benzodiazepine that has been used for the short-term treatment of insomnia, as a hypnotic/sedative agent, and as an oral pre-anesthetic agent. It is not available in the United States but is available in 64 other countries around the world. In Europe it is the most widely prescribed sedative/hypnotic drug. In the United States, current possession of this drug without a foreign prescription is illegal.

The abuse of Rohypnol has increased worldwide and has been reported on every continent in the world. This drug is used as a adjunctive agent for other drugs of abuse such as:

- Enhancing the "high" of low-quality heroin
- Mellowing the effects of cocaine
- Easing a user down from a crack or cocaine binge

In the United States, it is commonly used with alcohol to give a sense of well-being, reduce inhibitions, and promote amnesia. These properties make this drug useful for the purpose of "date rape."

Street names for Flunitrazepam include the following:

1. Roofies	7. Mind Erasers
2. Rophies	8. Forget Pill
3. Ropes	9. Trip and Fall
4. Roach-2	10. Ruffies
5. Rib	11. Duicitas (Candy)
6. Whiteys	12. Roches

9.3.5 Flunitrazepam and Metabolites in Urine for GC or GC-MS Confirmations Using a 200-mg CLEAN SCREEN Extraction Column (ZSDAU020 or ZCDAU020)

1. **Prepare sample—β-glucurondidase hydrolysis.**
   a. To 5 mL of urine add internal standard(s)* and 2 mL of β-glucuronidase solution.
   b. β-Glucuronidase solution contains 5000 FU/mL *Patella vulgata* in 0.1 M acetate buffer, pH = 5.0.
   c. Mix/vortex.
   d. Hydrolyze for 3 h at 65°C.
   e. Centrifuge for 10 min at 670g and discard pellet.
   f. Cool before proceeding.
2. **Condition CLEAN SCREEN extraction column.**
   1 × 3 mL of CH$_3$OH; aspirate.
   1 × 3 mL of DI H$_2$O; aspirate.
   1 × 1 mL of 0.1 M phosphate buffer, pH 6.0.
   Note: Aspirate at ≤3 in. Hg to prevent sorbent drying.
3. **Apply sample.**
   Load at 1 mL/min.
4. **Wash column.**
   1 × 2 mL of DI H$_2$O; aspirate.
   1 × 2 mL of 20% acetonitrile in 0.1 M phosphate buffer, pH 6.0; aspirate.

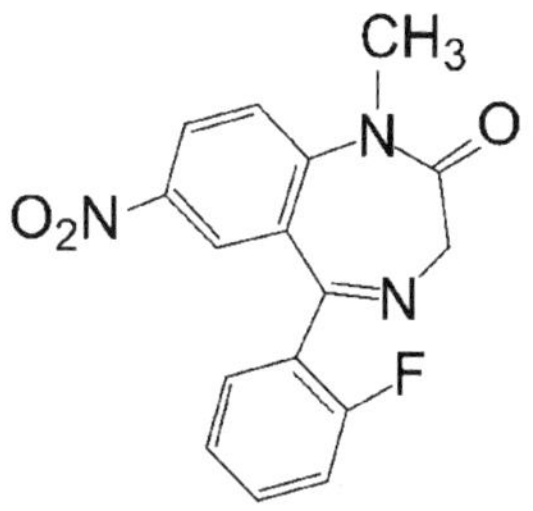

Fig. 5. Chemical structure of flunitrazepam.

Table 27

Generic name	Primary ion[b]	Secondary ion	Tertiary ion
Flunitrazepam	312	286	266
7-Aminoflunitrazepam	283	255	254
Desmethyl flunitrazepam	356	357	310
Oxazepam-D^5 [a]	462	463	
D^5-Oxazepam[a]			

[a]Internal standard.
[b]Quantitation ion.
GC conditions:
Column: DB5 or equivalent capillary column (15 m × 0.25 mm i.d. × 0.25 µm film)
Injector temperature = 250°C
Injector: Splitless mode
Temperature program 180°C to 275°C at 10°C/min then 275°C to 300°C at 25°C/min

Dry column (5 min at ≥10 in. Hg).
1 × 2 mL of hexane; aspirate.

5. Elute flunitrazepam, 7-aminoflunitrazepam, and desmethylflunitrazepam.
   1 × 3 mL of ethyl acetate; collect eluate at 1–2 mL/min.

6. Dry eluate.
   Evaporate to dryness at ≥40°C.

7. Derivatize.
   a. Add 50 µL of ethyl acetate and 50 µL MTBSTFA (with 1% TBDMCS).
   b. Overlay with N_2 and cap.
   c. Mix/vortex.
   d. React for 20 min at 90°C. Remove from heat source to cool.
Note: Do not evaporate MTBSTFA solution.

8. Quantitate.
   a. Inject 1–2 µL of sample onto chromatograph.
   b. Monitor the following ions (GC-MS):

9.4 TETRAHYDROCANNABINOL

Tetrahydrocannabinol (THC) is the most active pharmacological constituent found in the *Cannabis sativa* plant. Plant parts may contain up to 12% THC by weight. THC is administered by smoking or orally and will cause sedation, euphoria, temporal distortions and hallucinations (1).

Tetrahydrocannabinol is metabolized to two compounds: 11-hydroxy-THC and 8-β-hydroxy THC (Figure 6). Both metabolites are active; however, they do not significantly contribute to the acute effects of this drug. Additionally, another two inactive metabolites have been identified: 8-hydroxy-THC and 8, 11-dihydroxy-THC. A fifth metabolite, 11-carboxy-THC, has been identified and is produced by the oxidation of 11-hydroxy-THC (2).

About 70% of a dose of THC is excreted within 3 days in the feces (40%) and urine (30%). Unchanged THC is present in trace amounts in the urine, and 11-hydroxy-THC conjugate represents only 2% of the dose. The balance of the dose is excreted as conjugates of 11-carboxy-THC, and other unidentified acidic compounds persist in the urine for several weeks after a single dose (3-4). Passive inhalation of THC smoke has resulted in plasma THC levels and also urinary 11-carboxy-THC levels (5).

A number of useful methods have been developed for the determination of the parent drug and the metabolites from a number of biological matrices.

The key concept to remember is that extraction of cannabinols is accomplished by hydrophobic interaction. You can extract cannabinols on almost any hydrophobic phase of chain length C8 or longer. The key to clean extractions is the additional copolymeric constituents attached to the bonded phase packing. These constituents help remove the interferences that hinder the analysis.

9.4.1 Carboxy-THC in Urine Manual Method for GC or GC-MS Confirmations Using a 200-mg CLEAN SCREEN Extraction Column (ZSTHCO20 or ZCTHCO20)

1. **Prepare sample—base hydrolysis of glucuronides.**
   a. To 5 mL of urine add internal standard* and 200 μL of 10 N NaOH.
   b. Mix/vortex.
   c. Hydrolyze for 20 min at 60°C. Cool before proceeding.
   d. Adjust sample pH to 3.5 ± 0.5 with 2.0 mL of glacial acetic acid.
2. **Condition CLEAN SCREEN extraction column.**
   1 × 3 mL of CH_3OH; aspirate.
   1 × 3 mL of H_2O; aspirate.
   1 × 1 mL of 0.1 M HCl; aspirate.
   Note: Aspirate at ≤3 in. Hg to prevent sorbent drying.
3. **Apply sample.**
   Load at 1–2 mL/min.
4. **Wash column.**
   1 × 2 mL of DI H_2O; aspirate.
   1 × 2 mL of 0.1 M HCl/acetonitrile (70:30); aspirate.
   Dry column (5 min at ≥10 in. Hg).
   1 × 200 μL of hexane; aspirate.
5. **Elute carboxy-THC.**
   1 × 3 mL of hexane-ethyl acetate (50:50). Collect eluate at <5 mL/min.

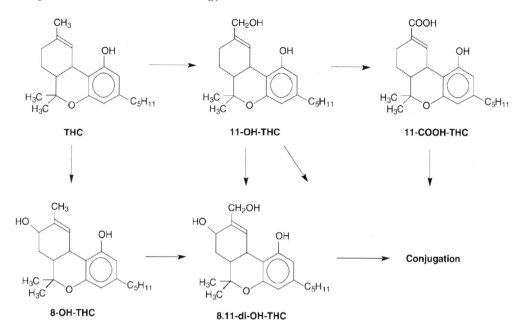

Fig. 6. Tetrahydrocannabinoid metabolism.

6. **Dry eluate.**
   Evaporate to dryness at ≤40°C.
7. **Derivatize.**
   a. Add 50 µL of ethyl acetate and 50 µL of BSTFA (with 1% TMCS).
   b. Overlay with nitrogen and cap.
   c. Mix/vortex.
   d. React 20 min at 70°C.
   e. Remove from heat source to cool.
   Note: Do not evaporate BSTFA.
8. **Quantitate.**
   Inject 1–2 µL of derivatized sample onto the GC-MS system.
   Monitor the following ions (mass selective detection):

9.4.2 Carboxy-THC in Urine Automated Method for GC or GC-MS Confirmations Using a 200-mg CLEAN SCREEN Extraction Column (CSTHC203 or CCTHC203)

1. **Prepare sample—base hydrolysis of glucuronides.**
   a. To 5 mL of urine add internal standarda and 200 µL of 10 *N* NaOH.
   b. Mix/vortex.
   c. Hydrolyze for 20 min at 60°C. Cool before proceeding.
   d. Adjust sample pH to 3.5 ± 0.5 with 2.0 mL of glacial acetic acid.
2. **Load sample into the RapidTrace module.**
   See Section 9.4.2.1 for the RapidTrace procedure.
3. **Remove prepared samples from the RapidTrace.**

Table 28

Analyte	Primary ion[b]	Secondary ion	Tertiary ion
Carboxy-Δ⁹ THC	371	473	488
D3 Carboxy-Δ⁹THC[a]	374	476	491

[a]Suggested internal standard for GC-MS: D3 Carboxy-Δ⁹THC
[b]Quantitation ion.
Source: UCT internal publication.

Table 29

Analyte	Primary ion[b]	Secondary ion	Tertiary ion
Carboxy-Δ⁹ THC	371	473	488
D3 Carboxy-Δ⁹THC[a]	374	476	491

[a]Suggested internal standard for GC-MS: D3 Carboxy-Δ⁹THC.
[b]Quantitation ion.
Source: UCT internal publication.

4. **Dry eluate.**
   Evaporate to dryness at ≤40°C using a TurboVap or equivalent evaporator.
5. **Derivatize.**
   a. Add 50 μL of ethyl acetate and 50 μL of BSTFA (with 1% TMCS).
   b. Overlay with nitrogen and cap.
   c. Mix/vortex.
   d. React for 20 min at 70°C.
   e. Remove from heat source to cool.
   Note: Do not evaporate BSTFA.
6. **Quantitate.**
   a. Inject 1–2 μL of derivatized sample onto the GC-MS system.
   b. Monitor the following ions (mass selective detection):

9.4.2.1 Settings for RapidTrace Analysis of Carboxy-THC

9.4.3 Carboxy-THC in Urine Manual Method for GC-MS Confirmations Using an 80-mg CLEAN SCREEN Reduced Solvent Volume Extraction Column (CSDAUA83)

1. **Prepare sample—base hydrolysis of glucuronides.**
   a. To 1 mL of urine add internal standarda and 100 μL of 10 *N* NaOH.
   b. Mix/vortex.
   c. Hydrolyze for 20 min 60°C. Cool before proceeding.
   d. Adjust sample pH to 3.5 ± 0.5 with approx 400 μL of glacial acetic acid.
2. **Condition CLEAN SCREEN extraction column.**
   1 × 500 μL of hexane-ethyl acetate (1:1).
   1 × 500 μL of CH_3OH; aspirate.
   1 × 500 μL of H_2O; aspirate.

Table 30

	Step	Source	Destination	mL	mL/min	Liq. Chk
1.	Condition	MeOH	Org	3	18	No
2.	Condition	H$_2$O	Aq.	3	18	No
3.	Condition	0.1 M HC1	Aq.	1	18	No
4.	Load	Sample	Bio.	4.0	1.2	No
5.	Load	Sample	Bio.	1.5	1.2	No
6.	Rinse	H$_2$O	Bio.	2.0	8.0	No
7.	Rinse	70:30	Org.	2.0	8.0	No
8.	Dry	Time = 5 min				
9.	Rinse	Hex	Org.	0.2	1.0	No
10.	Collect	Elute	Fractl	3.0	1.2	No
11.	Purge—cannula	MeOH	Cannula	3	30.	No
12.	Purge—cannula	H$_2$O	Cannula	3	30.	No

Load cannula depth = 0   Mix volume = .5
Mix cannula depth = 0   Mix speed = 30
Mix cycles = 2   Reagent mix cycles = 2

Table 31

Reagent setup

No.	Reagent	Abbreviation	Sip speed
1.	Water	H$_2$O	30
2.	Methanol	MEOH	30
3.	0.1 M HCl	0.1 M HCl	30
4.	0.1 M HCl - ACN	70:30	30
5.	Hexane	Hex	30
6.	Hex-EtAC 1:1	Elute	15
7.	Reagent 7	Reag7	30
8.	Reagent 8	Reag8	30
9.	Mixing vessel	Mixer	30
10.	Sample	Sample	30

Column air push volume = 0.4
Column air push volume speed multiplier = 2

Table 32

No.	Waste	Abbreviation
1.	Aqueous	Aq.
2.	Organic	Org.
3.	Biohazard	Bio.

Table 33

Analyte	Primary ion[b]	Secondary ion	Tertiary ion
Carboxy-Δ^9THC	371	473	488
D3 Carboxy-Δ^9THC[a]	374	476	491

[a]Suggested internal standard for GC-MS: D3 carboxy Δ^9THC.
[b]Quantitation ion.

  1×250 μL of 0.1 ^{M} HCl; aspirate.
  Note: Use gravity flow or minimal vacuum to condition the column.
3. **Apply sample.**
  Load at 1–2 mL/min.
4. **Wash colulmn.**
  1×500 μL of DI H_2O; aspirate.
  1×500 μL of 0.1 M HCl/acetonitrile (70:30); aspirate.
  Dry column (3 minutes at ≥10 in. Hg).
  1×100 μL of hexane; aspirate.
5. **Elute carboxyTHC.**
  2×750 μL of hexane-ethyl acetate (50:50).
6. **Dry eluate.**
  Evaporate to dryness at ≤40°C.
7. **Derivatize.**
  a. Add 50 μL of ethyl acetate and 50 μL of BSTFA (with 1% TMCS).
  b. Overlay with nitrogen and cap.
  c. Mix/vortex.
  d. React for 20 min at 70°C.
  e. Remove from heat source to cool.
  Note: Do not evaporate BSTFA.
8. **Quantitate.**
  a. Inject 1–2 μL of derivatized sample onto the GC-MS system.
  b. Monitor the following ions (mass selective detection):

The above example illustrates the use of a reduced solvent volume (RSV) SPE cartridge. There are many advantages to using a RSV column, including:

- A 75% reduction in the total liquid volume used for extraction.
  This factor may lower the costs per extraction, decrease solvent disposal costs and increase throughput.
- A 50% reduction in eluants volume results in faster drydown times and less chance of exposure to chemical fumes.

9.4.4 THC and Carboxy-THC in Whole Blood Manual Method for GC-MS Confirmations Using a 200-mg CLEAN SCREEN Extraction Column (ZSDAU020 or ZCDAU020)

1. **Prepare sample.**
  a. To 1 mL of whole blood sample add internal standard(s)* into a silanized screw-top test tube.

    b. Mix/vortex. Let stand up to 1 h.

    c. Add 2 mL of acetonitrile. Vortex, mix for 30 s and allow to sit for 3 min.

    d. Centrifuge at 670g for 10 min at maximum g-force.

    e. Decant into another silanized test tube and add 4 mL of 0.1 *M* acetate buffer, pH 4.5, to supernatant.

    f. Mix/vortex, centrifuge for 5 min and decant the supernatant into another silanized test tube. This step removes any blood fragments or foam.

2. Precondition CLEAN SCREEN extraction column.

    1 × 3 mL of hexane-ethyl acetate (75:25); aspirate.

3. Condition CLEAN SCREEN extraction column.

    1 × 3 mL of CH$_3$OH; aspirate.

    1 × 3 mL of DI H$_2$O; aspirate.

    1 × 1 mL of 0.1 *M* HCl; aspirate.

    Note: Use gravity flow or minimal vacuum.

4. Apply sample.

    Load at 1 mL/minute.

    Note: Use gravity flow or minimal vacuum.

5. Wash column.

    1 × 2 mL DI H$_2$O; aspirate.

    1 × 2 mL 0.1 *M* HCl - acetonitrile (70:30); aspirate.

    Dry columns (5 min at ≥10 in. Hg).

    1 × 200 µL of hexane.

    Note: Use gravity flow or minimal vacuum.

6. Elute THC and carboxy-THC.

    1 × 3 mL hexane-ethyl acetate (75:25).

    Note: Use gravity flow or minimal vacuum.

7. Dry eluate.

    Evaporate slowly to dryness at ≤40°C using a TurboVap or equivalent evaporator.

8. Derivatize.

    a. Add 50 µL of BSTFA (with 1% TMCS) and 50 µL of ethyl acetate.

    b. Overlayer with nitrogen gas and cap.

    c. Mix/vortex.

    d. React for 30 minutes at 70°C.

    e. Remove from heat source to cool.

    Note: Do not evaporate BSTFA solution.

9. Quantitate.

    a. Inject 2 µL of BSTFA sample onto chromatograph.

    b. Monitor the following ions (GC-MS):

9.4.5 THC and Carboxy-THC in Whole Blood: Automated Method for GC-MS Confirmations Using a 200-mg CLEAN SCREEN Extraction Column (CSDAU203 or CCDAU203)

1. Prepare sample.

    a. To 1 mL of whole blood sample add internal standard(s)a into a silanized screw-top test tube.

    b. Mix/vortex. Let stand up to 1 h.

    c. Add 2 mL of acetonitrile. Vortex for 30 s and allow to sit for 3 min.

    d. Centrifuge for 10 min at maximum rpm.

Tabe 34

Analyte	Primary ion[b]	Secondary ion	Tertiary ion
Carboxy-Δ^9THC	371	473	488
D3 Carboxy-Δ^9THC[a]	374	476	491
Tetrahydrocannabinol	303	315	386
D3 Tetrahydrocannabinol	306	318	389

[a]Suggested internal standards for GC-MS: D3 THC and D3 carboxy Δ^9THC.
[b]Quantitation ion.
Source: UCT internal publication.

Table 35

Analyte	Primary ion[b]	Secondary ion	Tertiary ion
Carboxy-Δ^9THC	371	473	488
D3 Carboxy-Δ^9THC[a]	374	476	491
Tetrahydrocannabinol	303	315	386
D3 Tetrahydrocannabinol[a]	306	318	389

[a]Suggested internal standards for GC-MS: D3 THC and D3 carboxyΔ^9THC.
[b]Quantitation ion.
Source: This method is taken from Stonebraker, W., et al. Robotic solid phase extraction and GC-MS analysis of THC in blood. *Am. Clin. Lab.* 17:18–29, 1998.

    e. Decant into another silanized test tube and add 4 mL of 0.1 *M* acetate buffer, pH 7.0 to supernatant.

    f. Mix/vortex, centrifuge for 5 min, and decant the supernatant into another silanized test tube. This step removes any blood fragments or foaming.

2. Load prepared sample onto the RapidTrace module.
See Section 9.4.5.1 for conditions.

3. Remove samples from the RapidTrace module.

4. Dry eluate.
Evaporate slowly to dryness at ≤40°C using a TurboVap or equivalent evaporator.

5. Derivatize.
    a. Add 50 μL of BSTFA (with 1% TMCS) and 50 μL of ethyl acetate.
    b. Overlay with nitrogen gas and cap tube.
    c. Mix/vortex.
    d. React for 30 min at 70°C.
    e. Remove from heat source to cool.
    Note: Do not evaporate BSTFA solution.

6. Quantitate.
    a. Inject 2 μL of BSTFA sample onto chromatograph.
    b. Monitor the following ions (GC-MS):

Table 36

	Step	Source	Destination	mL	mL/min	Liq. Chk
1.	Condition	Methanol	Org.	2.0	18	No
2.	Condition	H$_2$O	Aq.	2.0	18	No
3.	Condition	AC-MEOH	Org	2.0	18	No
4.	Load	Sample	Biohaz.	5.8	1.2	No
5.	Rinse	AC-MeOH	Aq.	1.0	6.0	No
6.	Dry	Time = 5 min				
7.	Collect	95:5	Practl	4.0	4.8	No
8.	Rinse	50:50	Org.	4.0	6.0	No
9.	Dry	Time = 5 min				
10.	Collect	75:25	Fract2	4.0	1.2	No
11.	Rinse	50:50	Org.	4.0	30	No
12.	Purge—cannula	methanol	Cannula	3.0	30	No
13.	Purge—cannula	H2O	Cannula	3.0	30	No
14.	Purge—cannula	H$_2$O	Cannula	3.0	30	No

Load cannula depth = 0.5   Mix volume = 2
Mix cannula depth = 0   Mix speed = .5
Mix cycles = 2   Reagent mix cycles = 2

Table 37

Reagent Setup

	No.	Reagent	Abbreviation	Sip speed
	1.	Water	H$_2$O	30
	2.	Methanol	MeOH	30
	3.	pH 7.0 Buffer-5% MeOH	AC-MeOH	30
	4.	Hexane-ET AC 95:5	95:5	30
	5.	Hexane-ET AC 75:25	75:25	15
	6.	MeOH-water 50:50	50:50	15
	7.	REAG 7		30
	8.	REAG 8		30
	9.	Mixing vessel	Mixer	30
	10.	Sample	Sample	30

Column air push volume = 2
Column air push volume speed multiplier = 2

Table 38

No.	Waste	Abbreviation
1.	Aqueous	Aqu.
2.	Biohazard waste	Biohaz.
3.	Organic waste	Org.

9.4.5.1 Setting for RapidTrace Analysis of THC in Whole Blood
9.4.5.2 GC-MS Conditions for THC

1. Instrument	HP Model 5980 GC with a Model 5971A mass selective detector used with a Model 7673 autosampler or equivalent instrument.
2. Column	HP5 or DB5 capillary column 30 m long x 0.25 mm x 0.25 µm film thickness.
3. Oven Conditions	200°C, hold for 1 min, ramp to 300°C at a rate of 15°C/min for a final hold time of 1.33 min. The total run time is 9.0 min.

4. Analytical Conditions
    a. The carrier gas was helium.
    b. Injector temperature = 250°C.
    c. Transfer line temperature = 280°C.
    d. The mass selective detector was operated in the selected ion monitoring mode with the photomultiplier.
    e. Set by increasing the autotune voltage +400–600 V above the autotune value.
    f. Selected ions were monitored at a dwell time of 25 ms.

9.5 COCAINE AND METABOLITES

Cocaine is found in the leaves of *Erythroxylon coca*, a plant that grows in South America. It is used therapeutically as a local anesthetic and as a drug of abuse for its stimulant properties. When self-administered the hydrochloride salt is used by nasal insufflation or intravenous administration. Commonly, the drug is used as the freebase ingested by smoking. Cocaine is rapidly inactivated in humans by the hydrolysis of one or more ester linkages. At the pH of water, the drug rapidly converts by hydrolysis to benzoylecgonine. In blood or plasma, the drug is readily hydrolyzed to ecgonine methyl ester by the enzyme cholinesterase. This reaction may be inhibited by the addition of fluoride or a cholinesterase inhibitor (1,2).

Benzoylecgonine is believed to arise spontaneously in vivo, as neither the liver nor serum esterases produce this compound. The further production of ecgonine methyl ester from benzoylecgonine may be the result of enzymatic hydrolysis (3).

Benzoylecgonine is the major metabolite of cocaine and is present in urine specimens 2–4 days after use and may be found without detection of the parent drug. The co-ingestion of ethanol with cocaine produces a characteristic metabolite, cocaethylene, that is pharmacologically active (Figure 8) (4).

We have developed a number of procedures for this drug and metabolites from different biological matrices.

9.5.1 Cocaine and Benzoylecgonine: Manual Method in Urine for GC or GC-MS Confirmations Using a 200-mg CLEAN SCREEN Extraction Column (ZSDAU020 or ZCDAU020)

1. Prepare sample.
    a. To 5 mL of urine add internal standard(s)[a] and 2 mL of 0.1 *M* phosphate buffer, pH 6.0.
    b. Mix/vortex.

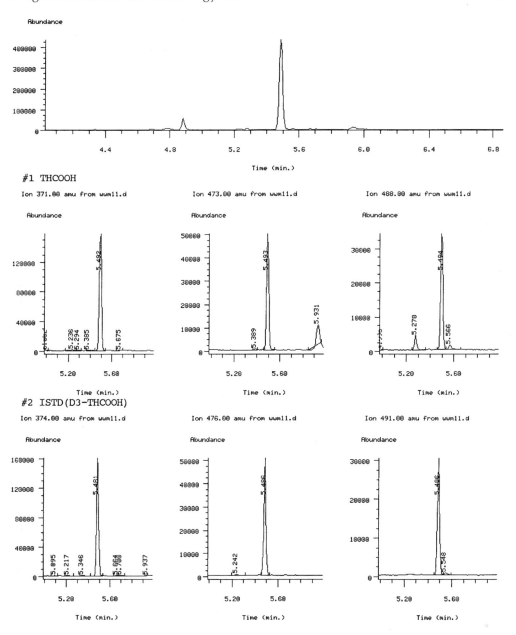

Fig. 7. Cannabinoid chromatography.

c. Sample pH should be 6.0 + 0.5. Adjust pH accordingly with 0.1 M monobasic or dibasic sodium phosphate.

2. **Condition CLEAN SCREEN extraction column.**

1 × 3 mL of CH_3OH; aspirate.

1 × 3 mL of DI H_2O; aspirate.

1 × 1 mL of 0.1 *M* phosphate buffer, pH 6.0; aspirate.

Note: Aspirate at ≤3 in. Hg to prevent sorbent drying.

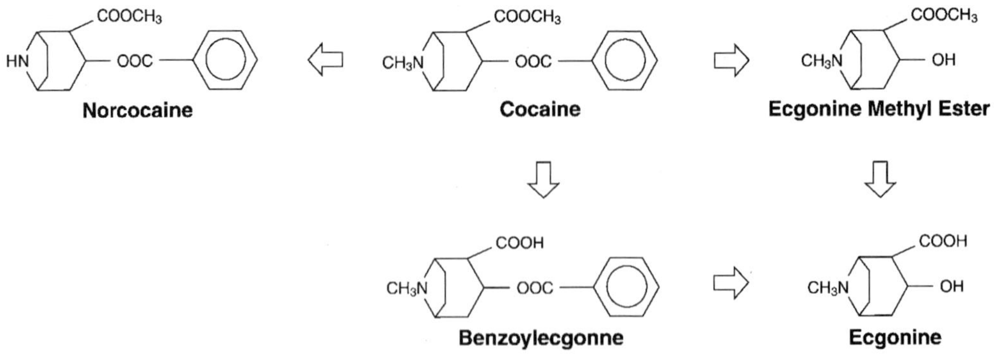

Fig. 8. Cocaine methabolism.

3. **Apply sample.**
   Load at 1–2 mL/min.
4. **Wash column.**
   1 × 2 mL of DI H$_2$O; aspirate.
   1 × 2 mL of 0.1 *M* HCl; aspirate.
   1 × 3 mL of methanol; aspirate.
   Dry column (5 min at ≥10 in. Hg).
5. **Elute cocaine and benzoylecgonine.**
   1 × 3 mL of methylene chloride-isopropanol-ammonium hydroxide (78:20:2).
   Collect eluate at 1–2 mL/min.
   Note: Prepare elution solvent daily. Add isopropanol to the ammonium hydroxide,
   mix; the pH of the elution solvent should be 11.0 or above.
6. **Dry eluate.**
   Evaporate to dryness at ≤40°C using a TurboVap or equivalent apparatus.
7. **Derivatize.**
   a. Add 50 µL of ethyl acetate and 50 µL of BSTFA (with 1% TMCS).
   b. Overlay with nitrogen gas and cap. Mix/vortex.
   c. React for 20 min at 70°C. Remove from heat source to cool.
   Note: Do not evaporate BSTFA solution.
8. **Quantitate.**
   a. Inject 1–2 µL of sample (in BSTFA solution) onto chromatograph.
   b. Monitor the following ions (GC-MS):

9.5.2 Cocaine and Benzoylecgonine: Automated Procedure in Urine for GC or GC-MS Confirmations Using a 200-mg CLEAN SCREEN Extraction Column (CSDAU203 or CCDAU203)

1. **Prepare sample.**
   a. To 5 mL of urine add internal standard(s)[a] and 2 mL of 0.1 *M* phosphate buffer, pH 6.0.
   b. Mix/vortex.
   c. Sample pH should be 6.0 ± 0.5. Adjust pH accordingly with 0.1 *M* monobasic or
      dibasic sodium phosphate.
2. **Place sample onto the RapidTrace.**
   See Subheading 9.5.2.1 for the procedure.
3. **Remove sample and evaporate eluate.**
   Evaporate to dryness at ≤40°C using a TurboVap or equivalent apparatus..

Table 39

Compound	Primary ion[b]	Secondary ion	Tertiary ion
Cocaine	182	198	303
D$_3$-Cocaine[a]	185	201	306
Benzoylecgonine-TMS	240	256	361
D$_3$-Benzoylecgonine-TMS[a]	243	259	364

[a]Suggested internal standards for GC-MS: D$_3$-cocaine, D$_3$-benzoylecgonine.
[b]Quantitation ion.

Table 40

Compound	Primary ion[b]	Secondary ion	Tertiary ion
Cocaine	182	198	303
D$_3$-Cocaine[a]	185	201	306
Benzoylecgonine-TMS	240	256	361
D$_3$-Benzoylecgonine-TMS[a]	243	259	364

[a]Suggested internal standards for GC-MS: D$_3$-Cocaine, D$_3$-benzoylecgonine.
[b]Quantitation ion.

4. **Derivatize.**
   a. Add 50 μL of ethyl acetate and 50 μL of BSTFA (with 1% TMCS).
   b. Overlay with nitrogen gas and cap. Mix/vortex.
   c. React for 20 min at 70°C. Remove from heat source to cool.
   Note: Do not evaporate BSTFA solution.
5. **Quantitate.**
   a. Inject 1–2 μL of sample (in BSTFA solution) onto the chromatograph.
   b. Monitor the following ions (GC-MS):

9.5.2.1 Settings for RapidTrace Analysis of Cocaine and Benzoylecgonine from Urine

9.5.2.2 GC-MS Analysis

1. **Instrumentation**
   The GC-MS system consisted of a Hewlett Packard 5971A mass selective detector, 7673 autosampler and a 5890 gas chromatograph fitted with a DB-5 capillary column (30 m long, x 0.25 mm i.d. x 0.25 μm film thickness).
2. **Analytical conditions**
   a. The method used selective ion monitoring (SIM) for three ions of each analyte.
   b. The injector port and transfer line was maintained at 250°C and 280°C, respectively.
   c. A 1–2 μL split less injection was performed with the following oven program:
   d. The initial temperature of 150°C was ramped at 25°C/min to 300°C and held for 1.5 min.
   e. The total run time was 7.5 min.
   f. The approximate retention time of cocaine was 4.0 min and benzoylecgonine was 4.4 min under these conditions.

Table 41

Step		Source	Destination	Volume	Flow[a]	Liq. Chk
1.	Condition	MeOH	Organic	3	18	no
2.	Condition	H₂O	Water	3	18	no
3.	Condition	Phosphate buffer, pH 6.0	Water	1	18	no
4.	Load	Sample	Bio.	4.0	1.2	no
5.	Load	Sample	Bio.	3.5	1.2	no
6.	Rinse	H₂O	Bio.	2	24	no
7.	Purge—Cannula	H₂O	Cannula	6	30	no
8.	Rinse	0.1 *M* HCl	Bio.	2	6	no
9.	Rinse	MeOH	Bio.	3	18	no
10.	Dry	Time = 5 min				
11.	Collect	Elute	Fract1	3	1.2	no
12.	Purge—Cannula	MeOH	Cannula	3	30	no
13.	Purge—Cannula	H₂O	Cannula	3	30	no

Load cannula depth = 0
Mix cannula depth = 0
Mix cycles = 2
Mix volume = 0 .5   Column air push volume = 2
Mix speed = 0.5   Column air push volume speed multiplier = 2
Reagent mix cycles = 2

Table 42

Reagent setup

No	Reagent	Abbreviation	Sip speed
1.	Water	H₂O	30
2.	Methanol	MeOH	30
3.	0.1 *M* Phosphate buffer, pH 6.0	pH 6	30
4.	0.1 *M* Acetate buffer	pH 4.5	30
5.	Hexane	Hexn	30
6.	Elution solvent[b]	Elute	15
7.	0.1 *M* Acetic acid	Acetic	30
8.	0.1 *M* Hydrochloric acid	HCl	30
9.	Mixing vessel	Mixer	15

[a]Flow in mL/min.

[b]The elution solvent for benzoylecgonine is methylene chloride-isopropanol-ammonium hydroxide (78:20:2). This solution is prepared daily.

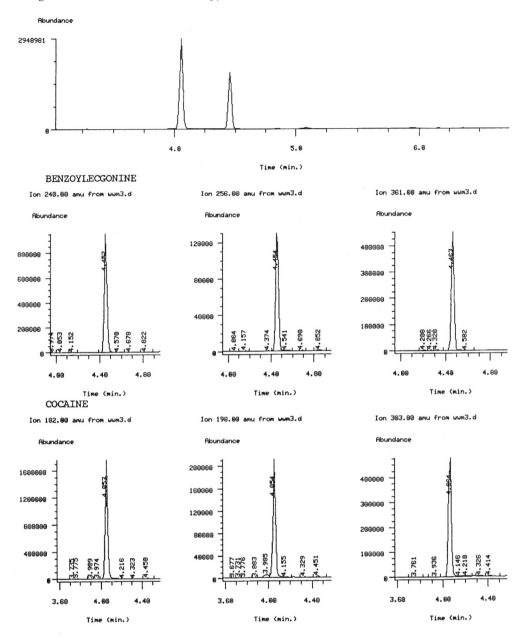

Fig. 9. Cocaine and benzoylecgonine chromatography.

9.5.3 Cocaine and Benzoylecgonine in Serum, Plasma, or Whole Blood: Manual Method for GC or GC-MS Confirmations Using 200-mg CLEAN SCREEN Extraction Column (ZSDAU020 or ZCDAU020)

1. **Prepare sample.**
   a. To 1 mL of sample (serum, plasma, or whole blood) add internal standard[a] and 4 mL of DI H_2O.
   b. Mix/vortex and let stand 5 min.
   c. Centrifuge for 10 min at 670g and discard pellet.
   d. Add 2 mL of 0.1 M phosphate buffer, pH 6.0. Mix/vortex.
   e. Sample pH should be 6.0 ± 0.5. Adjust pH accordingly with 0.1 M monobasic or dibasic sodium phosphate.
2. **Condition CLEAN SCREEN extraction column.**
   1 × 3 mL of CH_3OH; aspirate.
   1 × 3 mL of DI H_2O; aspirate.
   1 × 1 mL of 0.1 M phosphate buffer, pH 6.0; aspirate.
   Note: Aspirate at ≤3 in. Hg to prevent sorbent drying.
3. **Apply sample.**
   Load at 1–2 mL/min.
4. **Wash column.**
   1 × 2 mL of DI H_2O; aspirate.
   1 × 2 mL of 0.1 M HCl; aspirate.
   1 × 3 mL of CH_3OH; aspirate.
   Dry column (5 min at ≥10 in. Hg).
5. **Elute cocaine and benzoylecgonine.**
   1 × 3 mL of CH_2Cl_2–IPA–NH_4OH (78:20:2); collect eluate at 1–2 mL/min.
   Note: Prepare elution solvent daily. Add IPA–NH_4OH, mix, then add CH_2Cl_2 (pH 11.0–12.0).
6. **Dry eluate.**
   Evaporate to dryness at ≤40°C.
7. **Derivatize.**
   a. Add 50 μL of ethyl acetate and 50 μL of BSTFA (with 1% TMCS).
   b. Overlay with nitrogen gas and cap. Mix/vortex.
   c. React for 20 min at 70°C. Remove from heat source to cool.
   Note: Do not evaporate BSTFA solution.
8. **Quantitate.**
   Inject 1–2 μL of sample (in BSTFA solution) onto chromatograph.
   Monitor the following ions (GC-MS):

9.5.4 Cocaine and Benzoylecgonine in Serum, Plasma, or Whole Blood: Automated Method for GC or GC-MS Confirmations Using a 200-mg CLEAN SCREEN Extraction Column (CSDAU203 or CCDAU203)

1. **Prepare sample.**
   a. To 1 mL of sample (serum, plasma, or whole blood) add internal standard[a] and 4 mL of DI H_3O.
   b. Mix/vortex and let stand 5 min.

Table 43

Compound	Primary ion[b]	Secondary ion	Tertiary ion
Cocaine	182	198	303
D$_3$-Cocaine[a]	185	201	306
Benzoylecgonine-TMS	240	256	361
D$_3$-Benzoylecgonine-TMS[a]	243	259	364

[a]Suggested internal standards for GC-MS: D$_3$-cocaine, D$_3$-benzoylecgonine.
[b]Quantitation ion.

    c. Centrifuge for 10 min at 670*g* and discard pellet.

    d. Add 2 mL of 0.1 *M* phosphate buffer, pH 6.0. Mix/vortex.

    e. Sample pH should be 6.0 ± 0.5. Adjust pH accordingly with 0.1 *M* monobasic or dibasic sodium phosphate.

2. Load sample onto the RapidTrace module.

    See Section 9.5.4.1 for the RapidTrace procedure.

3. Remove samples and dry eluate.

    Evaporate to dryness at ≤40°C using a TurboVap or equivalent.

4. Derivatize.

    a. Add 50 µL of ethyl acetate and 50 µL of BSTFA (with 1% TMCS).

    b. Overlay with nitrogen gas and cap. Mix/vortex.

    c. React for 20 min at 70°C on a heater block.

    d. Remove from heat source to cool.

    Note: Do not evaporate BSTFA solution.

5. Quantitate.

    a. Inject 1–2 µL sample (in BSTFA solution) onto the chromatograph.

    b. Monitor the following ions (GC-MS):

9.5.4.1 Settings for RapidTrace Analysis of Cocaine and Benzoylecgonine in Serum, Plasma, or Whole Blood

9.5.5 Cocaine and Benzoylecgonine in Serum, Plasma, or Whole Blood for HPLC Using a 200-mg CLEAN SCREEN Extraction Column (ZSDAU020 or ZCDAU020)

1. Prepare sample.

    a. To 1 mL of sample add internal standard(s) and 4 mL of DI H$_2$O (5.0 ≤ pH ≤ 7.0).

    b. Whole blood: Mix/vortex and let stand 5 min.

    c. Centrifuge for 10 min at 670*g* and discard pellet.

    d. Add 2 mL of 0.1 *M* phosphate buffer, pH 6.0. Mix/vortex.

    e. Sample pH should be 6.0 ± 0.5. Adjust pH accordingly with 0.1 *M* monobasic or dibasic sodium phosphate.

2. Condition CLEAN SCREEN extraction column.

    1 × 3 mL of CH$_3$OH; aspirate.

    1 × 3 mL of DI H$_2$O; aspirate.

    1 × 1 mL of 0.1 *M* phosphate buffer, pH 6.0; aspirate.

    Note: Aspirate at ≤3 in. Hg to prevent sorbent drying.

Table 44

Compound	Primary ion[b]	Secondary ion	Tertiary ion
Cocaine	182	198	303
D3-Cocaine[a]	185	201	306
Benzoylecgonine-TMS	240	256	361
D3-Benzoylecgonine-TMS[a]	243	259	364

[a]Suggested internal standards for GC-MS: D3-cocaine, D3-benzoylecgonine.
[b]Quantitation ion.

Table 45

Step		Source	Destination	Volume	Flow[a]	Liq. Chk
1.	Condition	MeOH	Organic	3	18	no
2.	Condition	H2O	Water	3	18	no
3.	Condition	Phosphate buffer, pH 6.0	Water	1	18	no
4.	Load	Sample	Bio.	1.2	no	
5.	Load	Sample	Bio.	3.5	1.2	no
6.	Rinse	H2O	Bio.	2	24	no
7.	Purge—cannula	H2O	Cannula	6	30	no
8.	Rinse	0.1 M HCl	Bio.	2	6	no
9.	Rinse	MeOH	Bio.	3	18	no
10.	Dry	Time = 5 minutes				
11.	Collect	Elute	Fract1	3	1.2	no
12.	Purge—cannula	MeOH	Cannula	3	30	no
13.	Purge—cannula	H2O	Cannula	3	30	no

Load cannula depth = 0   Column air push volume = 2
Mix cannula depth = 0   Column air push volume speed multiplier = 2
Mix cycles = 2   Mix speed = 0.5
Mix volume = 0.5   Reagent mix cycles = 2

Table 46

Reagent setup

No.	Reagent	Abbreviation	Sip speed
0.	Vent	VENT	30
1.	Water	H2O	30
2.	Methanol	MeOH	30
3.	0.1 M Phosphate buffer, pH 6.0	pH 6	30
4.	0.1 M Acetate Buffer	pH 4.5	30
5.	Hexane	Hexn	30
6.	Elution solvent[b]	Elute	30
7.	0.1 M Acetic acid	Acetic	30
8.	0.1 M HCl	HC1	30
9.	Mixing vessel	MIXER	15

[a]Flow in mL/min.
[b]The elution solvent for benzoylecgonine is methylene chloride-isopropanol-ammonium hydroxide (78:20:2). This solution is prepared daily.

3. Apply sample.
Load at 1–2 mL/min.

4. Wash column.
1 × 2 mL of DI H$_2$O; aspirate.
1 × 2 mL of 0.1 *M* HCl; aspirate.
1 × 3 mL of CH$_3$OH; aspirate.
Dry column (5 min at ≥10 in. Hg).

5A.   *Elute cocaine and benzoylecgonine.
1 × 3 mL of CH$_2$Cl$_2$–IPA–NH$_4$OH (78:20:2); collect eluate at 1–2 mL/min.
Note: Prepare elution solvent daily. Add IPA–NH$_4$OH, mix, then add CH$_2$Cl$_2$, pH 11.0–12.0.

5B.   *Elute cocaine and benzoylecgonine.
1 × 2 mL of CH$_3$OH–NH$_4$OH (98:2); collect eluate at 1–2 mL/min.
Note: Prepare elution solvent daily.
Add 3 mL of DI H$_2$O and 500 µL of CH$_2$Cl$_2$ to eluate.
Mix/vortex 10 s. Centrifuge if necessary to separate layers.
Aspirate and discard aqueous (upper) layer.

6. Concentrate.
a. Evaporate to dryness at ≤ 40°C.
b. Reconstitute in mobile phase for injection into HPLC.

---

*Choose *either* 5A or 5B.

9.5.6 Extraction of Cocaine and Its Metabolites from Meconium for GC or CG-MS Analysis Using CLEAN SCREEN Extraction Columns (ZSDAU020 OR ZCDAU020)

1. Prepare sample.
   a. Vortex 0.5–1 g of meconium and 2 mL of CH3OH.
   b. Centrifuge and transfer the supernatant to a clean tube.
   c. To each tube add 3 mL of 0.1 *M* phosphate buffer, pH 6.0, and internal standard,a and vortex.
   d. Matrix must be more aqueous than organic for good retention to occur.
2. Condition CLEAN SCREEN® extraction column.
   2 × 3 mL of CH$_3$OH; aspirate.
   1 × 3 mL of DI H$_2$O; aspirate.
   1 × 3 mL of 0.1 *M* phosphate buffer, pH 6.0; aspirate.
   Note: Aspirate at ≤ 3 in. Hg to prevent sorbent drying.

3. Apply sample.
Load at 1- 2 mL/min. Allow to dry.

4. Wash column.
1 × 1 mL of DI H$_2$O; aspirate.
1 × 1 mL of 0.1 *M* HC1; aspirate.
1 × 3 mL of CH$_3$OH; aspirate.
Dry column (5 min at ≤10 in. Hg).

5. Elute isolates.
Note: Prepare elution solvent daily. Add IPA–NH$_4$OH, mix, then add CH$_2$Cl$_2$, pH 11.0–12.0.

6. Evaporate.
Evaporate the elution solvent to dryness *without heating*.

Table 47

Compound	Primary ion[b]	Secondary ion	Tertiary ion
Cocaine	182	198	303
D₃-Cocaine[a]	185	201	306
Benzoylecgonine-TMS	240	256	361
D₃-Benzoylecgonine-TMS[a]	243	259	364

[a]Suggested internal standards for GC-MS: D_3=cocaine, D_3=benzoylecgonine.
[b]Quantitation ion.

7. Derivatize.
   a. Add 50 µL of ethyl acetate and 50 µL of BSTFA (with 1% TMCS).
   b. Overlay with nitrogen gas and cap. Mix/vortex.
   c. React for 20 min at 70°C. Remove from heat source to cool.
   Note: Do not evaporate BSTFA solution.
8. Quantitate.
   Inject 1–2 µL of sample onto the chromatograph.
   Monitor the following ions (GC-MS):

9.6 LYSERGIC ACID DIETHYLAMIDE

Lysergic acid diethylamide (LSD) is a very potent psychoactive drug (Figure 10) that has

been abused over the past three decades. LSD has become increasingly popular with the adolescent population, where its use exceeds that of cocaine. LSD is not considered to be highly toxic; however, the psychotic effects of this drug can cause the user to commit irrational acts that can lead to serious injury or death. Factors that have contributed to its continued use include availability, low cost, and difficulty to detect.

The determination of this drug in biological fluids has been complicated by its low dose (40–120 µg/dose), extensive biotransformation of the drug with only about 1% of the dose excreted as unchanged drug, low volatility of the parent drug, surface adsorption, and inherent instability of the drug in light heat and acid.

Presented are methods that have been used for the determination of LSD from urine and whole blood.

9.6.1 Lysergic Acid Diethylamide (LSD) in Serum, Plasma, or Whole Blood for GC or GC-MS Confirmations Using a 200-mg CLEAN SCREEN Extraction Column (ZSDAU020 or ZCDAU020)

1. Prepare sample.
   a. To 1 mL of serum, plasma, or whole blood add 4 mL of deionized water and internal standard.[a]
   b. Mix/vortex and let stand 5 min.
   c. Centrifuge for 10 min at 670*g* and discard pellet.
   d. Add 2 mL 100 m*M* phosphate buffer, pH 6.0.

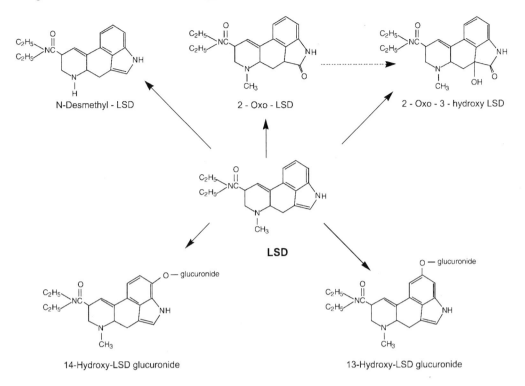

N-Desmethyl - LSD   2 - Oxo - LSD   2 - Oxo - 3 - hydroxy LSD

LSD

14-Hydroxy-LSD glucuronide   13-Hydroxy-LSD glucuronide

Fig. 10. Metabolism of LSD.

   e. Mix/vortex.

   f. Sample pH should be 6.0 ± 0.5. Adjust pH accordingly with 100 mM monobasic or dibasic sodium phosphate.

2. Condition CLEAN SCREEN® extraction column.

1 × 3 mL of CH$_3$OH; aspirate.

1 × 3 mL of DI H$_2$O; aspirate.

1 × 1 mL of 100 mM phosphate buffer, pH 6.0; aspirate.

Note: Aspirate at ≤3 in. Hg. to prevent sorbent drying.

3. Apply sample.

Load at 1 mL/min.

4. Wash column.

1 × 3 mL of DI H$_2$O; aspirate.

1 × 1 mL of 100 mM acetic acid; aspirate.

1 × 3 mL of CH$_3$OH; aspirate.

Dry column (5 min at ≥10 in Hg).

5. Elute LSD.

1 × 3 mL of CH$_2$Cl$_2$–IPA–NH$_4$OH (78:20:2); collect eluate at 1 mL/min.

Note: Prepare elution solvent daily. Add IPA–NH$_4$OH, mix, then add CH$_2$Cl$_2$, pH 11.0–12.0.

6. Dry eluate.

Evaporate to dryness at ≤40°C.

7. Derivatize.

   a. Add 20 µL of ethyl acetate and 20 µL of BSTFA (with 1% TMCS).

   b. Overlay with nitrogen gas and cap. Mix/vortex.

   c. React for 20 min at 70°C. Remove from heat source to cool.

   Note: Do not evaporate BSTFA solution.

8. Quantitate.

   Inject 1–3 µL of sample onto the chromatograph.

   Monitor the following ions (GC-MS):

   LSD: 395[b], 293, 268

   D[3]-LSD[a]:298[b], 296, 271

---

[a]Suggested internal standard for GC-MS: D[3]-LSD.
[b]Quantitation ion.

9.6.2 Lysergic Acid Diethylamide (LSD) in Urine for GC or GC-MS Confirmations Using a 200-mg CLEAN SCREEN® Extraction Column (ZSDAU020 or ZCDAU020)

1. Prepare sample.

   a. To 5 mL of urine add internal standard[a] and 2 mL of 100 mM phosphate buffer, pH 6.0.

   b. Mix/vortex.

   c. Sample pH should be 6.0 + 0.5. Adjust pH accordingly with 100 mM monobasic or dibasic sodium phosphate.

2. Condition CLEAN SCREEN extraction column.

   1 × 3 mL of CH_3OH; aspirate.

   1 × 3 mL of DI H_2O; aspirate.

   1 × 1 mL of 100 mM phosphate buffer, pH 6.0; aspirate.

   Note: Aspirate at ≤3 in. Hg. to prevent sorbent drying.

3. Apply sample.

   Load at 1 mL/min.

4. Wash column.

   1 × 3 mL of DI H_2O; aspirate.

   1 × 1 mL of 100 mM acetic acid; aspirate.

   1 × 3 mL of CH_3OH; aspirate.

   Dry column (5 min at ≥10 in. Hg).

5. Elute LSD.

   1 – 3 mL of CH_2Cl_2–IPA–NH_4OH (78:20:2); collect eluate at 1–2 mL/min.

   Note: Prepare elution solvent daily. Add IPA–NH_4OH, mix, then add CH_2Cl_2, pH 11.0–12.0.

6. Dry eluate.

   Evaporate to dryness at ≤40°C.

7. Derivatize.

   a. Add 20 µL of ethyl acetate and 20 µL of BSTFA (with 1% TMCS).

   b. Overlay with nitrogen gas and cap. Mix/vortex.

   c. React for 20 min at 70°C. Remove from heat source to cool.

   Note: Do not evaporate BSTFA solution.

8. Quantitate.

   a. Inject 1–3 µL of sample onto chromatograph.

   b. Monitor the following ions (GC-MS):

LSD: 395[b], 293, 268
D3-LSD:[a] 398[b], 296, 271

---

[a]Suggested internal standard for GC-MS: D[3]-LSD.
[b]Quantitation ion.

9.7. DETERMINATION OF OPIATES USING OXIME-TMS DERIVATIVES

The determination of opiates in body fluids is a challenging task because of the variety of different opiates available and the structural similarity of these compounds. In addition, multiple common metabolic pathways exist for these compounds, making interpretation of the results difficult. (For example, codeine can form morphine and morphine can form normorphine.) Differences in individual metabolism may also confound the analyst. Numerous analytical methods have been developed to address these problems (e.g., structural similarities, isomerism, chromatographic issues). In most cases derivatization chemistries have been tried; however, each chemistry brings another set of problems. The following method utilizes a dual derivatization that eliminates the problem of keto-enol tautomerization. The opiate is first reacted with hydroxylamine to form the oxime and then, upon isolation, is derivatized with MSTFA (Figure 11). Advantages to this method are better chromatographic resolution and higher mass fragmentation patterns that gives better confirmation and quantitation (Figure 12).

A second method has been presented using enzymatic digestion with propyl derivatives formed from the use of propionic anhydride. Advantages of this method are that the derivatives are (1) exceptionally stable (up to 5 d), (2) conditions mild enough for thebaine (a marker for poppy seed ingestion) to be determined and (3) the quantitation of 6-monoacetyl morphine (the major metabolite of heroin) can be done. The determination of 12 opiates has been performed using this method.

Table 48 shows a list of commonly found peripherally modified morphine derivatives.

Note: For the propylation derivatization to work effectively you must use a very pure proprionic anhydride that has no acetic anhydride in it. Acetic anhydride can be an impurity in proprionic anhydride resulting from its manufacturing process. The process of acetic anhydride will cause the formation of 6MAM from morphine and give an indication of the presence of heroin. If you find a consistent percentage of 6MAM in your samples, check your proprionic anhydride. There are high purity proprionic anhydride sources available. Check your proprionic anhydride for the presence of acetic anhydride before using it if you are going to use this method.

9.7.1 Opiates in Urine-Oxime-TMS Procedure: Manual Method for GC or GC-MS Confirmations Using a 200-mg CLEAN SCREEN Extraction Column (ZSDAU020 or ZCDAU020)

1. **Prepare sample acid hydrolysis of glucuronides.**
    a. To 2 mL of urine add internal standard(s)[a] and 400 µL of concentrated HC1.
    b. Add 200 µL of 10% hydroxylamine solution.
    c. Mix/vortex.
    d. Heat to 90°C for 20 min in a heating block or autoclave for 15 min on a liquid cycle.

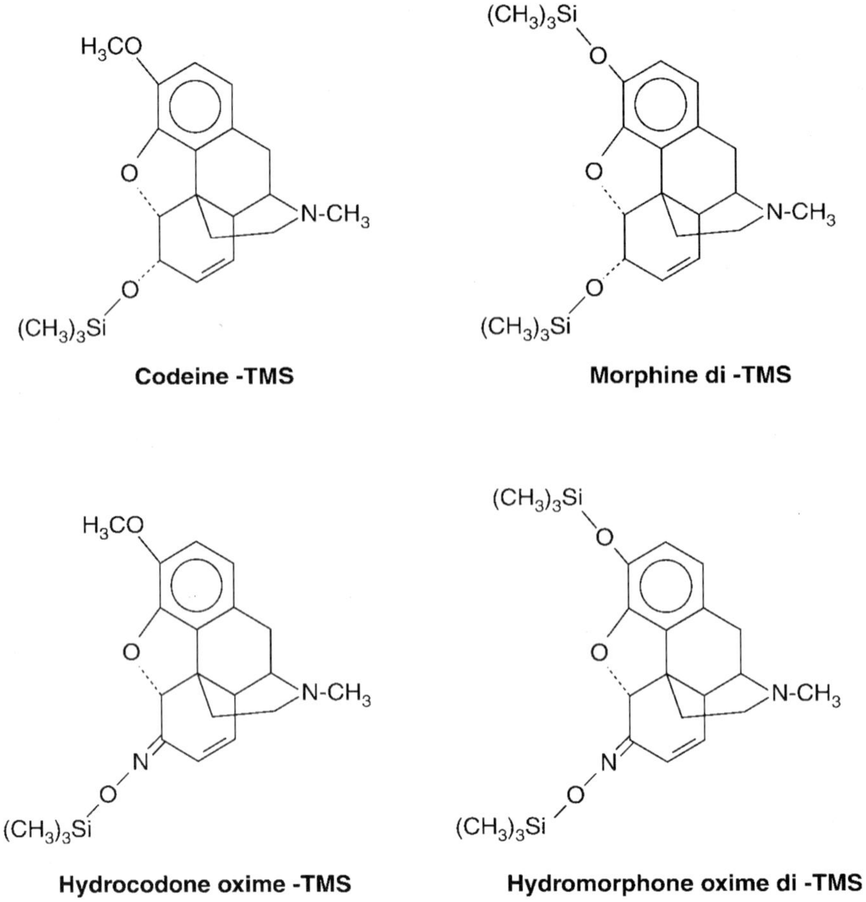

Codeine -TMS

Morphine di -TMS

Hydrocodone oxime -TMS

Hydromorphone oxime di -TMS

Fig. 11. Opiate TMS oxime structures.

    e. Cool before proceeding.

    f. Centrifuge for 10 min at 2000 rpm and discard pellet.

    g. Add 500 µL of 50% ammonium hydroxide. Mix/vortex.

    h. Adjust sample pH to 6.0–7.0 by dropwise addition of 50% ammonium hydroxide.

2. Condition CLEAN SCREEN extraction column.

    1 × 3 mL of methanol; aspirate.

    1 × 3 mL of DI H_2O; aspirate.

    1 × 3 mL of 0.1 *M* phosphate buffer, pH 6.0; aspirate.

    Note: Aspirate at ≤3 in. Hg to prevent sorbent drying.

3. Apply sample.

    Load at 1–2 mL/min.

4. Wash column.

    1 × 3 mL of DI H_2O; aspirate.

    1 × 3 mL of 0.1 *M* acetate buffer, pH 4.5; aspirate.

    1 × 3 mL of methanol; aspirate.

    Dry column (5 min at ≥10 in. Hg).

A TMS derivatives

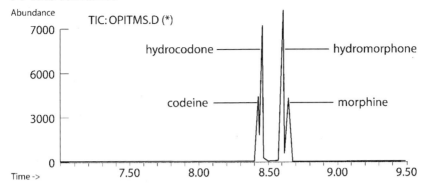

B Oxime TMS derivatives

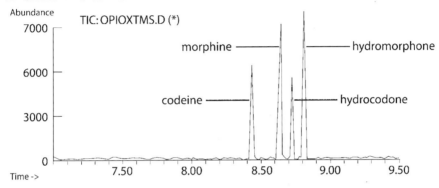

Fig. 12. Peripherally modified morphine derivatives.

5. **Elute opiates.**
   1 × 3 mL methylene chloride-isopropanol-ammonium hydroxide (78:20:2).
   Collect eluate at 1–2 mL/min.
   Note: Prepare elution solvent daily.
   Add isopropanol to the ammonium hydroxide, mix, and then add methylene chloride.
   Check the pH of the elution solution; it should be at pH = 11.0 or higher.
6. **Dry eluate.**
   Evaporate to dryness at ≤40°C using a TurboVap® or equivalent.
7. **Derivatize.**
   a. Add 100 μL of ethyl acetate and 50 μL of MSTFA.
   b. Overlayer with nitrogen gas and cap. Mix/vortex.
   c. React for 20 min at 85°C in a heat block.
   d. Remove from heat source to cool.
   Note: Do not evaporate MSTFA solution.
8. **Quantitate.**
   a. Inject 1–2 μL of derivatized sample onto the chromatograph.
   b. Monitor the following ions:

Table 48
Peripherally Modified Morphine Derivatives

Opiate	R =	$\Delta^{7,8}$	X =	Y=	Relative Potency (Morphine = 1)	Uses and Comments
Morphine	H	Yes	H,α–OH	H	1	Strong analgesic
Codeine	CH$_3$	Yes	H,α–OH	H	0.15	Mild analgesic, antitussive
Ethylmorphine	C2H5	Yes	H,α–OH	H	0.1	Ophthalmologic (chemotic) use
Heroin	CH$_3$CO	Yes	H,α–OOCCH$_3$	H	4	Potent analgesic, strong addiction potential
Hydromorphone (Dilaudid)	H	No	O	H	5	Less sedative, shorter acting vs morphine
Hydrocodone (Dicoadid)	CH$_3$	No	O	H	0.7	Orally effective analgesic and antitussive
Oxymorphone (Numorphan)	H	No	O	OH	10	Strong analgesic
Oxycodone (Eucodal)	CH$_3$	No	O	OH	1	Orally effective analgesic and antitussive
Dihydrocodeine	CH$_3$	No	H,α–OH	H	0.3	Weak analgesic, faster acting than morphine, hypotensive

9.7.2 Opiates in Urine-Oxime-TMS Procedure: Automated Method for GC or GC-MS Confirmations Using a 200-mg CLEAN SCREEN Extraction Column (CSDAU203 or CCDAU203)

1. **Prepare sample acid hydrolysis of glucuronide.**
   a. To 2 mL of urine add internal standard(s)[a] and 400 μL of concentrated HCl.
   b. Add 200 μL 10% hydroxylamine solution.
   c. Mix/vortex.
   d. Heat to 90°C for 20 min in a heating block or autoclave for 15 min on a liquid cycle.
   e. Cool before proceeding.
   f. Centrifuge for 10 min at 670g and discard pellet.

Table 49

Compound	Retention Time	Primary ion[b]	Secondary ion	Tertiary ion
D$_3$-Codeine oxime TMS[a]	6.9	374	359	346
Morphine oxime TMS	7.3	236	414	429
D$_3$-Morphine oxime TMS[a]	7.3	239	417	432
Hydrocodone oxime TMS	7.46	386	371	329
Hydromorphone oxime TMS	7.66	355	429	444
Oxycodone-oxime TMS	7.99	474	459	401
Oxmorphone-oxime TMS	7.91	459	287	532

[a]Suggested internal standards for GC-MS: D$_3$-codeine, D$_3$-morphine.
[b]Quantitation ion.

Table 50

Compound	Retention time	Primary ion[b]	Secondary ion	Tertiary ion
D$_3$-Codeine oxime TMS[a]	6.9	374	359	346
Morphine oxime TMS	7.3	236	414	429
D$_3$-Morphine oxime TMS[a]	7.3	239	417	432
Hydrocodone oxime TMS	7.46	386	371	329
Hydromorphone oxime TMS	7.66	355	429	444
Oxycodone-oxime TMS	7.99	474	459	401
Oxmorphone-oxime TMS	7.91	459	287	532

[a]Suggested internal standards for GC-MS: D$_3$-codeine, D$_3$-morphine.
[b]Quantitation ion.

    g. Add 500 μL of 50% ammonium hydroxide. Mix/vortex.

    h. Adjust sample pH to 6.0–7.0 by dropwise addition of 50% ammonium hydroxide.

2. **Place samples onto RapidTrace.**

   See Subheading 9.7.2.1 for settings.

3. **Remove samples and evaporate eluate.**

   Evaporate to dryness at ≤40°C using a TurboVap or equivalent.

4. **Derivatize.**

   a. Add 100 μL of ethyl acetate and 50 μL of MSTFA.

   b. Overlay with nitrogen gas and cap. Mix/vortex.

   c. React 20 min at 85°C in a heater block.

   d. Remove from heat source to cool.

   Note: Do not evaporate MSTFA solution.

5. **Quantitate.**

   a. Inject 1 to 2 μL of derivatized sample onto the chromatograph.

   b. Monitor the following ions:

Table 51

Step		Source	Destination	mL	mL/min	Liq. Chk
1.	Condition	MeOH	Org	3	18	No
2.	Condition	H_2O	Aq.	3	18	No
3.	Condition	pH 6.0	Aq.	3	18	No
4.	Load	sample	Bio	3.4	1.2	No
5.	Rinse	H_2O	Aq.	3	12	No
6.	Purge–cannula	H_2O	Cannula	6	35	No
7.	Rinse	pH 4.5	Aq.	3	12	No
8.	Rinse	MeOH	Aq.	3	12	No
9.	Dry	Time = 5 min				
10.	Collect	Elute	Fract1	4	1.2	No
11.	Purge—cannula	MeOH	Cannula	4	30	No
12.	Purge—cannula	H_2O	Cannula	4	30	No

Load cannula depth = 0   Mix volume = 0.5
Mix cannula depth = 0   Mix speed = 30
Mix cycles = 2   Reagent mix cycles = 2

Table 52

Reagent setup

No.	Reagent	Abbreviation	Sip speed
1.	Water	H_2O	30
2.	Methanol	MEOH	30
3.	Phosphate buffer	pH 6	30
4.	Acetate buffer	pH 4.5	30
5.	Hexane	Hexn	30
6.	MeCl–IPA–NH_4OH (78:20:2)	Elute	15
7.	0.1 *M* acetic acid	Acetic	30
8.	Reagent 8	Reag8	30
9.	Mixing vessel	Mixer	15
10.	Sample	Sample	15

Column air push volume = 0.4
Column air push volume speed multiplier = 4

9.7.2.1 Settings for RapidTrace Analysis of Opiates in Urine Using the Oxime-TMS Procedure

9.7.2.2 GC-MS Analysis

1. Instrumentation

The GC-MS system consisted of a Hewlett Packard 5971 A mass selective detector, 7673 autosampler, and a 5890 gas chromatograph fitted with a Selectra® CC-1 capillary column (comparable to a HP1 or DB1) 15 m long, 0.25 mm i.d. and 0.25 μm film thickness.

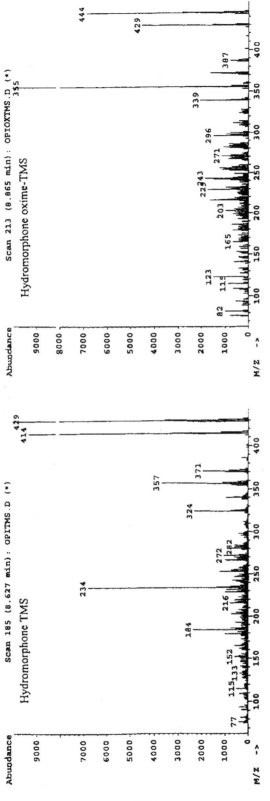

Fig.13. Mass fragmentation pattern—hydromorphone.

223

Table 53

No.	Waste	Abbreviation
1.	Aqueous	Aq.
2.	Organic Solvent	Org.
3.	Biohazardous	Bio.

2. Analytical Conditions

a. The MS mode was selective ion monitoring (SIM) for three ions of each analyte.

b. The injector port and transfer line was maintained at 230°C and 280°C, respectively.

c. A 1–2 μL sample injection using the split less mode was performed with the following oven conditions:

d. An initial temperature of 140°C was increased to 230°C at a rate of 30°C/min and then raised to 250°C at a rate of 5°C/min and to 290°C at a rate of 40°C/min and held for 1 min.

e. The total run time was 9 min. An example of a separation is given in Figure 12.

9.7.3 6-Monoacetyl Morphine, Thebaine, and Opiates Using Propyl Derivatives

The confirmation and identification of opiates in biological matrices often may lead to more questions than answers. The presence of codeine and morphine may be indicative of pain therapy, heroin abuse, or poppy seed ingestion. Several recent studies have proposed using 6-acetylmorphine as the primary marker for heroin abuse (1,2). Heroin is metabolized to 6-acetylmorphine within minutes after the drug enters the body; this is either conjugated or further metabolized to morphine (1–4).

Thebaine is a marker for poppy seed ingestion. Poppy seeds contain varying concentrations of morphine, codeine, thebaine, and other compounds (Figure 14). Thebaine undergoes considerable degradation with exposure to heat, especially in the acidic conditions used in derivatization with BSTFA (5). We have developed a method to simultaneously detect and quantify 6-acetylmorphine, thebaine, and 10 other opiates in urine using automated SPE. This method utilizes enzyme hydrolysis, SPE with a Zymark RapidTrace system, and derivatization followed by GC-MS analysis.

9.7.4 Opiates in Human Urine-Propyl Derivatives: Manual Method for GC or GC-MS Confirmations Using a 200-mg CLEAN SCREEN® Extraction Column (ZSDAU020 or ZCDAU020)

1. Prepare sample-enzymatic hydrolysis of glucuronides:

a. To 4 mL of urine, add internal standard(s)[a] and 3 mL of 0.1 *M* phosphate buffer, pH 6.0 and 12,500 U of β-glucuronidase from limpets (in pH 6.0 phosphate buffer).

b. Heat to 60°C for three hours; cool.

2. Condition CLEAN SCREEN extraction column.

1 × 2 mL of methanol; aspirate.

1 × 2 mL of DI H$_2$O; aspirate.

1 × 2 mL of 0.1 *M* phosphate buffer, pH 6.0; aspirate.

Note: Aspirate at ≤3 in. Hg to prevent sorbent drying.

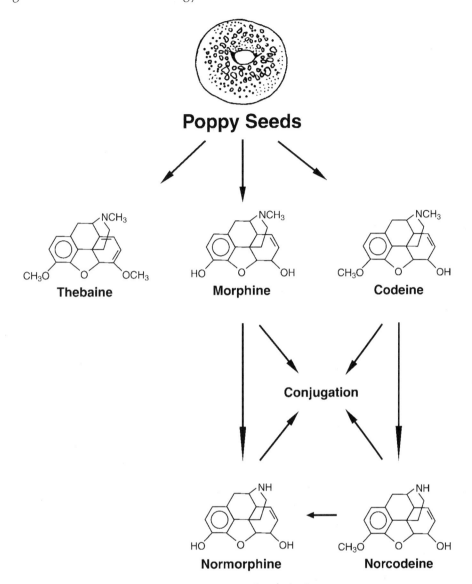

Fig. 14. Poppy seed metabolism.

3. **Apply sample.**
   Load at 1–2 mL/min.
4. **Wash column.**
   1 × 3 mL of DI H_2O; aspirate.
   1 × 3 mL of 0.1 *M* acetate buffer, pH 4.5; aspirate.
   1 – 3 mL of methanol; aspirate.
   Dry column (5 min at ≥10 in. Hg).
5. **Elute opiates.**
   1 × 2 mL ethyl acetate-isopropanol-ammonium hydroxide (84:12:4).
6. **Dry eluant.**
   Evaporate to dryness at ≤40°C using a TurboVap or equivalent.

Table 54
Propyl Derivatives of Opiates

Compound	Rel ret time[b] (ratio)	Primary ion	Secondary ion	Tertiary ion
Hydrocodone[a]	0.81	299	242	214
Thebaine[a]	0.84	311	296	312
D[3]-Codeine	0.89	358	285	232
Codeine	0.89	355	282	229
Oxycodone	0.90	371	314	298
Heroin[a]	0.91	327	369	268
Hydromorphone	0.94	285	341	228
6-Monoacetyl morphine (6MAM)	0.96	327	268	382
Oxymorphone	0.99	357	300	413
D[3]-Morphine	1.00	344	271	400
Morphine	1.00	341	268	397
Naloxone	1.04	327	383	328
Nalorphine	1.05	367	350	294
Norcodeine	1.11	223	224	397
Normorphine	1.20	210	383	236

[a]Does not derivatize under these conditions.
[b]Relative retention time-based upon D[3] morphine retention time.

7. **Derivatize.**
    a. Add 200 µL of a 1:1 solution of propionic anhydride-pyridine.
    b. Make this solution fresh daily.
    c. Mix/vortex.
    d. React for 60 min at 40°C in a heater block.
    e. Remove from heat source to cool.
    f. Evaporate to dryness at ≤40°C using a TurboVap or equivalent.
    g. Reconstitute the residue with 50 µL of ethyl acetate-methanol (70:30).
    h. Transfer the solution to a limited-volume insert for GC-MS analysis.

9.7.5 Opiates in Urine-Propyl Procedure: Automated Method for GC or GC-MS Confirmations Using a 200-mg CLEAN SCREEN Extraction Column (CSDAU203 or CCDAU203)

1. **Prepare sample—enzymatic hydrolysis of glucuronides.**
    a. To 4 mL of urine, add internal standard(s)[a], and 3 mL of 0.1 *M* phosphate buffer, pH 6.0., and 12,500 U of β-glucuronidase from limpets (made in pH 6.0 phosphate buffer).
    b. Heat to 60°C for 3 h; cool.
2. **Place sample onto the RapidTrace.**
    See Section 9.7.3.1 for RapidTrace conditions.
3. **Remove samples and evaporate.**
    Evaporate to dryness at ≤40°C using a TurboVap or equivalent.

4. **Derivatize.**
   a. Add 200 μL of a 1:1 solution of propionic anhydride-pyridine.
   b. Make this solution fresh daily.
   c. Mix/vortex.
   d. React for 60 minutes at 40°C in a heater block.
   e. Remove from heat source to cool.
   f. Evaporate to dryness at ≤40°C using a TurboVap or equivalent.
   g. Reconstitute the residue with 50 μL of ethyl acetate-methanol (70:30).
   h. Transfer the solution to a limited-volume insert for GC-MS analysis.

5. **Quantitate.**
   a. Inject 1–2 μL of derivatized sample onto the chromatograph.
   b. Monitor the ions in Table 54.

9.7.5.1 Setting for RapidTrace Analysis of Opiates in Urine Using Propyl Derivative Method

9.7.6 Free (Unbound) Opiates in Serum, Plasma, or Whole Blood for GC or GC-MS Confirmations Using a 200-mg CLEAN SCREEN Extraction Column (ZSDAU020 or ZCDAU020)

1. **Prepare sample.**
   a. To 1 mL of sample add internal standard(s)[a] and 4 mL of DI H_2O (5 ≤ pH ≤ 7.0).
   b. For whole blood: Mix/vortex and let stand 5 min.
   c. Centrifuge for 10 min at 670g and discard pellet.
   d. Add 2 mL of 0.1 M phosphate buffer, pH 6.0. Mix/vortex.
   e. Sample pH should be 6.0 ± 0.5. Adjust pH accordingly with 0.1 M monobasic or dibasic sodium phosphate.

2. **Condition CLEAN SCREEN extraction column.**
   1 × 3 mL of CH_3OH; aspirate.
   1 × 3 mL of DI H_2O; aspirate.
   1 × 1 mL of 0.1 M phosphate buffer, pH 6.0; aspirate.
   Note: Aspirate at ≤3 in. Hg to prevent sorbent drying.

3. **Apply sample.**
   Load at 1 mL/min.

4. **Wash column.**
   1 × 2 mL of DI H_2O; aspirate.
   1 × 2 mL of 0.1 M acetate buffer, pH 4.5; aspirate.
   1 × 3 mL of CH_3OH; aspirate.
   Dry column (5 min at ≥10 in. Hg).

5. **Elute opiates.**
   1 × 3 mL of CH_2Cl_2–IPA–NH_4OH (78:20:2); collect eluate at 1–2 mL/min.
   Note: Prepare elution solvent daily. Add IPA–NH_4OH, mix, then add CH_2Cl_2, pH 11.0–12.0.

6. **Dry eluate.**
   Evaporate to dryness at ≤40°C.

7. **Derivatize μL of ethyl acetate and 50 μL of BSTFA (with 1% TMCS).**
   b. Overlay with nitrogen gas and cap. Mix/vortex.
   c. React for 20 min at 70°C. Remove from heat source to cool.
   Note: **Do not evaporate BSTFA solution.**

Table 55

Step		Source	Destination	Volume	Flow	Liq. Chk.
1.	Condition	MeOH	Organic	3	12	No
2.	Condition	H₂O	Water	3	12	No
3.	Condition	Phosphate buffer, pH 6.0	Water	2	12	No
4.	Load	Sample	Bio.	5	1.2	No
5.	Load	Sample	Bio.	3.7	1.2	No
6.	Purge—cannula	Water	Cannula	6	8	No
7.	Rinse	Acetate, pH 4.5	Bio.	1	8	No
8.	Rinse	MeOH	Bio.	3	8	No
9.	Dry	Time = 5 minutes				
10.	Collect	Elute	Fract1	3	1.2	No
11.	Purge—cannula	MeOH	Cannula	3	30	No
12.	Purge—cannula	H₂O	Cannula	3	30	No

Load cannula depth = 0   Mix volume = 0.5
Mix cannula depth = 0   Mix speed = 0.5
Mix cycles = 2   Reagent mix cycles = 2
                          Column air push volume = 2
                          Column air push volume speed multiplier = 2

Table 56

Reagent setup

No.	Reagent	Abbreviation	Sip speed
0.	Vent	Vent	30
1.	Water	H₂O	30
2.	Methanol	MeOH	30
	3.0. 1 *M* phosphate buffer, pH 6.0	pH 6	30
4.	0.1 *M* acetate buffer, pH 4.5	pH 4.5	30
5.	Hexane	Hexn	30
6.	Elution solvent[b]	Elute	30
7.	0.1 *M* Acetic acid	Acetic	30
8.	0.1 *M* HCl	HCl	30
9.	Mixing vessel	Mixer	30

[a]Flow in mL/min.

[b]The elution solvent for opiate/propyl is ethyl acetate-isopropanol-ammonium hydroxide (84:12:4). This solution is prepared daily.

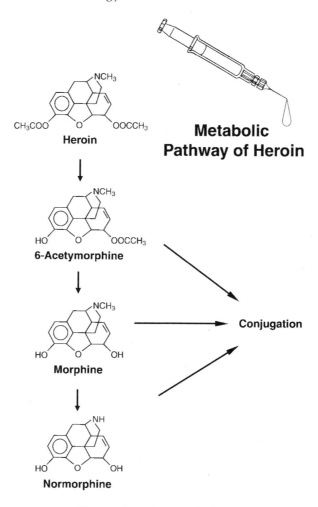

Metabolic Pathway of Heroin

Fig. 15. Heroin metabolism.

8. Quantitate.
   a. Inject 1–2 µL of sample onto chromatograph.
   b. Monitor the following ions (GC-MS):

9.7.6.1 GC-MS Analysis

Instrumentation

The GC-MS system consisted of a Hewlett Packard 5971A mass selective detector, 7673 Autosampler, and a 5890 gas chromatograph fitted with a Selectra® CC-5 capillary column (comparable to a HP5 or DB5) 30 m long, 0.25 mm i.d. and 0.25 µm film thickness.

Analytical Conditions

The method used selected ion monitoring (SIM) for three ions of each analyte. The dwell times were set to allow approximately 2.5 cycles per second. The injection port and transfer line were maintained at 250°C and 280°C, respectively. The initial oven temperature was 100°C with an isocratic hold for 1 min following a 2 µL injec-

Table 57

Compound	Primary ion[b]	Secondary ion	Tertiary ion
TMS-Codeine	371	234	343
TMS-D$_3$-Codeine[a]	374	237	346
TMS-Morphine	429	287	324
TMS-D$_3$-Morphine[a]	432	290	327

[a]Suggested internal standards for GC-MS: D$_3$-codeine, D$_3$-morphine
[b]Quantitation ion.

Table 58

Derivatized Drug	Retention Time		Major Ions in Spectra	
	TMS	HOX-TMS	TMS	HOX-TMS
Codeine	8.43	8.43	371*,356,343,234	371*, 356, 343, 234
Morphine	8.67	8.67	429, 414, 401, 236*	429, 414, 401, 236*
Hydrocodone	8.47	8.77	371*, 356, 313, 234	386*, 371, 329, 297
Hydromorphone	8.63	8.86	429*, 414, 371, 357	444, 429, 355*, 339
Oxycodone	8.65	9.07	459*, 444, 368, 312	474*, 459, 401, 385
Oxymorphone	8.84	9.14	517*, 502, 412, 355	532*, 517, 459, 287

*Quantitation ion.

tion. The oven is ramped to 250°C at 25°C/min and a 2.00-min hold was followed by a ramp to 290°C at 10°C/min and a 0.5-min hold. The oven was then ramped to 325°C at 25°C/min and held for 3.1 min. The total run time was 18.00 min. The analyses, ions, and relative retention times are listed in Table 58. Figure 16 shows a chromatogram of an extracted 25-ng/mL urine standard.

Recovery

The average recovery of each analyte was calculated by comparing areas under the curve for the base ion for the extracted and unextracted standards. The average recovery for each analyte was over 85% (range 85–104) with the exception of nalorphine (53%). Thebaine averaged a 97.5% recovery even without derivatization. 6-monoacetylmorphine (6MAM) averaged 100.5% recovery.

Linearity

All of the analyses were linear from 12.5 to 1000 ng/mL with the exception of thebaine, naloxone, and oxycodone. They were limited to 25–1000 ng/mL.

Stability

Propyl derivatives have been reported stable for >5 d (6).

Sensitivity

This assay has adequate sensitivity and selectivity for all of the analyses tested. Many analyses could be detected and quantified at lower concentrations than the lowest concentration tested (12.5 ng/mL).

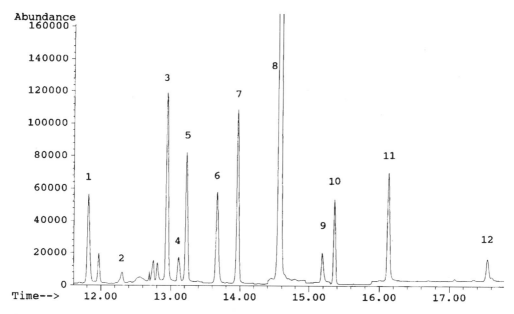

Fig. 16. Chromatography of propyl opiates. Chromatogram of 25 mg/mL extracted urine standard.

9.8 PHENCYCLIDINE

Phencyclidine (1-phenylcyclohexylpiperidine, PCP), originally used as a horse tranquilizer, is now a popular drug of abuse. This drug is structurally related to ketamine and was thought to have human use as an intravenous anesthetic. This drug can be administered by smoking, nasal insufflation, oral intake, or intravenous injection. Its primary effects are lethargy, hallucinations, loss of coordination, and disorientation. Its street names include *angel dust, embalming fluid, rocket fuel, supergrass,* and *killer weed.* It normally comes in a white crystalline powder form; however, a liquid form is PCP base dissolved in ether, which is a highly flammable solvent. It also has been sprayed onto leafy materials such as oregano, marijuana, mint, or parsley and ingested by smoking.

Currently, a number of designer (street) drugs have been synthesized by similar chemical reactions. They include phenylcyclohexylpyrrolidine (PHP), phenylcyclopentylpiperidine (PCPP), and thienylcylohexylpiperidine (TCP) (Figure 17). Blood levels for PCP vary from 0.007 to 0.24 mg/L (1). The plasma half-life has been estimated at 11–13 h (2) and 7- 46 h (3). In cases of severe poisoning a half-life of 1–4 d may occur (4). The metabolism of PCP indicates two identified inactive metabolites: 4-phenyl-4 piperdinocylohexanol and 1-(1-phenylcyclohexyl)-4-hydroxypiperdine, which is metabolized to glucuronide conjugates that are found in the urine (Figure 18). Intravenous dosing indicated that 30%–50% of the dose was found in the urine as unchanged PCP within 72 h (5). One problem in the ingestion of the street variety of PCP is that the starting precursor, 1-piperidinocyclohexanecarbonitrile, found in 20% of samples, can release cyanide in vivo. This can have serious toxicity issues (6–8). The following SPE extraction procedure works with recovery of above 95% and has also been successfully used for the designer drugs shown in Figure 17.

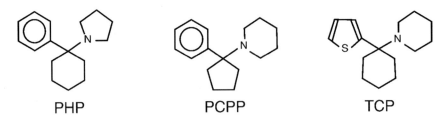

Fig. 17. Phencyclidine metabolism in humans.

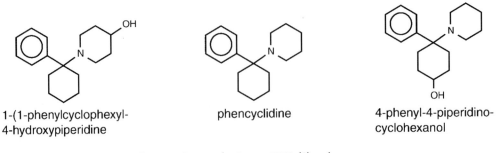

1-(1-phenylcyclohexyl-   phencyclidine   4-phenyl-4-piperidino-
4-hydroxypiperidine   cyclohexanol

Fig. 18. Street designer PCP-like drugs.

9.8.1 Phencyclidine in Urine for GC or GC-MS Confirmations Using a 200-mg CLEAN SCREEN Extraction Column (ZSDAU020 or ZCDAU020) (9)

1. **Prepare sample.**
   a. To 5 mL of urine add internal standard(s)[a] and 2 mL of 0.1 *M* phosphate buffer, pH 6.0.
   b. Mix/vortex.
   c. Sample pH should be 6.0 ± 0.5. Adjust pH accordingly with 0.1 *M* monobasic or dibasic sodium phosphate.
2. **Condition CLEAN SCREEN extraction column.**
   1 × 3 mL of methanol; aspirate.
   1 × 3 mL of DI H$_2$O; aspirate.
   1 × 1 mL of 0.1 *M* phosphate buffer, pH 6.0; aspirate.
   Note: Aspirate at ≤3 in. Hg to prevent sorbent drying.
3. **Apply sample.**
   Load at 1–2 mL /min.
4. **Wash column.**
   1 × 3 mL of DI H$_2$O; aspirate.
   1 × 1 mL of 0.1 *M* acetic acid; aspirate.
   1 × 3 mL of methanol; aspirate.
   Dry column (5 min at ≥10 in. Hg).
5. **Elute phencyclidine.**
   1 × 3 mL of methylene-chloride-isopropanol-ammonium hydroxide (78:20:2).
   Collect eluate at 1–2 mL/min.
   Note: Prepare this solution fresh daily.
   Add isopropanol and ammonium hydroxide first, mix, and then add the methylene chloride. The pH of this solution should be 11.0 or higher.

Table 59

Compound	Primary ion[c]	Secondary ion	Tertiary ion
Phencyclidine	200	91	242
D[5]-Phencyclidine[a]	205	96	247
Ketamine[b]	180	209	152

[a]Suggested internal standard for GC-MS: D[5]-phencyclidine.
[b]Suggested internal standard (non-GC-MS): ketamine.
[c]Quantitation ion.

Table 60

Compound	Primary ion[c]	Secondary ion	Tertiary ion
Phencyclidine	200	91	242
D[5]-Phencyclidine[a]	205	96	247
Ketamine[b]	180	209	152

[a]Suggested internal standard for GC-MS: D[5]-phencyclidine.
[b]Suggested internal standard (non GC-MS): ketamine.
[c]Quantitation ion.

6. **Dry eluate.**
   a. Evaporate to dryness at ≤40°C using a TurboVap or equivalent.
   b. Remove immediately on completion.
   c. Reconstitute with 100 μL of ethyl acetate.
7. **Quantitate.**
   Inject 1 to 2 μL of sample onto the GC-MS.
   Monitor the following ions (GC-MS):

9.8.2 Phencyclidine in Urine Automated Method for GC or GC-MS Confirmations Using a 200-mg CLEAN SCREEN Extraction Column (CSDAU203 or CCDAU203)

1. **Prepare sample.**
   a. To 5 mL of urine add internal standard(s)[a] and 2 mL of 0.1 M phosphate buffer, pH 6.0.
   b. Mix /vortex.
   c. Sample pH should be 6.0 ± 0.5. Adjust pH accordingly with 0.1 M monobasic or dibasic sodium phosphate.
2. **Load sample onto the RapidTrace module.**
   See Section 9.8.2.1 for conditions.
3. **Remove sample and dry eluate.**
   a. Evaporate to dryness at <40°C using a TurboVap or equivalent.
   b. Remove immediately on completion.
   c. Reconstitute with 100 μL of ethyl acetate.
4. **Quantitate.**
   a. Inject 1–2 μL of sample onto the GC-MS.
   b. Monitor the following ions (GC-MS):

Table 61

Step		Source	Destination	mL	mL/min	Liq. chk
1.	Condition	MeOH	Org.	3	18	No
2.	Condition	H₂O	Aq.	2	18	No
3.	Condition	pH 6.0	Aq.	1	18	No
4.	Load	Sample	Bio.	4.0	1.0	No
5.	Load	Sample	Bio.	3.4	1.0	No
6.	Purge—cannula	H₂O	Cannula	6	30	No
7.	Rinse	H₂O	Bio.	3	12	No
8.	Rinse	0.1 MHAc	Aq.	1	12	No
9.	Rinse	MeOH	Org.	3	12	No
10.	Dry	Time = 5 min				
11.	Collest	Elute	Fract1	1	1.2	No
12.	Purge—cannula	MeOH	Cannula	4	30	No
13.	Purge—cannula	H₂O	Cannula	4	30	No

Load cannula depth = 0   Mix volume = 0.5
Mix cannula depth = 0   Mix speed = 30
Mix cycles = 2   Reagent mix cycles = 2

Table 62

Reagent setup

No.	Reagent Name	Abbreviation	Sip speed
1.	Water	H₂O	30
2.	Methanol	MeOH	30
3.	Phosphate buffer	pH 6.0	30
4.	Acetate buffer	pH 4.5	30
5.	Hexane	Hexn	30
6.	MeCl–IPA–NH₄OH (78:20:2)	Elute	15
7.	0.1 *M* Acetic acid	Acetic	30
8.	Reagent 8	Reag8	30
9.	Mixing vessel	Mixer	15
10.	Sample	Sample	15

Column air push volume = 0.2
Column air push volume speed multiplier = 2

Table 63

No.	Waste	Abbrev
1.	Aqueous	Aq.
2.	Organic	Org.
3.	Biohazardous	Bio.

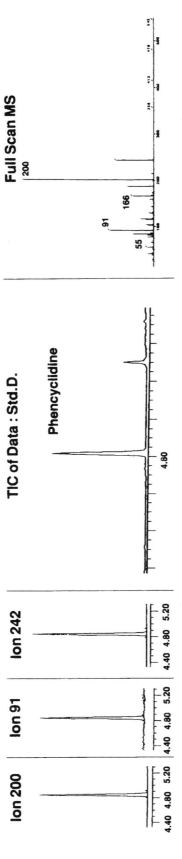

Fig. 19. Phencclidine chromatography.

9.8.2.1 Settings for RapidTrace Analysis of Phencyclidine in Urine
9.8.2.2 GC-MS Analysis

1. Instrumentation

The GC-MS system consisted of a Hewlett Packard 5971A mass selective detector, 7673 autosampler and 5890 gas chromatograph fitted with a Selectra® CC-5 capillary column (comparable to a DB-5 or HP-5) 30 m long, 0.25 i.d. and 0.25 μm film thickness.

2. Analytical Conditions

The method used selective ion monitoring (SIM) for three ions of each analyte. The injection port and transfer line were maintained at 250°C and 280°C, respectively. A 1–2 μL splitless injection was performed with the following oven program:

a. The initial temperature was set at 120°C with an isothermal hold of 2 min.

b. The oven is ramped at 20°C/min to 300°C with a hold of 1 min.

c. The total run time is 12 min.

d. The approximate retention time for D5-phencyclidine and phencyclidine was 5 min.

REFERENCES

[1] Worldwide Monitoring—Application Brochure. United Chemical Technologies, Inc., 1992.

[2] Clouette, R., Brendler, J., Wimbush, G., and Garrdott, J. The determination of amphetamine, methamphetamine and other phenylalkylamines in blood and urine by a dual derivatization method. SOFT Poster #48, 1997.

[3] RapidTrace Procedure Book. United Chemical Technologies, Inc., 1999.

[4] Thurman, E., Pedersen, M., Stout, R., and Martin, T. Distinguishing sympathomimetic amines from amphetamine and methamphetamine in urine by gas chromatography/mass spectroscopy. J. Analyt. Toxicol. 16:19–28, 1992.

[5] Melgar, R., and Kelly, R. A novel GC/MS derivatization method for amphetamines. J. Analyt. Toxicol. 17:399–402, 1993.

[6] Thompson, W., and Dasgupta, A. Microwave-induced rapid preparation of fluoro derivatives of amphetamine, methamphetamine and 3,4-methylenedioxymethamphetamine for GC-MS confirmation assays. Clin. Chem. 40:1703–1706, 1994.

[7] Paul, B., Past, M., and McKinley, R. Amphetamine as an artifact of methamphetamine during periodate degradation of interfering ephedrine, pseudoephedrine and phenylpropanolamine: An improved procedure for the accurate quantitation of amphetamines in urine. J. Analyt. Toxicol. 18: 331–336, 1994.

[8] El Sohly, M. A procedure for eliminating interferences from ephedrine and related compounds. In the GC/MS analysis of amphetamine and methamphetamine J. Analyt. Toxicol. 16:109–111, 1992.

[9] Coty, J., Valtier, S., and Stillman, S. Amphetamine and fenproporex levels following multidose administration of fenproporex J. Analyt. Toxicol. 23:187–194, 1999.

[10] Coty, J., and Valtier, S. A gas chromatographic-mass spectroscopy method for the quantitation of Clobenzorex. J. Analyt. Toxicol. 23:603–608, 1999.

[11] Coty, J. Metabolic precursor to amphetamine and methamphetamine. Forensic Sci. Rev. 5:109–127, 1993.

[12] Helmlin, H., Bracher, K., and Bourquin, D. Analysis of 3,4 methylenedioxymethamphetamine (MDMA) and its metabolites in plasma and urine by HPLC-DAD and GC-MS. J. Analyt. Toxicol. 20:432–440, 1996.

[13] Product application paper: The quantification of barbiturates in human urine By GC-MS with an automate solid phase extraction system. United Chemical Technologies, Inc., 1999.

[14] Applications Manual. United Chemical Technologies, Inc., 1992 version.

[15] RapidTrace Application Manual. United Chemical Technologies, Inc., 1999 version.

[16]*Product Application Paper.* Reduced sample volume extraction of barbiturates. United Chemical Technologies, Inc., 1999.

[17]Lemberger, L., and Rubin, A. The physiologic disposition of marihuana in man. Life Sci. 17:1637–1642, 1975.

[18]Perez-Reyes, M., Owens, S., and DiGuiseppi, S. The clinical pharmacology and dynamics of marihuana cigarette smoking. J. Clin. Pharmacol. 21:201–207, 1981.

[19]Kanter, S., and Hollister, L. Marihuana metabolites in urine of man. Res. Commun. Chem. Path. Pharm. 17:421- 431, 1997.

[20]Wall, M., Sadler, B., and Brine, D. Metabolism, disposition, and kinetics of delta-9-tetrahydrocannabinol in men and Women. Clin. Pharmaceut. Ther. 34:352–363, 1983.

[21]Cone, E., and Johnson, R. Contact highs and urinary cannabinoid excretion after passive exposure to marijuana smoke. Clin. Pharmaceut. Ther. 40:247–257, 1986.

[22]Stewart, D., Inaba, T., Tang, B., and Kalow, W. Hydrolysis of cocaine in human plasma by cholinesterase. Life Sci. 20:1557–1564, 1977.

[23]Baselt, R. Stability of cocaine in biological fluids. J. Chromatogr. 268:502–505, 1983.

[24]Stewart, D., Inaba, T., Lucassen, M., Kalow, W. Cocaine metabolism: Cocaine and norcocaine hydrolysis by liver and serum esterases. Clin. Pharmacol. Ther. 25:464–468, 1979.

[25]Jatlow, P. Cocaethylene :A neuropharmacologically active metabolite associated with concurrent cocaine-ethanol ingestion. Life Sci. 48:1787–1794, 1991.

[26]Broussard, L., Presley, L., Pittman, T., Clouette, R., and Wimbish, G. Simultaneous identification and quantification of codeine, morphine, hydrocodone, and hydromorphone in urine as trimethylsilyl and oxime derivatives by gas chromatography-mass spectrometry. Clin. Chem. 43:1029–1032, 1997.

[27]Clouette, R., Wimbish, G. Improved chromatographic separation of opiates as TMS derivatives by formation of the oxime-TMS derivatives of hydrocodone and hydromorphone. J. Analyt. Toxicol. 20:77–82, 1996.

[28]Jones, C., Chaney, G., and Mastorides, S. Simultaneous analysis of Opiates in urine by SPE and GC-MS with stabilization of keto-opiates via conversion to the oxime derivative. J. Analyt. Toxicol. 21:86–92, 1997.

[29]Glass, L., Ingalls, S., Schilling, C., and Hoppel, C. Atypical urinary opiate excretion pattern. J. Analyt. Toxicol. 21:509–513, 1997.

[30]Fuller, D., and Anderson, W. A simplified procedure for the determination of codeine, free morphine and 6 acetyl morphine in urine. J. Analyt. Toxicol. 16:315–318, 1982.

[31]Basalt, R., and Cravey, R. *Disposition of Toxic Drugs and Chemicals in Man*, 4th edit. Chemical Toxicology Institute pp. 366–370, 1995.

[32]Cone, E., Welch, P., Mitchell, J., and Paul, B. Forensic drug testing for opiates I, detection of 6 acetyl morphine (6MAM) in urine as an indicator of recent heroin exposure: Drug and assay considerations and detection times. J. Analyt. Toxicol. 15:1–7, 1991.

[33]Cassella, G., Wu, A., Shaw, B., Hill, D. The analysis of thebaine in urine for the detection of poppy seed consumption. J. Analyt. Toxicol. 21:376–383, 1997.

[34]Soper J.W. A single step GC-MS procedure for quantitation of 6 monoacetylmorphine, coupled with simultaneous quantitation (6) and/or detection (8) of 14 additional opiate compounds, following derivatization with propionic anhydride. Proc. Am. Acad. Forensic Sci. 2:215–216, 1996.

[35]Pierce, D. S. Detection and quantitation of phencyclidine in blood by use of ($^2H_5$) phencyclidine and selected ion monitoring applied to nonfatal cases of phencyclidine intoxication. Clin. Chem. 22:1623–1626, 1976.

[36]Marshman, J., Ramsay, M., and Sellers, E. Quantitation of phencyclidine in biological fluids and application to human overdose. Toxicol. Appl. Pharmaceut. 35:129–136, 1976.

[37]Cook, C., Brine, D., and Jeffcoat, A. Phencyclidine disposition after intravenous and oral doses. Clin. Pharmaceut. Ther. 31:625–634, 1982.

[38]Done, A., Aronow, R., Miceli, J., Lin, D. Pharmacokinetic observations in the treatment of phencyclidine poisoning, a preliminary report management of the poisoned patient. (Rumack, B. and Temple, A., eds.), Princeton, NJ: Scientific Press, pp. 79–102, 1997.

[39]Wall M. E. Phencyclidine metabolism and disposition in man following a 100 μg intravenous dose. Res. Commun. Substance Abuse 2:161–172, 1982.

[40]Cone, E., Vaupel, D., and Buchwald, W. Phencyclidine: detection and measurement of toxic precursors and analogs in illicit samples. J. Analyt. Toxicol. 4:119–123, 1980.

[41]Marshman, J., Ramsay, M., Sellers, E. Quantitation of phencyclidine in biological fluids and application to human overdose. Toxicol. Appl. Pharmaceut. 35:129–136, 1976.

[42]Soine, W., Vincek, W., and Agee, D. Phencyclidine contaminants generate cyanide. N. Eng, J. Med. 301:438–444, 1979.

[43]UCT Internal Publication.

Selected Readings:

Amphetamines and Related Drugs

Brenneisen, K., and Mathys, K. Determination of S- (-) cathinone and its main metabolite R,S (-) norephedrine in human plasma by high-performance liquid chromatography. Liquid Chromatog. 14:271–286, 1991.

Cody, J. Determination of methamphetamine enantiomer ratios in urine by gas chromatography mass spectrometry. Chromatography 580:77–95, 1995.

Dong-Seok, L. Determination of phenylalkylamines, narcotic analgesics and beta-blockers by gas chromatography mass spectroscopy. J. Analyt. Toxicol. 14:77-83, 1990.

Ellerbe, P., Long, T., and Welch, M. The determination of amphetamine and methamphetamine in a lyophilized human urine reference material. J. Analyt. Toxicol. 17:165–169, 1993.

Fisher, D., and Bourque, A. Quantification of amphetamine in urine: Solid-phase extraction, polymeric reagent derivatization and reversed phase chromatography. Chromatography 614:142–147, 1993.

Foster, B., Gilbert, D., Hutchaleelaha, A., and Mayersohn, M. Entiomeric determination of amphetamine and methamphetamine in urine by precolumn derivatization with Marfey's reagent and HPLC. J. Analyt. Toxicol. 22:265–269, 1998.

Kunsman, G., Jones, R., Levine, B., and Smith, M. Methylephedrine concentrations in blood and urine specimens. J. Analyt. Toxicol. 22:310–313, 1998.

Lee, M., Yu, S., and Lin, C. Solid phase extraction in amphetamine and methamphetamine analysis of urine. J. Analyt. Toxicol. 21:278–282, 1997.

Mc Cambly, K., Kelly, R., Johnson, T., Johnson, J., and Brown, W. Robotic solid phase extraction of amphetamines from urine for analysis by gas chromatography-mass spectrometry. J. Analyt. Toxicol. 21:438–444, 1997.

Patel, R., Beson, J., and Hometchko, D. Solid phase extraction of amphetamine and methamphetamine using polymeric supports and heranesulfonic exanesulfonic acid. LC-GC 6:152–165, 1992.

Poklis, A., Still, J., Slattum, P., Edinboro, L. Urinary excretion of d-amphetamine following oral doses in humans: Implications for urine drug testing. J. Analyt. Toxicol. 22:481–486, 1998.

Thurman, E., Pedersen, M., Stout, R., Martin, T. Distinguishing sympathomimetic amines from amphetamine and methamphetamine in urine by gas chromatography/mass spectroscopy. J. Analyt. Toxicol. 16:19–27, 1992.

Urry, F., Kushnir, M., Nelson, G., McDowell, M., and Jennison, T. Improving ion mass ratio performance at low concentrations in methamphetamine GC-MS assay through internal standard selection. J. Analyt. Toxicol. 20:592–595, 1996.

Wu, A., Wong, S., and Johnson, K. The conversion of ephedrine to methamphetamine and methamphetamine-like compounds during and prior to gas chromatography. Biol. Mass Spectrom. 21:278–284, 1992.

Valtier, S., and Cody, J. Evaluation of internal standards for the analysis of amphetamine and methamphetamine. J. Analyt. Toxicol. 19:375–381, 1995.

Wu, A. Inigbinde, T., and Wong, S. Identification of methamphetamines and over-the counter sympathomimetic amines by full scan GC ion trap MS with electron impact and chemical ionization. J. Analyt. Toxicol. 16:137–141, 1992.

Zhou, X., and Krull, S. Direct enantiomeric analysis of amphetamine in plasma by simultaneous solid phase extraction and chiral derivatization. Chromatographia 35:153–160, 1993.

Amphetamine and Methamphetamine Designer Analogs

Giroud, C., Augsburger, M., Rivier, L., and Mangin, P. 2C-B: A new psychoactive phenylethylamine recently discovered in ecstasy tablets sold on the Swiss black market. J. Analyt. Toxicol. 22:345–354.

Helmlin, H., Bracher, K., Bourquin, D., and Vonlanthen, D. Analysis of 3, 4-methylenedioxymethamphetamine (MDMA) and its metabolites in plasma and urine by HPLC-DAD and GC-MS. J. Analyt. Toxicol. 20:422–430, 1996.

Juraldo, C.,Gimenez, M., Soriano, T., Menendez, M., and Repetto, M. Rapid analysis of amphetamine, methamphetamine MDA and MDMA using solid phase micro extraction, direct on-fiber derivatization and analysis by GC-MS. J. Analyt. Toxicol. 24:11–15, 2000.

Kunsman, G., Levine, B., Kuhlman, J., and Jones, R. MDA-MDMA concentrations in urine samples. J. Analyt. Toxicol. 20:517–521, 1996.

Thompson, W., and Dasgupta, A. Microwave induced rapid preparation of fluoro derivatives of amphetamine, methamphetamine and 3, 4 methylenedioxymethamphetamine for GC-MS confirmation assays. Clin. Chem. 40:1703–1706, 1994.

Brzezinka, B., Bold, P., and Budzikiewicz, H. A screening method for the rapid detection of barbiturates in serum by means of tandem mass spectrometry. Biol. Mass Spectrom. 22:346–350, 1993.

Colbert, D., Smith, D., Landon, J., and Sidki, A. Single reagent polarization fluoroimmunoassay for barbiturates in urine. Clin. Chem. 30:1765–1767, 1984.

Joern, W. Unexpected volatility of barbiturate derivatives: An extractive alkylation procedure for barbiturates and benzoylecgonine. J. Analyt. Toxicol. 18:423–427, 1994.

Mule, S., Casella, G. Confirmation and quantitation of barbiturates in human urine by GC-MS. J. Analyt. Toxicol. 13:13–16, 1989.

Pocci, R., Dixit, V., and Dixit, V. Y. Solid-phase extraction and GC/MS confirmation of barbiturates from human urine. J. Analyt. Toxicol. 16:45–48, 1990.

Smith, F., and Pomposini, D. Detection of phenobarbital in bloodstains, semen, seminal stains, saliva, saliva stains perspiration stains and hair. J. Forensic Sci. 26:582–586, 1981.

Berrueta, L., Gallo, B., and Vicente, F. Analysis of oxazepam in urine using solid-phase extraction and high-performance liquid chromatography with fluorescence detection by post-column derivatization. J. Chromatogr. 616:344–348, 1993.

Casas, M., Berueta, L., Gallo, B., and Vicente, F. Solid phase extraction of 1, 4-benzodiazepines from biological fluids. J. Pharmaceut. Biomed. Analysis 1:277–284, 1993.

DeMeglio, D., and Locke, K. A bonded phase extraction procedure for the separation of benzodiazepines from tricyclic antidepressants. UCT internal publication.

Ferrara, S., Tedeschi, L., Frison, G., and Castagna, F. Solid-phase extraction and HPLC-UV confirmation of drugs of abuse in urine J. Analyt. Toxicol. 16:217–222, 1992.

Glass, L., Ingalls, S., and Hoppel, C. Factors affecting enzymatic hydrolysis, mixed mode solid phase extractions and GC-MS analysis of urinary nordiazepam, oxazepam, temazepam and α hydroxyalprazolam. Poster—SOFT 97, 1997.

Hall, M., Robinson, C., and Brissie, R. High-performance liquid chromatography of alprazolam in postmortem blood using solid-phase extraction. J. Analyt. Toxicol. 19:511–513, 1995.

He, W., Parissis, N., and Kiratzdis, T. Determination of benzodiazepines in forensic samples by HPLC with photodiode detection. J. Forensic Sci. 43:1061–1067, 1998.

Hold, K., Crouch, D., Rollins, D., and Wilkins, D. Determination of aprazolam and α
    hdroxyalprazolam in human plasma by gas chromatography/negative-ion chemical ioniza-
    tion mass spectrometry. J. Mass Spectrom. 31: 1033–1039, 1996.

Lambert, W., Meyer, E., Xue-Ping, Y., and De Leenheer, A. Screening, identification and
    quantitation of benzodiazepines in postmortem samples by HPLC with photodiode array
    detection. J. Analyt. Toxicol. 19:35–40, 1995.

Moore, C., Long, G., and Marr, M. Confirmation of benzodiazepines in urine as trimethylsilyl
    derivatives using gas chromatography-mass spectroscopy.
J. Chromatogr. B: Biomed. Appl. 655:132–137, 1994.

West, R., and Ritz, D. GC/MS analysis of five common benzodiazepine metabolites in urine as
    tert butyl dimethyl silyl derivatives. J. Analyt. Toxicol. 17:114–116, 1993.

Cirimele, V., and Kintz, P. Testing human hair for flunitrazepam and 7 aminoflunitrazepam by
    GC-MS-NCI. Forensic Sci. Int. 84:189–200, 1997.

Deinl, I., Frazelius, C., and Angeraier, L. On line immuno-affinity extraction and HPLC analy-
    sis of flunitrazepam and its main metabolites in serum. J. Analyt. Toxicol. 23:598–602,
    1999.

Deinl, I., Mahr, G., and Von Meyer, L. Determination of flunitrazepam and its major metabolite
    in serum and urine by HPLC after mixed mode solid-phase extraction.
J. Analyt. Toxicol. 22:197–202, 1998.

El Sohly, M., Feng, S., Salamone, S., and Wu, R. A sensitive GC-MS procedure for the analysis
    of flunitrazepam and its metabolites in urine. J. Analyt. Toxicol. 21:61–67, 1997.

Greenblatt, D. Automated electron capture gas chromatographic analysis of flunitrazepam in
    plasma. J. Analyt. Toxicol. 21:341–345.

He, W., and Parissis, N. Simultaneous determination of flunitrazepam and its metabolites in
    plasma and urine by HPLC/DAD after solid phase extraction. J. Pharmaceut. Biomed.
    Analysis 16:707–715, 1997.

LeBeau, M., Montgomery, M., Wagner, J., and Miller, M. Analysis of bio-fluids for flunitrazepam
    and metabolites by electrospray LC-MS. J. Forensic Sci. 45:1133–1141, 2000.

Ngyen, H., and Nan, D. Rapid method for the solid-phase extraction and GC-MS analysis of
    flunitrazepam and its major metabolites in urine. J. Analyt. Toxicol. 24:37–45, 2000.

Negrusz, A., Moore, C., Deitermann, D. Highly sensitive micro-plate enzyme immuno-assay
    screening and NCI-GC-MS confirmation of flunitrazepam and its major metabolite 7-
    aminoflunitrazepam in hair. J. Analyt. Toxicol. 23:429–435, 1999.

O'Dell, L., Chaney, G., Darpino, Telepchak, M. Evaluation of reduced solvent volume solid-
    phase extraction cartridges with with analysis by gas chromatography-mass spectroscopy
    for determination of 11-nor-9 carboxy Δ^9 THC in urine. J. Analyt. Toxicol. 21:433–437,
    1997.

Baker, T., Harry, J., Russell, J., and Myers, R. Rapid method for the GC-MS confirmation of
    11-nor-carboxy-Δ^9-tetahydrocannabinol in urine. J. Analyt. Toxicol. 8:255–259, 1994.

Blanc, J., Manneh, V., Ernst, R.. Adsorption losses from urine-based cannabinoid calibrators
    during routine use. Clin. Chem. 39:1705–1712, 1993.

Brunk, S. False negative GC/MS assay for carboxy THC due to ibuprofen interference.
    J. Analyt. Toxicol. 12:290–291, 1988.

Cirimele, V., Sachs, H., Kintz, P., and Mangin, P. Testing human hair for cannabis. III Rapid
    screening procedure for the simultaneous identification of Δ^9-tetrahydrocannabinol, can-
    nabinol, and cannabidiol. J. Analyt. Toxicol. 20:13–16, 1996.

Clouette, R., Jacob, M., Koteel, P., and Spain, M. Confirmation of 11 nor-Δ^9-tetrahydrocannab-
    inol in urine as its t-butyldimethylsilyl derivative using GC/MS. J. Analyt. Toxicol. 17:1–
    4, 1993.

Congost, M., De la Torre, R., and Segura, J. Optimization of the quantitative analysis of the
    major cannabis metabolite in urine by GC/MS. Biomed. Environ. Mass Spectrom. 16:367–
    372, 1998.

Foltz, R., McGinnis, K., Chinn, D. Quantitative measurement of Δ^9-tetrahydrocannabinol and two major metabolites in physiological specimens using capillary column gas chromatography/negative ion chemical ionization mass spectrometry. Biomed. Mass Spectrom.10:316–323, 1983.

Goldberger, B., and Cone, E. Confirmatory tests for drugs in the workplace by GC/MS. J. Chromatogr. A, 674:73–86, 1994.

Hall, B., Satterfield-Dover, M., Parikh, A., and Brodbelt, J. Determination of cannabinoids in water and human saliva by solid-phase microextraction and quadrupole ion trap GC/MS. Analyt. Chem. 70:1788–1796, 1998.

Huang, W., Moody, D., and Foltz, R. Simultaneous determination of Δ^9-tetrahydrocannabinol and 11-nor-9-carboxy-Δ^9tetrahydrocannabinol in human plasma by solid-phase extraction. and gas chromatography negative ion chemical ionization mass spectrometry. Presented at the SOFT/TIAFT Conference, Albuquerque, NM, 1998.

Joem, W. Surface adsorption of the urinary marijuana carboxy metabolite: The problem and a partial solution. J. Analyt. Toxicol.16:401– 440, 1992.

Johnson, J., Jennison, T., Peat, M., and Foltz, R. Stability of Δ^9-tetrahydrocannabinol (THC), 11-hydroxy-THC, and 11-nor-9-carboxy-THC in blood and plasma. J. Analyt. Toxicol. 8:202–204, 1984.

Lindgren, J. Quantification of Δ^9-tetrahydrocannabinol in tissues and body fluids. Arch. Toxicol. 6:74–80, 1988.

Kemp, P., Abukhalaf, I., Manno, J. Cannabinoids in humans.

II The influence of three methods of hydrolysis on the concentration of THC and two metabolites in urine. J. Analyt. Toxicol.19:292–298, 1995.

Kemp, P., Abukhalaf, I., Manno, B., Manno, J. Cannabinoid concentrations detected in human urine by GC/MS are influenced by the method of hydrolysis used. Presented at the TIAFT-SOFT, Tampa, FL, 1994.

Kemp, P., Abukhalaf, I., Manno, J. Cannabinoids in humans. 1. Analysis of Δ^9-tetrahydrocannabinol and six metabolites in plasma and urine using GC/MS. J. Analyt. Toxicol. 9:285–289, 1995.

Kintz, P., Cirimele, V., and Mangin, P. Testing human hair for cannabis. 11. Identification of THC-COOH by GC/NCI-MS as a unique proof. J. Forensic Sci. 40:619–622, 1995.

Lemm, U., Tenczer, J., and Baudisch, H. Antibody-mediated extraction of the main tetrahydrocannabinol metabolite from human urine and its identification by GC/MS in the sub-nanogram range. J. Chromatogr. 342:393–398, 1985.

McBurney, L., Bobbie, B., and Sepp, L. GC/MS and EMIT analysis for Δ^9-tetrahydrocannabinol metabolites in plasma and urine of human subjects. J. Analyt. Toxicol. 10:56–64, 1986.

Moeller, M., Doerr, G., and Warth, S. Simultaneous quantitation of delta-9-tetrahydrocannabinol (THC) and 11-nor-9-carboxy Δ^9-tetrahydrocannabinol (THC-COOH) in serum by GC/MS using deuterated internal standards and its application to a smoking study and forensic cases. J. Forensic Sci. 37:969–983, 1992.

Moore, C., Lewis, D., Becker, J., and Leikin, J. The determination of 11 -nor-Δ^9-tetrahydrocannabinol-9-carboxylic acid in meconium. J. Analyt. Toxicol. 20:50–54, 1996.

Odell, L., Rymut, K., Chaney, G., Darpino, T., and Telepchak, M. Evaluation of reduced solvent volume solid-phase extraction columns with analysis by GC/MS for the determination of 11-nor-9-carboxy-Δ^9-THC in urine. J. Analyt. Toxicol. 21:433–437, 1997.

Singh, J., and Johnson, L. Solid-phase extraction of THC metabolite from urine using the Empore disk cartridge prior to analysis by GC-MS. J. Analyt. Toxicol. 21:384–387, 1997.

Stonebraker, W., Lamoreaux, T., Bebault, M. Robotic solid-phase extraction and GC/MS analysis of THC in blood. Am. Clin. Lab. 17:18–29, 1998.

Szirmai, M., Beck, O., Stephansson, N., and Halldin, M. A GC/MS study of three major acidic metabolites of Δ^9-tetrahydrocannabinol J. Analyt. Toxicol. 20:573–578, 1996.

Wimbish, G., and Johnson, K. Full spectral GC/MS identification of Δ^9-carboxy-tetrahydro-cannabinol in urine with the Finnigan ITS 40. J. Analyt. Toxicol. 14:292–295, 1990.

Aderjan, R., Schmitt, G., Wu, M., and Meyer, C. Determination of cocaine and benzoylecgonine by derivatization with Iodomethane-D3 or PFPA/HFIP in human blood and urine. J. Analyt. Toxicol. 17:51–55, 1993.

Cone, E., Yousefnejad, D., Hilisgrove, M., Holicky, B., and Darwin, W. Passive inhalation of cocaine. J. Analyt. Toxicol. 19:399–411, 1995.

Cone, E. Pharmacokinetics and pharmacodynamics of cocaine. J. Analyt. Toxicol. 19:459–478, 1995.

Cone, E., Darwin, W. Rapid assay of cocaine, opiates and metabolites by gas chromatography-mass spectrometry. J. Chromatogr. 16:43–61, 1992.

Cone, E., Oyler, J., and Darwin, W. Cocaine disposition in saliva following intravenous, intranasal, and smoking. J. Analyt. Toxicol. 21:465–475, 1992.

Cone, E., Yousefnejad, D., Darwin, W., and Maguire, T. Testing human hair for drugs of abuse. 11. Identification of unique cocaine metabolites in hair of drug abusers. J. Analyt. Toxicol. 15:250–252, 1991.

Cone, E., Kato, K., Hillsgrove, M. Cocaine excretion in the semen of drug users. J. Analyt. Toxicol. 20:139–140, 1996.

Cone, E., Hilisgrove, M., and Darwin, W. Simultaneous measurement of cocaine, cocaethylene, their metabolites, and "crack" pyrolysis products by gas chromatography-mass spectrometry. Clin. Chem. 40:129 - 130, 1994.

Crouch, D., Alburges, M., Spanbauer, A., Rollins, D., and Moody, D. Analysis of cocaine and its metabolites from biological specimens using solid-phase extraction and positive ion chemical ionization mass spectrometry. J. Analyt. Toxicol.19:352–358, 1995.

Farre, M., de la Torre, R., Llorente, M. Alcohol and cocaine interactions in humans. J. Pharmacol. Exp. Ther. 266:1364–1373, 1993.

Harkey, M., Henderson, G., and Zhou, C. Simultaneous quantitation of cocaine and its major metabolites in human hair by gas chromatography-chemical ionization mass spectroscopy. J. Analyt. Toxicol. 15:260–265, 1991.

Henderson, G., Harkey, M., Zhou, C., and Jones, R. Cocaine and metabolite concentrations in the hair of South American coca chewers. J. Analyt. Toxicol. 16:199–201, 1992.

Jain, L., Meyer, W., Moore, C. Detection of fetal cocaine exposure by analysis of amniotic fluid. Obstet. Gynecol. 81:787–790, 1993.

Jennison, T., Wozniak, E., Jones, C., and Urryl, F. The reliability of a solid-phase extraction system for the analysis of benzoylecgonine in urine. J. Chromatogr. Sci. 32:2–6, 1994.

Kato, K., Hilisgrove, M., Weinhold, L., Gorelick, D., Darwin, W., and Cone, E. Cocaine and metabolite excretion in saliva under stimulated and non-stimulated conditions. J. Analyt. Toxicol. 17:338–341, 1993.

Martinez, F., Poet, T., Pillai, R. Cocaine metabolite (benzoylecgonine) in hair and urine of drug users. J. Analyt. Toxicol. 17:138–142, 1993.

Moller, M., Fey, P., and Rimbach, S. Identification and quantitation of cocaine and its metabolites benzoylecgonine and ecgonine methyl ester, in hair of Bolivian coca chewers by gas chromatography/ mass spectroscopy. J. Analyt. Toxicol. 16:291–296, 1992.

Moore, C., Browne, S., Tebbett, I., Negrusz, A. Determination of cocaine and its metabolites in brain tissue using high-flow solid phase extraction columns and high-performance liquid chromatography. Forensic Sci. Int. 53:215–219, 1992.

Moore, C., Browne, S., Tebbett, I., Negrusz, A., Meyer, W., and Jaine, L. Determination of cocaine and benzoylecgonine in human amniotic fluid by using high flow solid phase extraction columns and HPLC. Forensic Sci. Int. 56:177–181, 1993.

Moore, C., Browne, S., Tebbett, I., Negrusz, A., Meyer, W., and Jaine, L. Determination of cocaine and its major metabolite, benzoylecgonine, in amniotic fluid, umbilical cord blood, umbilical cord tissue, and neonatal urine: A case study. J. Analyt. Toxicol. 17:62–65, 1993.

Murphy, L., Olsen, G., and Konkol, R. Quantitation of benzoyl-norecgonine and other cocaine metabolites in meconium by high-performance liquid; chromatography. J. Chromatogr. 613:330–335, 1993.

Nakashima, K., Okamoto, M., Yoshida, K. Preparation of a fluorescent derivative of benzoylecgonine and preliminary studies of its application to the analysis of urine. J. Chromatogr. 584:275–279, 1992.

Oyler, J., Darwin, W., Preston, K., Suess, P., and Cone, E. Cocaine disposition in meconium from newborns of cocaine-abusing mothers and urine of adult drug users. J. Analyt. Toxicol. 20:453–462, 1996.

Paul, B., Dreka, C., Summers, J., Smith, M. One-step esterification of benzoylecgonine with dimethylformamide-dipropylacetal or dimethylformamide-disopropylacetal in the presence of urine. J. Analyt. Toxicol. 20:506–508, 1996.

Ripple, M., Golberger, B., Caplan, Y., Blitzer, M., and Schwartz, S. Detection of cocaine and its metabolites in human amniotic fluid. J. Analyt. Toxicol. 16:328–381, 1992.

Roy, I., Jefferies, T., Threadgill, M., and Dewar, G. Analysis of cocaine, benzoylecgonine, ecgonine methyl ester, ethylcocaine and norcocaine in human urine using HPLC with post column ion-pair extraction and fluorescence detection. Pharmaceut. Biomed. Analysis 10:223–227, 1990.

Schramm, W., Craig, P., Smith, R., Berger, G. Cocaine and benzoylecgonine in saliva, serum, and urine. Clin. Chem. 36:481–485, 1993.

Winecker, R., Goldberger, B., Tebbett, I. Detection of cocaine and its metabolites in amniotic fluid and umbilical cord tissue. J. Analyt. Toxicol. 21:97–104, 1997.

Wu, A., Onigbinde, T., Johnson, K., and Wimbish, G. Alcohol-specific cocaine metabolites in serum and urine of hospitalized patients. J. Analyt. Toxicol. 16:132–136, 1997.

Paul, B., Mitchell, J., and Burbage, R. Gas chromatographic electron-impact mass fragmentometric determination of lysergic acid diethylamide in urine. J. Chromatogr. 529:103–112, 1990.

Poch, G., Klette, K., Hallare, D., Manglicmot, M. Detection of metabolites of lysergic acid diethylamide (LSD) in human urine specimens: 2-Oxo-3-hydroxy-LSD, a prevalent metabolite of LSD. J. Chromatogr. B 724:23–33, 1999.

Poch, G., Klette, K., and Anderson, C. The quantitation of 2-oxo-3-hydroxylysergic acid diethylamide (O-H-LSD) in human urine specimens, a metabolite of LSD: Comparative analysis using liquid chromatography-selected ion monitoring mass spectroscopy and liquid chromatography-ion trap mass spectroscopy. J. Analyt. Toxicol. 24:170–179, 2000.

Sklerov, J., Kalasinsky, K., and Ehorn, C. Detection of lysergic acid diethylamide (LSD) in urine by gas chromatography-ion trap tandem mass spectroscopy. J. Analyt. Toxicol. 23:474–478, 1999.

Besner, J., Band, C., Rondeau, J., Yamlahi, L., Caille, G., Varin, F., and Stewart, J. Determination of opiates and other basic drugs by high-performance liquid chromatography with electrochemical detection. Pharmaceut. Biomed. Analysis 7:1811–1814, 1989.

Bouquillon, A., Freeman, D., and Moulin, D. Simultaneous solid-phase extraction and chromatographic analysis of morphine and hydromorphone in plasma. J. Chromatogr. 577:354–357, 1992.

Chad, G., Gulati, A., Bhat, R., Tebbett, I. High-performance liquid chromatographic determination of morphine, morphin-3-glucuronide and morphine-6-glucuronide. J. Chromatogr. 571:263–270, 1991.

Cone, E., Holicky, B., Grant, T., Darwin, W., and Goldberger, B. Pharmacokinetics and pharmacy of intranasal "snorted" heroin. J. Analyt. Toxicol. 17:327–337, 1993.

Soares, M., Seabra, V., De Lourdes, M., and Bastos, A. Comparative study of different extractive procedures to quantify morphine in urine by HPLC-UV. J. Liq. Chromatogr. 15:1533–1545, 1992.

Goldberger, B., Cone, E., Grant, T., Caplan, Y., Levine, B., and Smialek, J. Disposition of heroin and its metabolites in heroin-related deaths. J. Analyt. Toxicol. 18:22–28, 1994.

Goldberger, B., Darwin, W., Grant, T., Allen, A., Caplan, Y., and Cone, E. Measurement of heroin and its metabolites by isotope-dilution electron-impact mass spectrometry. Clin. Chem. 39:670–675, 1993.

Hanisch, P., and Meyer, L. Determination of the heroin metabolite 6-monoacetylmorphine in urine by high performance liquid chromatography with mass spectroscopy. J. Analyt. Toxicol. 17:220–223, 1993.

Heybrook, W., Caulfield, W., Johnston, A., Turner, P. Automatic on-line extraction coupled with electrochemical detection as an improved method for the HPLC co-analysis of codeine and morphine in plasma and gastric juice. Pharmaceut. Biomed. Analysis 8:1021–1027, 1990.

Hold, K., Wilkins, D., Crouch, D., Rollins, D., and Maes, R. Detection of stanzolol in hair by negative ion chemical ionization mass spectrometry. J. Analyt. Toxicol. 20:345–349, 1996.

Jenkins, A., Oyler, J., and Cone, E. Comparison of heroin and cocaine concentrations in blood and plasma. J. Analyt. Toxicol. 19:359–374, 1995.

Kuhlman, J., Magluilo, J., Cone, E., and Levine, B. Simultaneous assay of buprenorphine and norbuprenorphine by negative chemical ionization tandem mass spectrometry. J. Analyt. Toxicol. 20:229–235, 1996.

Kuhlman, J., Lalani, S., Magluilo, J., Levine, B., Darwin, W., Johnson, R., and Cone, E. Human pharmacokinetics of intravenous, sublingual and buccal buprenorphine. J. Analyt. Toxicol. 20:369–378, 1996.

Milne, R., Nation, R., Reynolds, G., Somogyi, A., Van Crugten, V. High performance liquid chromatographic determination of morphine and its 3- and 6-glucuronide metabolites. J. Chromatogr. 565:457–464, 1991.

O'Neal, C., and Poklis, A. Simultaneous determination of acetylcodeine, monoacetylmorphine, and other opiates in urine by GC-MS. J. Analyt. Toxicol. 21:427–439.

Papadoyannis, I., Zotou, A., Samanidou, V., Theodoridis, G., and Zougrou, F. Comparative study of different solid phase extraction cartridges the simultaneous RP-HPLC analysis of morphine and codeine. J. Liq. Chromatogr. 16:3017–3040, 1992.

Zaromb, S., Alcaraz, J., Lawson, D., and Woo, C. Detection of airborne cocaine and heroin by high-throughput liquid-absorption preconcentration and liquid chromatography. J. Chromatogr. 643:107–115, 1993.

Bailey, D., and Guba, J. Measurement of phencyclidine in saliva. J. Analyt. Toxicol. 4: 311–313, 1980.

Grieshaber, A., Constantino, A., and Lappas, N. Stability of phencyclidine in stored blood samples. J. Analyt. Toxicol. 22:515–524, 1998.

Stevenson, C., Cibull, D., Platoff, G., Bush, D., Gere, J. Solid phase extraction of phenyclidine from urine followed by capillary gas chromatography/mass spectrometry. J. Analyt. Toxicol. 16:337–339, 1992.

Tai, S., Christensen, R., Coakley, K., Ellerbe, P., Long, T., Welch, M. Certification of phencyclidine in lyophilized human urine reference materials. J. Analyt. Toxicol. 20: 43–49, 1996.

Chapter 10

Selected Solid Phase Extraction Applications in Drug Analysis

The following chapters will outline specific analytical methods that have been published or have been developed in the laboratory for selected drugs, highlighting the use of solid phase extraction.

The format for presenting these data will be the same as that in previous chapters.

10.1 ANALYSIS OF β BLOCKERS AND AGONISTS

The discovery of β-receptors on human cells has led to significant developments in the area of pharmacological agents. β-adrenergic antagonists, termed β blockers have had significant therapeutic impact in the treatment of cardiac arrhythmias, hypertension, and anxiety. β_2-agonists are useful as bronchodilators and in the treatment of asthma. All β-adrenergic drugs (agonists and antagonists) have been banned by the International Olympic Committee and the International Sports Federation because of their sympathomimetic activity. The analysis of these agents is difficult, owing to the extensive metabolism of these agents with similar structures and metabolisms. The first application of this isolation was done in the area of equine testing for horse racing, using an XtrackT large-particle-size DAU sorbent. This sorbent would allow the viscous horse urine to pass through without plugging the column. A number of methods are presented. A summary of chromatographic data for the methaneboronate derivatives of β-adrenergic agents is shown in Table 1. Table 3 shows similar data for TMS derivatives of β-agonists.

From: *Forensic Science and Medicine:*
Forensic and Clinical Applications of Solid Phase Extraction
Edited by: M. J. Telepchak, T. F. August, and G. Chaney © Humana Press Inc., Totowa, NJ

Table 1
β-Adrenergic Agents: Methaneboronate Derivatives

β-blockings agents	Mol Weight	Relative retention time	Percent Recovery from SPE	Primary[b] ion	Secondary ion	Tertiary ion
Carteolol	316	1.2	96%	301	316	218
Metoprolol	291	1.59	97%	276	291	140
Nadolol	357	1.91	97%	342	357	217
Alprenolol	273	1.17	97%	258	273	138
Timolol	340	1.904	94%	340	325	152
Acebutolol	360	2.17	91%	246	299	360
Bisoprolol	349	1.31	101%	230	334	349
Betaxolol	331	1.32	98%	316	331	246
Oxprenolol	289	1.34	94%	274	289	218
Pindolol	272	1.85	99%	272	257	124
Atenolol	290	1.93	92%	275	290	164
Propranol	283	1.77	92%	283	268	128
Labetalol	376	2.24	93%	271	229	361, 376
Sotalol	296	1.906	94%	281	296	239
Isoproterenol[a]	259	1.0		202	244	259

[a]Internal standard.
[b]Quantitation ion.

10.1.1 β-Blockers (β-Adrenergic Agents) in Urine for GC-MS Confirmations Using 200-mg CLEAN SCREEN Extraction Column (ZSDAU020 or ZCDAU020)

1. **Condition CLEAN SCREEN® extraction column.**
    1 × 3 mL of methanol; aspirate.
    1 × 3 mL of deionized water; aspirate.
    1 × 3 mL of 0.1 M acetate buffer, pH 4.7.
    Note: Aspirate at ≤3 in. Hg to prevent sorbent drying.
2. **Apply sample.**
    a. Take 1 mL of urine and add 2 mL of 0.1 M acetate buffer, at pH 4.7.
    b. Load at 1–2 mL/ min.
3. **Wash column.**
    1 × 1 mL of methanol.
    1 × 2 mL of deionized water; aspirate.
    1 × 2 mL of 20% 0.1 M acetate buffer, pH 4.7; aspirate.
    Dry column (5 min at ≥10 in. Hg).
    2 × 1 mL acetone-methanol (1:1); aspirate.
4. **Elute β-blockers.**
    1 × 1 mL of dichloromethane-isopropanol-ammonium hydroxide (82:16:2).
    Collect the eluate by gravity feed.
    Note: Prepare elution solvent fresh daily.

5. Dry eluate.

Evaporate to dryness at ≤40°C.

6. Derivatize.

Derivatization solution:

a. Methaneboronic acid at 5 mg/mL prepared in dry ethyl acetate (use molecular sieve).

b. Store this solution at –20°C (freezer conditions) until use.

Reaction mixture:

a. Add 100 µL of the methaneboronic acid solution (*see* derivatization solutions above).

b. Mix/vortex.

c. React 15 min at 70°C. Remove from heat source to cool.

Note: Do not evaporate this solution.

7. Analysis.

Inject 1–2 µL of sample (derivatized solution).

Reference

Branum, G., Sweeney, S., Palmeri, A., Haines, L., Huber, C. The feasibility of the detection and quantitation of β adrenergic blockers by solid phase extraction and subsequent derivatization with methaneboronic acid. J Analyt. Toxicol. 22:135–141, 1998.

10.1.2 β-Blockers (β₂-Agonists) in Urine for GC-MS Confirmations Using 200-mg CLEAN SCREEN Extraction Column (ZSDAU020 or ZCDAU020)

1. Condition CLEAN SCREEN extraction column.

1 × 3 mL of methanol; aspirate.

1 × 3 mL of deionized water; aspirate.

1 × 3 mL of 0.1 *M* acetate buffer, pH 4.7.

Note: Aspirate at ≤3 in. Hg to prevent sorbent drying.

2. Apply sample.

a. Take 1 mL of urine and add 2 mL of 0.1 *M* acetate buffer, pH 4.7.

b. Load at 1–2 mL/min.

3. Wash column.

1 × 1mL of methanol.

1 × 2 mL of deionized water; aspirate.

1 × 2 mL 20% 0.1 *M* acetate buffer, pH 4.7; aspirate.

Dry column (5 min at ≥10 in. Hg).

2 × 1 mL acetone-methanol (1:1); aspirate.

4. Elute β blockers.

1 × 1mL dichloromethane-isopropanol-ammonium hydroxide (82:16:2).

Collect the eluate by gravity feed.

Note: Prepare elution solvent fresh daily.

5. Dry eluate.

Evaporate to dryness at ≤40°C.

6. Derivatize.

Derivatization solution:

a. Methaneboronic acid at 5 mg/mL prepared in dry ethyl acetate (use molecular sieve).

b. Store this solution at –20°C (freezer conditions) until use.

Reaction mixture:

a. Add 100 µL of the methaneboronic acid solution (*see* derivatization solution above).

b. Mix/vortex.

Table 2

Compound	Primary ion	Secondary ion	Tertiary ion
Carisoprodol	260	245	158
Meprobamate	144	114	83
Hexobarbital[a]	221	157	236

[a]Internal standard.

c. React 15 min at 70°C. Remove from heat source to cool.
Note: Do not evaporate this solution.
7. **Analyze.**
Inject 1–2 μL of sample (derivatized solution).

10.2 CARISOPRODOL AND ITS METABOLITES IN URINE BY GC-MS ANALYSIS USING A 200-MG CLEAN SCREEN EXTRACTION COLUMN (ZSDAU020 OR ZCDAU020)

1. **Prepare sample.**
    a. To 0.5 mL of sample add internal standard and 2 mL of 0.1 *M* phosphate buffer, pH 6.0.
    b. Add 2 mL of 0.1 *M* phosphate buffer, pH 6.0.
    c. Sample pH should be 6.0 ± 0.5. Adjust pH accordingly with 0.1 *M* monobasic or dibasic sodium phosphate.
2. **Condition 200-mg CLEAN SCREEN extraction column.**
    1 × 3 mL of CH₃OH; aspirate.
    1 × 3 mL of DI H₂O; aspirate.
    1 × 2 mL of 0.1 *M* phosphate buffer, pH 6.0; aspirate.
    Note: Aspirate at ≤3 in. Hg to prevent sorbent drying.
3. **Apply sample.**
    Load at 1–2 mL/min.
4. **Wash column.**
    1 × 4 mL of DI H₂O; aspirate.
    1 × 2 mL of 1.0 *M* acetic acid; pH 4.5.
    Dry column (5 min at ≥10 in. Hg).
    Dry inside of column using cotton-tipped application stick.
    1 × 3 mL of hexane; aspirate.
    Dry column (5 min at ≥10 in. Hg).
5. **Elute carisoprodol and metabolites.**
    1 × 4 mL of CH₂Cl₂–IPA–NH₄OH (78:20:2); collect the eluate at 1–2 mL/min.
6. **Dry eluate.**
    Evaporate to dryness at ≤40°C.
7. **Quantitate.**
    a. Reconstitute the dried sample with 100 μL of derivatization grade acetonitrile.
    b. Inject 1–2 μL of sample onto chromatograph.
    c. Monitor the following ions (GC-MS):

Table 3
TMS Derivatives of β_2-Agonists

β_2-Agonists	Molecular weight time	Retention time (min) (AMU)	Primary[b] ion	Secondary ion	Tertiary ion
Salbutamol tris-TMS	445	4.8	369	86 (67%)	350 (8%)
Clenbuterol mono-TMS	349	4.6	86	262 (20%)	243 (7%)
Terbutylene tris-TMS	441	4.5	356	86 (87%)	426 (4%)
Fenoterol tetra-TMS	591	7.2	322	412 (63%)	356 (39%) 236 (34%)
Isoprenaline tris-TMS	427	4.7	355	72 (72%)	356 (68%) 357 (30%) 412 (4%)
Bamethane[a] bis-TMS	353	4.0	267	86 (67%)	338 (4%)

[a]Bamethane is used as the internal standard (500 ng/mL).
[b]Quantitation ion.

10.3 CLONAZEPAM AND 7-AMINOCLONAZEPAM IN URINE FOR GC-MS CONFIRMATIONS USING A 200-MG CLEAN SCREEN EXTRACTION COLUMN (ZSDAU020 OR ZCDAU020)

1. **Prepare sample: β-glucuronidase hydrolysis.**
   a. To 2 mL of urine add internal standard(s)[a] and 1 mL of β-glucuronidase solution.
   b. β-glucuronidase solution contains 5000 FU/mL of *Patella vulgata* in 0.1 *M* phosphate buffer, pH 6.0.
   c. Mix/vortex. Hydrolyze for 3 h at 65°C using a tube heater block.
   d. Cool before proceeding.
2. **Condition CLEAN SCREEN extraction column.**
   1 × 3 mL of methanol; aspirate.
   1 × 3 mL of deionized water; aspirate.
   1 × 1 mL 0.1 M phosphate buffer, pH 6.0.
   Note: Aspirate at ≤3 in. Hg to prevent sorbent drying.
3. **Apply sample.**
   Load at 1–2 mL/min.
4. **Wash column.**
   1 × 2 mL of deionized water; aspirate.
   1 × 2 mL 20% acetonitrile in 0.1 *M* phosphate buffer, pH 6.0; aspirate.

Table 4

Compound	Primary Ion[b]	Secondary ion	Tertiary ion
Clonazepam	372	374	326
7-Aminoclonazepam	342	344	399
Oxazepam-D[5a]	462	464	463

[a]Suggested internal standard for GC-MS: oxazepam-D[5].
[b]Quantitation ion.
Source: UCT internal publication.

Dry column (5 min at ≥10 in. Hg).
1 × 2 mL of hexane; aspirate.

5. **Elute clonazepam and 7-aminoclonazepam.**

1 × 3 mL of ethyl acetate with 2% NH_4OH: collect eluate at 1–2 mL/min.
Note: Prepare fresh daily.

6. **Dry eluate.**

Evaporate to dryness at ≤40°C.

7. **Derivatize.**

a. Add 50 µL of ethyl acetate and 50 µL of MTBSTFA (with 1% TBDMCS).
b. Mix/vortex.
c. React 20 min at 90°C. Remove from heat source to cool.
Note: Do not evaporate MTBSTFA solution.

8. **Analysis.**

a. Inject 1–2-µL sample (MTBSTFA solution)
b. Principal ions (mass selective detection):

10.4 DHEA, TESTOSTERONE, AND EPITESTOSTERONE IN URINE FOR GC OR GC-MS ANALYSIS USING A 200-MG CLEAN-THRU® EXTRACTION COLUMN (ZCDAU020)

1. **Prepare sample.**

a. Pipet 5 mL of urine into 16 × 100 mm borosilicate glass test tubes.
b. Add internal standard, adjust sample pH to 5.5–6.5 using concentrated sodium phosphate monobasic or dibasic. Mix sample.
c. Centrifuge samples at 1509*g* for 5 min.

2. **Condition CLEAN SCREEN extraction column.**

1 × 3 mL of CH_3OH; aspirate.
1 × 3 mL of DI H_2O; aspirate.
1 × 3 mL of 0.1 *M* phosphate buffer, pH 6.0.

3. **Apply sample.**

a. Pour supernatant onto the column.
b. Allow to flow via gravity.

4. **Wash column.**

1 × 3 mL of DI H_2O; aspirate.
Dry column (10 min at ≥10 mm Hg).

5. **Elute steroids.**

1 × 3 mL of methanol.

Table 5

Compound	Primary ion[b]	Secondary ion
Testosterone	432	417
Epitestosterone	432	417
DHEA	432	417
16α Hydroxytestosterone[a]	520	

[a]Suggested internal standard at 20 ng/mL.
[b]Quantitation ion.
Source: UCT internal publication.

6. **Enzymatic hydrolysis.**
   a. Dry eluates under a stream of nitrogen after which 2 mL of 0.2 M phosphate buffer, pH 7.0, and 250 u of β-glucuronidase are added, vortex mixed, and allowed to incubate at 50°C for 1 h. Samples are then cooled, and the pH adjusted to 10.0-11.0 using a 1:1 mixture of N_2HCO_3–Na_2CO_3.

7. **Addition cleanup.**
   a. Add 5 mL of *n*-butyl chloride to each sample.
   b. Cap the tubes are capped and shake vigorously for 10 min, then centrifuge at 3000 rpm for 5 mins.
   c. Transfer the organic layer to clean test tubes and dry under a stream of nitrogen.
   d. Place the dried sample in a desiccator and further dry under vacuum for 30 min.

8. **Derivatize.**
   a. Add 50 μL of MSTF–NH_4–dithioerythritol. (1000:2:5, v/w/w) and incubate at 70°C for 20 min.
   b. Centrifuge sample at 3000 rpm for 1 min. and transfer directly to GC injector vials.

9. **Quantitate.**
   Inject 1 μL of sample onto the GC-MS:

10.5 FENTANYL AND ANALOGS IN URINE FOR *GC* OR *GC-MS* CONFIRMATIONS USING A 200-MG *CLEAN SCREEN* EXTRACTION COLUMN *(ZSDAU020 OR ZCDAU020)*

1. **Prepare sample.**
   a. To 5 mL of sample add internal standard[a] and 2 mL of 0.1 M phosphate buffer, pH 6.0.
   b. Mix/vortex.
   c. Sample pH should be 6.0 ± 0.5. Adjust pH accordingly with 0.1 M monobasic or dibasic sodium phosphate.

2. **Condition CLEAN SCREEN extraction column.**
   1 × 3 mL of CH_3OH; aspirate.
   1 × 3 mL of DI H_2O; aspirate.
   1 × 1 mL of 0.1 M phosphate buffer, pH 6.0; aspirate.
   Note: Aspirate at ≤3 in. Hg to prevent sorbent drying.

3. **Apply sample.**
   Load at 1 mL/min.

Table 6

Compound	Primary ion[b]	Secondary ion	Tertiary ion
Fentanyl	245	146	189
D[5]-Fentanyl[a]	250	151	194
a-Methylfentanyl	259	203	146
p-Fluorofentanyl	263	164	207
3-Methylfentanyl	259	160	203
Thienfentanyl	245	146	189
Sufentanil	289	140	
Carfentanil	303	187	
Lofentanil	317	201	289
Alfentanil	289	268	222

[a]Suggested internal standard for GC-MS: D_5-fentanyl.
[b]Quantitation ion.
Source: UCT internal publication working with the Philadelphia Medical Examiner's Office.

4. **Wash column.**
   1 × 3 mL of DI H_2O; aspirate.
   1 × 1 mL of 0.1 *M* acetic acid; aspirate.
   1 × 3 mL of CH_3OH; aspirate.
   Dry column (5 min at ≥10 in. Hg).

5. **Elute fentanyls.**
   1 × 3 mL of CH_2Cl_2–IPA–NH_4OH (78:20:2); collect eluate at 1–2 mL/min.
   Note: Prepare elution solvent daily. Add IPA–NH_4OH, mix, then add CH_2Cl_2, pH 11.0–12.0.

6. **Concentrate.**
   a. Evaporate to dryness at ≤40°C.
   b. Reconstitute with 50 μL of ethyl acetate.

7. **Quantitate.**
   a. Inject 1–2 μL of sample onto the chromatograph.
   b. Monitor the following ions (GC-MS):

10.6 FLUNITRAZEPAM, 7-AMINOFLUNITRAZEPAM, AND DESMETHYLFLUNITRAZEPAM IN URINE FOR GC-MS CONFIRMATION USING A 200-MG CLEAN SCREEN EXTRACTION COLUMN (ZSDAU020 OR ZCDAU020)

1. **Prepare sample: β-glucuronidase hydrolysis.**
   a. To 5 mL of urine add internal standard(s) and 1 mL of β-glucuronidase. β-glucuronidase solution contains 5000 FU/mL *Patella vulgata* in 0.1 *M* phos phate buffer, pH 6.0.
   b. Mix/vortex. Hydrolyze for 3 h at 65°C.
   c. Cool before proceeding.

Table 7

Compound	Primary ion[b]	Secondary ion	Tertiary ion
Flunitrazepam	312	286	266
7-Aminoflunitrazepam	283	255	254
Demethylflunitrazepam	356	357	310
Oxazepam-D^5[a]	462	464	463

[a]Suggested internal standard for GC-MS: oxazepam-D^5.
[b]Quantitation ion
Source: UCT internal publication.

2. **Condition CLEAN SCREEN extraction column.**
   1 × 3 mL of methanol; aspirate.
   1 × 3 mL of deionized water; aspirate.
   1 × 1 mL of 0.1 *M* phosphate buffer, pH 6.0.
   Note: Aspirate at ≤3 in. Hg to prevent sorbent drying.
3. **Apply sample.**
   Load at 1–2 mL/min.
4. **Wash column.**
   1 × 2 mL of DI H$_2$O; aspirate.
   1 × 2 mL of 20% acetonitrile in 0.1 *M* phosphate buffer, pH 6.0; aspirate.
   Dry column (5 min at ≥10 in. Hg).
   1 × 2 mL of hexane; aspirate.
5. **Elute flunitrazepam, 7-aminoflunitrazepam and desmethylflunitrazepam.**
   1 × 3 mL of ethyl acetate with 2% NH$_4$OH; collect eluate at 1–2 mL/min.
   Note: Prepare fresh daily.
6. **Dry eluate.**
   Evaporate to dryness at ≤40°C.
7. **Derivatize.**
   a. Add 50 µL of ethyl acetate and 50 µL of MTBSTFA (with 1% TBDMCS).
   b. Mix/vortex.
   c. React for 20 min at 90°C. Remove from heat source to cool.
   Note: Do not evaporate MTBSTFA solution.
8. **Analysis.**
   a. Inject 1–2 µL of sample (in MTBSTFA solution)
   b. Principal ions (mass selective detection):

10.7 FLUOXETINE AND NORFLUOXETINE

Fluoxetine is a bicyclic antidepressant, currently being marketed as Prozac® by Eli Lilly and Company and is used in the treatment of depression. In 1988, fluoxetine was introduced as an alternative to the currently prescribed tricyclic and tetracyclic antidepressants. It has been reported as having fewer side effects than other antidepressants. Fluoxetine hydrochloride, or N-methy-8-[4-(trifluoromethyl) phenoxy] benzenepropanamine, has also undergone investigation as a treatment for obsessive-compulsive disorder.

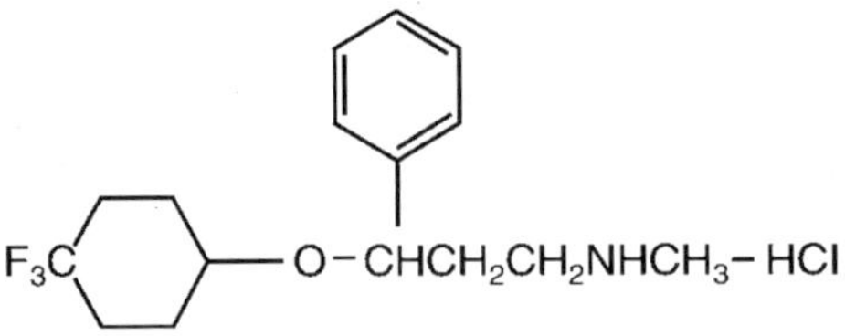

$C_{17}H_{18}F_3NO\cdot HCl$

Molecular Weight: 345.79
Solubility:
H2O   =14 mg/mL
MeOH =250 mg/mL
$CHCl_3$ =125 mg/mL
Stability at 25°C to 50°C
24 months

PROZAC
Fluoxetine hydrochloride
(1)-N-methyl-3-phenyl-3-[(a,a,a-trifluoro-p-tolyl)-oxy]
Propylamine hydrochloride

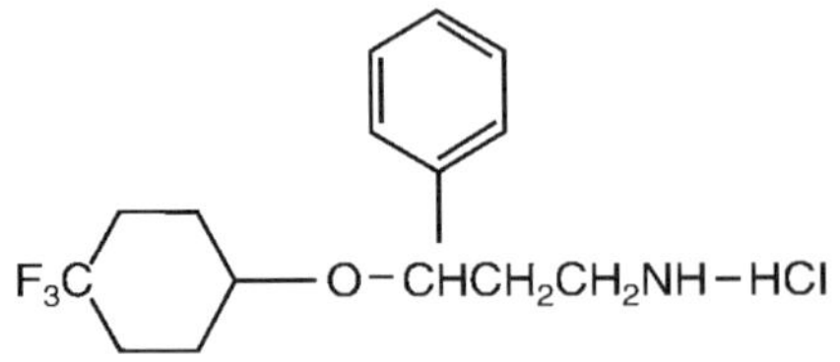

$C_{16}H_{15}F_3NO\cdot HCl$

Molecular Weight: 330.79
Solubility:

PROZAC METABOLITE DEMETHYLATED
Metabolite hydrochloride
3-phenyl-3-[(a,a,a-trifluoro-p-tolyl)-oxy] Propylamine hydrochloride

Fig. 1. The chemical structures opf fluoxetine and its metabolite.

Fluoxetine is believed to function by inhibiting presynaptic reuptake of serotonin resulting in enhanced serotoninergic neurotransmission. This is the same mechanism by which the tricyclic antidepressants function. The drug exhibits similar therapeutic effects as to amitriptyline, imipramine, and doxepin when used to treat unipolar depression. However, fluoxetine has been shown to produce fewer side effects, such as milder anticholinergic symptoms, and it does not alter normal cardiac conductivity. Metabolism of fluoxetine occurs mainly by *n*-desmethylation of the side chain, which results in the formation of a primary amine, referred to as norfluoxetine. The metabolite is pharmacologically active, in that it too can block the reuptake of serotonin (Fig. 1).

The therapeutic dosage for fluoxetine is 20–60 mg/d and it is metabolized in the liver to norfluoxetine and other unidentified pharmacologically inactive metabolites. Therapeutically monitored levels are observed at 40–450 ng/mL for both fluoxetine and norfluoxetine, separately.

Section 10.7.1 describes an extraction procedure of fluoxetine and norfluoxetine using a CLEAN SCREEN bonded phase column. The column extraction provides an extremely clean sample with high recoveries of fluoxetine and norfluoxetine. The CLEAN SCREEN extraction method takes about 20 min for 24 samples. Quantitative analysis can be accomplished by HPLC, GC, or GC-MS. The method described uses GC-MS, using the pentafluoropropionic anhydride derivative to enhance the chromatography and ion fragmentation pattern. The total run time is 6 min per injected sample.

Table 8

Compound	Primary ion[b]	Secondary ion	Tertiary ion
Fluoxetine	117	190	294
Norfluoxetine	117	176	280
Protriptyline[a]	191	409	119

[a]Internal standard: protriptyline.
[b]Quantitation ion.
Source: UCT internal publication. *See* Figure 2.

Expected therapeutic levels are 40–450 ng/mL in plasma or serum. Assay sensitivity is approx 20 ng/mL. The method is accurate and reproducible, making it a method of choice for therapeutic monitoring of fluoxetine and norfluoxetine.

10.7.1 Fluoxetine and Norfluoxetine in Serum, Plasma, or Whole Blood: Application for GC or GC-MS Analysis Using a 200-mg CLEAN SCREEN Extraction Column (ZSDAU020 OR ZCDAU020)

1. **Prepare sample.**
   a. To 1 mL of sample add internal standarda and 4 mL of DI H_2O.
   b. Add 2 mL of 0.1 M phosphate buffer, pH 6.0.
   c. Mix/vortex. Sample pH should be 6.0 ± 0.5. Adjust pH accordingly with 0.1 M monobasic or dibasic sodium phosphate.
2. **Condition 200-mg CLEAN SCREEN extraction column.**
   1 × 3 mL of CH_3OH; aspirate.
   1 × 3 mL of DI H_2O; aspirate.
   1 × 1 mL of 0.1 M phosphate buffer, pH 6.0; aspirate.
   Note: Aspirate at ≤3 in. Hg to prevent sorbent drying.
3. **Apply sample.**
   Load at 1–2 mL/min.
4. **Wash column.**
   1 × 3 mL of DI H_2O; aspirate.
   1 × 3 mL of 1.0 M acetic acid; aspirate.
   1 × 3 mL of CH_3OH; aspirate.
   Dry column (5 min at ≥10 in. Hg).
5. **Elute fluoxetine, norfluoxetine, and internal standard.**
   1 × 3 mL of CH_2Cl_2–IPA–NH_4OH (78:20:2); collect the eluate at 1–2 mL/min.
6. **Dry eluate.**
   Evaporate to dryness at ≤40°C.
7. **Derivatize.**
   a. Add 100 μL of ethyl acetate and 50 μL of PFPA.
   b. Fill tube with nitrogen gas cap; vortex.
   c. Derivatize at 90°C for 30 min.
   d. Evaporate to dryness at ≤40°C.

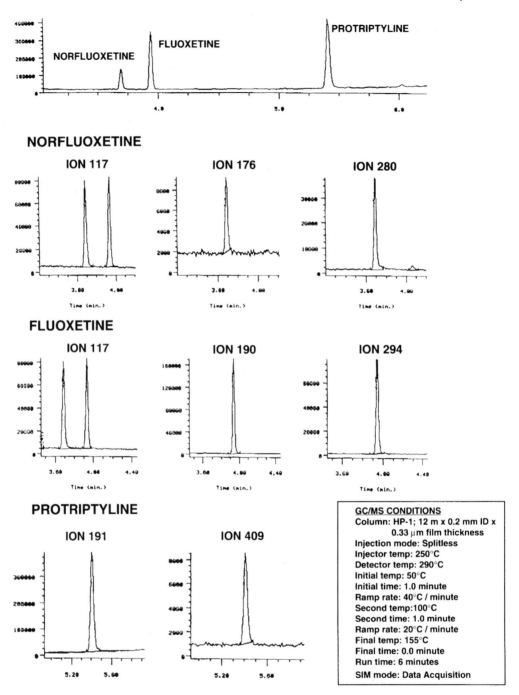

Fig. 2. Fluoxetine and norfluoxetine (100 ng/mL) extracted from plasma analyzed GC-MS.

8. Reconstitute and inject.
   a. Reconstitute with 200 µL of ethyl acetate.
   b. Inject 2 µL.
9. Quantitate.
Monitor the following ions (mass selective detection):

10.8 GABAPENTIN IN SERUM, PLASMA, OR WHOLE BLOOD FOR GC OR GC-MS ANALYSIS USING A 200-MG CLEAN-UP® C18 EXTRACTION COLUMN

1. Prepare sample.
   a. Place 500 µL of sample, calibrator, or control into a 10 × 25 mm disposable glass test tube and add 25 µL of internal standarda (5.0 mg/L). Vortex tube.
   b. Add 500 µL of 20% acetic acid and vortex tube again.
2. Condition SPE column.
   1 × 3 mL of CH_3OH; aspirate.
   1 × 3 mL of DI H_2O; aspirate.
   1 × 3 mL of 0.1 *N* HCl aspirate.
3. Apply sample.
   Load at 1–2 mL/min.
4. Wash column.
   1 × 3 mL of DI H_2O; aspirate.
   1 × 3 mL of ethyl acetate.
   1 × 3 mL of hexane.
   Dry column (5 min at ≥10 in. Hg) or until column is dry.
5. Elute.
   1 × 1 mL of 2% NH_4OH in MeOH.
6. Evaporated to dryness at 40°C in a water bath.
7. Derivatize.
   a. Add 50 µL of MTBSTFA + 1% tBDMCS reagent to the residue.
   b. Cap tube and put into a water bath at 70°C for 30 min.
   c. Remove and allow to cool for 5–10 min.
8. Quantitate.
   Inject 1–2 µL onto the chromatograph.

ªInternal standard: 1-aminomethyl-1-cycloheptyl acetic acid.

Reference

Wolf II, C., Sady, J., and Pokalis, A. Determination of gabapentin in serum using solid phase extraction and gas-liquid chromatography. J. Analyt. Toxicol. 20:498–501, 1996.

10.9 KETAMINE IN URINE FOR OR GC OR GC-MS CONFIRMATIONS USING A 200-MG CLEAN SCREEN EXTRACTION COLUMN (ZSDAU020 OR ZCDAU020)

1. Prepare sample.
   a. To 5 mL of urine add internal standard[a] and 2 mL of 0.1 *M* phosphate buffer, pH 6.0.
   b. Mix/vortex.
   c. The sample pH should be 6.0 ± 0.5. Adjust pH accordingly with 0.1 *M* monobasic or dibasic sodium phosphate.

Table 9

Compound	Primary ion[b]	Secondary ion	Tertiary ion
Ketamine	180	209	152
Hexobarbital[a]	221	157	156

[a]Internal standard.
[b]Quantitation ion.
Source: UCT internal publication.

2. Prepare CLEAN SCREEN extraction column.
  1 × 3 mL of CH_3OH; aspirate.
  1 × 3 mL of DI H_2O; aspirate.
  1 × 1 mL of 0.1 *M* phosphate buffer, pH 6.0; aspirate.
  Note: Aspirate at ≤3 in. Hg to prevent sorbent drying.
3. Apply sample.
  Load at 1 mL/min.
4. Wash column.
  1 × 3 mL of DI H_2O; aspirate.
  1 × 1 mL of 0.1 *M* acetic acid; aspirate.
  Dry column (5 min at ≥10 in. Hg).
  1 × 2 mL of hexane; aspirate.
5. Elute ketamine.
  1 × 3 mL of dichloromethane-isopropanol-ammonium chloride (78:20:2).
  Collect eluants at 1–2 mL/min using minimal vacuum.
  Note: Make the elution solvent fresh daily.
6. Dry eluate.
  a. Evaporate to dryness at ≤40°C.
  b. Reconstitute with 100 μL of methanol.
7. Quantitate.
  a. Inject 1–2 μL onto the chromatograph.
  b. Monitor the following ions (mass selective detection):

10.10 LIDOCAINE AND IBUPROFEN IN URINE FOR OR *GC* OR *GC-MS* CONFIRMATIONS USING A 200-MG CLEAN SCREEN EXTRACTION COLUMN *(XRDAH 503 OR XRDAH 506)*

1. Prepare sample.
  a. To 5 mL of urine add internal standard[a] and 2 mL of 0.1 *M* acetate buffer, pH 4.5.
  b. Mix/vortex.
  c. The sample pH should be 4.5 ± 0.5.
2. Prepare CLEAN SCREEN extraction column.
  1 × 5 mL of CH_3OH; aspirate.
  1 × 5 mL of DI H_2O; aspirate.
  1 × 3 mL of 0.1 *M* phosphate buffer, pH 6.0; aspirate.
  Note: Aspirate at ≤ 3 in. Hg to prevent sorbent drying.
3. Apply sample.
  Load at 1 mL/min.

Table 10

Compound	Primary ion[b]	Secondary ion	Tertiary ion
Lidocaine	86	234 (5%)	87 (5%)
Ibuprofen	163	161 (98%)	206 (20%)
Hexobarbital[a]	221	157 (30%)	236 (5%)

[a]Internal standard: deuterated barbiturate or hexobarbital.
[b]Quantitation ion.
Source: UCT internal publication.

4. **Wash column.**
   1 × 5 mL of DI H_2O; aspirate.
   1 × 3mL of 0.1 $_M$ acetic acid; aspirate.
   Dry column (5 min at ≥10 in. Hg).
   1 × 5 mL of hexane; aspirate.
5. **Elute ibuprofen (acid neutral drug).**
   a. Place the collection rack with tubes into the manifold.
   b. 1 × 5 mL of hexane-ethyl acetate (70:30).
   c. Collect eluate at <3 mL/min using minimal vacuum.
   Note: Make elution solvent fresh daily.
6. **Wash column.**
   a. Remove the collection rack.
   b. Wash the columns with 1 × 5 mL of methanol.
   c. Dry column (5 min at >10 mm Hg).
7. **Elute lidocaine.**
   a. Return the collection rack into the manifold.
   b. 1 × 5 mL ethyl acetate-ammonium hydroxide (96:4).
   c. Collect eluants at 1–2 mL/min.
   Note: Prepare the elution solvent fresh daily.
8. **Dry eluate.**
   a. Combine both extracts together.
   b. Evaporate to dryness at ≤40°C.
   c. Reconstitute with 100 µL of ethyl acetate.
7. **Quantitate.**
   a. Inject 1–2 µL onto the chromatograph.
   b. Monitor the following ions (mass selective detection):

10.11 METHAQUALONE IN URINE FOR GC OR GC-MS CONFIRMATIONS USING A 200-MG CLEAN SCREEN EXTRACTION COLUMN (ZSDAU020 OR ZCDAU020)

1. **Prepare sample.**
   a. To 5 mL of urine add internal standarda and 2 mL of 0.1 *M* phosphate buffer, pH 6.0.
   b. Mix/vortex.
   c. The sample pH should be 6.0 ± 0.5. Adjust pH accordingly with 0.1 *M* monobasic or dibasic sodium phosphate.

Table 11

Compound	Primary ion[b]	Secondary ion	Tertiary ion
Methaqualone	235	250	233
Hexobarbital[a]	221	157	156

[a]Internal standard.
[b]Quantitation ion.
Source: UCT internal publication.

2. **Prepare CLEAN SCREEN extraction column.**
   1 × 3 mL of CH_3OH; aspirate.
   1 × 3 mL of DI H_2O; aspirate.
   1 × 1 mL of 0.1 *M* phosphate buffer, pH 6.0; aspirate.
   Note: Aspirate at ≤3 in. Hg to prevent sorbent drying.
3. **Apply sample.**
   Load at 1 mL/min.
4. **Wash column.**
   1 × 3 mL of DI H_2O; aspirate.
   Dry column (5 min at ≥10 in. Hg).
   1 × 2 mL of hexane; aspirate.
5. **Elute methaqualone.**
   1 × 3 mL of hexane-ethyl acetate (50:50); collect eluate a ≤5 mL/min.
6. **Dry eluate.**
   a. Evaporate to dryness at ≤40°C.
   b. Reconstitute with 100 µL ethyl acetate.
7. **Quantitate.**
   a. Inject 1–2 µL onto the chromatograph.
   b. Monitor the following ions (mass selective detection):

Caution: At pH 6.0 methaqualone behaves like an un-ionized neutral drug and comes off in the neutral fraction. If the sample pH drops below 4.5 some of the methaqualone will elute in the basic fraction. At pH 2.5 (the pK_a of methaqualone) you will see one-half of the drug in the neutral fraction and one-half in the basic fraction. This is exactly what the theory predicts will happen.

10.12 METHADONE IN URINE FOR *GC* OR *GC-MS* CONFIRMATIONS USING A 200-MG CLEAN SCREEN EXTRACTION COLUMN (*ZSDAU020* OR *ZCDAU020*)

1. **Prepare sample.**
   a. To 5 mL of urine add internal standard(s)[a] and 2 mL of 0.1 *M* phosphate buffer, pH 6.0.
   b. Mix/vortex.
   c. The sample pH should be 6.0 ± 0.5. Adjust pH accordingly with 0.1 *M* monobasic or dibasic sodium phosphate.

Table 12

Compound	Primary ion[b]	Secondary ion	Tertiary ion
Methadone	72	91	165
Methadone D[3a]	75	94	168
Phenyltoloxamine[a]	58		

[a]Internal standard.

[b]Quantitation ion.

Source: UCT internal publication.

2. **Condition CLEAN SCREEN extraction column.**
   1 × 3 mL of CH_3OH; aspirate.
   1 × 3 mL of DI H_2O; aspirate.
   1 × 2 mL of 0.1 *M* phosphate buffer, pH 6.0; aspirate.
   Note: Aspirate at ≤3 in. Hg to prevent sorbent drying.
3. **Apply sample.**
   Load at 1–2 mL/min.
4. **Wash column.**
   1 × 3 mL of DI H_2O; aspirate.
   1 × 1 mL of 0.1 *M* acetic acid; aspirate.
   1 × 3 mL of CH_3OH; aspirate.
   Dry column (5 min at ≥10 in. Hg).
5. **Elute methadone.**
   1 × 3 mL of CH_2Cl_2–IPA–NH_4OH (78:20:2); collect eluate at 1–2 mL/min.
   Note: Prepare elution solvent daily. Add IPA–NH_4OH, mix, then add CH_2Cl_2, pH 11.0–12.0.
6. **Concentrate.**
   a. Evaporate to dryness at ≤40°C.
   b. Reconstitute with 100 µL of ethyl acetate.
7. **Quantitate.**
   a. Inject 1–2 µL onto the chromatograph.
   b. Monitor the following ions (mass selective detection):

10.13 NICOTINE AND COTININE

10.13.1 Nicotine and Cotinine in Urine for GC or GC–MS Confirmations Using a 200-mg CLEAN SCREEN Extraction Column (ZSDAU020 or ZCDAU020)

1. **Prepare sample.**
   a. To 5 mL of urine add internal standard(s)[a] and 2 mL of 0.1 *M* acetic acid solution.
   b. Mix/vortex.
2. **Condition CLEAN SCREEN extraction column.**
   1 × 3 mL of CH_3OH; aspirate.
   1 × 3 mL of DI H_2O; aspirate.
   1 × 2 mL of 0.1 *M* acetic acid; aspirate.
   Note: Aspirate at ≤3 in. Hg to prevent sorbent drying.

Table 13

Compound	Primary ion[b]	Secondary ion	Tertiary ion	Other
Nicotine	84	133	162	
Cotinine	98	119	176	

[a]D3 Cotinine and D4 nicotine are available as deuterated internal standards.
[b]Quantitation ion.

3. **Apply sample.**
   Load at 1 mL/min.
4. **Wash column.**
   1 × 3 mL of DI H_2O; aspirate.
   1 × 1 mL of 1.0 M acetic acid; aspirate.
   Dry column (5 min at ≥10 in. Hg).
   1 × 2 mL of hexane; aspirate.
   1 × 4 mL pf hexane-ethyl acetate (50:50); aspirate.
   1 × 1 mL of methanol; aspirate.
5. **Elute basic drugs.**
   Place a collection rack into the manifold with sample tubes.
   1 × 3 mL of CH_2Cl_2–IPA–NH_4OH (78:20:2); collect eluate at 1 mL/min.
   Note: Prepare elution solvent daily. Add IPA–NO_4OH, mix, then add CH_2Cl_2, pH 11.0–12.0.
6. **Concentrate.**
   a. Evaporate to dryness at ≤40°C.
   b. Take care not to overheat or overevaporate.
   c. Reconstitute with 100 µL of methanol.
7. **Quantitate.**
   a. Inject 1–2 µL onto the chromatograph.
   b. Monitor the following ions (GC-MS):

Gas Chromatography Conditons
Column: RTx5, DB-5, or HP-5 or equivalent column (30 m × 0.25 mm id × 0.25 µm film).
Temperature program: 60°C, hold 2 min then ramp to 250°C at 25°C /min; then hold for 1 min; then to 300°C at 25°C/min.
Injection Temperature: 250°C Transfer line: 280°C
Purge time = 1 min splitless mode
Source: UCT internal publication.

10.13.2 Nicotine and Cotinine in Serum for GC or GC-MS Confirmations Using a 200-mg CLEAN SCREEN Extraction Column (ZSDAU020 or ZCDAU020)

1. **Prepare sample.**
   a. To 2 mL of serum, plasma, or whole blood add internal standard(s)[a] and 2 mL of 0.1 M acetic acid solution.
   b. Mix/vortex.

Table 14

Compound	Primary ion[b]	Secondary ion	Tertiary ion
Nicotine	84	133	162
Cotinine	98	119	176

[a]D^3-cotinine and D^4-nicotine are available as deuterated internal standards.
[b]Quantitation ion.

2. **Condition CLEAN SCREEN extraction column.**
   1×3 mL of CH_3OH; aspirate.
   1×3 mL of DI H_2O; aspirate.
   1×1 mL of 1.0 *M* acetic acid; aspirate.
   Note: Aspirate at ≤3 in. Hg to prevent sorbent drying.
3. **Apply sample.**
   Load at 1 mL/min.
4. **Wash column.**
   1×3 mL of DI H_2O; aspirate.
   1×1 mL of 0.1 *M* acetic acid; aspirate.
   Dry column (5 min at ≥10 in. Hg).
   1×2 mL of hexane; aspirate.
   1×4 mL of hexane-ethyl acetate (50:50); aspirate.
   1×1 mL of methanol; aspirate.
5. **Elute basic drugs.**
   Place a collection rack into the manifold with sample tubes.
   1×3 mL of CH_2Cl_2–IPA–NH_4OH (78:20:2); collect eluate at 1 mL/min.
   Note: Prepare elution solvent daily. Add IPA–NO_4OH, mix, then add CH_2Cl_2, pH 11.0–12.0.
6. **Concentrate.**
   a. Evaporate to dryness at ≤40°C.
   b. Take care not to overheat or overevaporate.
   c. Reconstitute with 100 µL of methanol.
7. **Quantitate.**
   a. Inject 1–2 µL onto the chromatograph.
   b. Monitor the following ions (GC-MS):

Gas Chromatography Conditions
Column: RTx5, DB-5, or HP-5 or equivalent column (30 m × 0.25 mm i.d. × 0.25 µm film)
Temperature program: 60°C; hold 2 min then ramp to 250°C at 25°C /min; then hold for 1 min; then to 300°C at 25°C/min.
Injection temperature: 250°C
Transfer line: 280°C
Purge time = 1 min splitless mode

Table 15

Compound	Primary ion[b]	Secondary ion	Tertiary ion	Other
Propoxyphene	58	115	208	250, 265
Propoxyphene D[5a]	63	120	213	255, 270

[a]Internal standard.
[b]Quantitation ion.

10.14 PROPOXYPHENE IN URINE FOR GC OR GC-MS CONFIRMATIONS USING A 200-MG CLEAN SCREEN EXTRACTION COLUMNS (DAU020 OR ZCDAU020)

1. **Prepare sample.**
   a. To 5 mL of urine add internal standard(s)[a] and 2 mL of 0.1 M phosphate buffer, pH 6.0.
   b. Mix/vortex.
   c. Sample pH should be 6.0 ± 0.5. Adjust pH accordingly with 0.1 M monobasic or dibasic sodium phosphate.
2. **Condition CLEAN SCREEN extraction column.**
   1 × 3 mL of CH_3OH; aspirate.
   1 × 3 mL of DI H_2O; aspirate.
   1 × 2 mL of 0.1 M phosphate buffer, pH 6.0; aspirate.
   Note: Aspirate at ≤3 in. Hg to prevent sorbent drying.
3. **Apply sample.**
   Load at 1 mL/min.
4. **Wash column.**
   1 × 3 mL of DI H_2O; aspirate.
   1 × 1 mL of 0.1 M acetic acid; aspirate.
   1 × 3 mL of CH_3OH; aspirate.
   Dry column (5 min at ≥10 in. Hg).
5. **Elute propoxyphene.**
   1 × 3 mL of CH_2Cl_2–IPA–NH_4OH (78:20:2); collect eluate at 1 mL/min.
   Note: Prepare elution solvent daily. Add IPA–NO_4OH, mix, then add CH_2Cl_2, pH 11.0–12.0.
6. **Concentrate.**
   a. Evaporate to dryness at ≤40°C.
   b. Reconstitute with 100 μL of ethyl acetate.
7. **Quantitate.**
   a. Inject 1–2 μL onto the chromatograph.
   b. Monitor the following ions (GC-MS):

Note: Because of problems in the determination of norpropoxyphene, the primary metabolite of dextroproxyphene, base catalyst of the sample by addition of one drop of 35% sodium hydroxide solution to the urine sample and then after mixing bring the pH to 6.0 for SPE extraction. This step interconverts the norpropoxyphene to norpropoxypheneamide, a more stable compound. For more information see

Table 16

Compound	Primary ion[b]	Secondary ion	Tertiary ion
Psilocin-TMS	290	348	73 (291)

[a]Internal standard.
[b]Quantitation ion.

Amalfitano, G., Bessard, J., Vincent, F., Esseric, H., Bessard, G. Gas chromatographic quantitation of dextropropoxyphene and morpropoxyphene in urine after solid-phase extraction. J. Analyt. Toxicol. 20:547–554, 1996.
  Source: UCT internal publication.

10.15 Psilocin in Urine for GC or GC-MS Confirmations Using a 200-mg CLEAN SCREEN Extraction Column (ZSDAU020 or ZCDAU020)

1. **Prepare sample.**
    a. To 5 mL of urine add internal standard and 2 mL of 0.1 M phosphate buffer, pH 6.0.
    b. Mix/vortex.
    c. Add 12,500–25,000 U of β-glucuronidase; mix/vortex.
    d. Place the sample into a water bath at 45°C for 90 min.
    e. Remove from the bath and allow to cool.
    f. Centrifuge at 1509g for 10 min.
    g. Use the clear filtrate (discard the plug) for SPE.
2. **Prepare CLEAN SCREEN extraction column.**
    1 × 3 mL of CH_3OH; aspirate.
    1 × 2 mL of DI H_2O; aspirate.
    1 × 2 mL of 0.1 M phosphate buffer, pH 6.0; aspirate.
    Note: Aspirate at ≤3 in. Hg to prevent sorbent drying.
3. **Apply sample.**
    Load at 1 mL/min.
4. **Wash column.**
    1 × 3 mL of DI H_2O; aspirate.
    1 × 2 mL of 20% acetonitrile in water; aspirate.
    1 × 1 mL 0.1 M acetic acid; aspirate.
    Dry column (3 min at ≥10 in. Hg).
    1 × 2 mL of hexane; aspirate.
    1 × 3 mL of hexane-ethyl acetate (50:50).
    1 × 3mL of methanol.
    Dry column (3 min at >10 in. Hg)
5. **Elute psilocin.**
    1 × 3 mL of dichloromethane-isopropanol-ammonium hydroxide (78:20:2).
    Collect eluant at 1 mL/min.
    Note: Prepare elution solvent daily.
6. **Dry eluate.**
    Evaporate to dryness at ≤35°C.

7. Derivatize.
    a. Reconstitute with 50 μL of MSTFA.
    b. Cap the sample tube and place it into a heater block at 70°C for 20 min.

8. Quantitate.
    a. Inject 1–2 μL onto the chromatograph.
    b. Monitor the following ions (mass selective detection):

Gas Chromatography Conditions

HP Model 5890 GC with a 5970 MSD
Column: DB-5 (25 m × 0.32 mm i.d. × 0.17 μm film thickness
Carrier gas: Helium (5 psi head pressure)
Injection size: 1 μL splitless mode
Injection temperature: 275°C
Detector temperature: 300°C
Temperature program: 70°C, hold 1 min then ramp to 240°C at 20°C/min; hold for 2 min.

Reference: Grieshaber, A., Moore, K., Levine, B., and Smith, M. The detection of psilocin in human urine. Presented at the TRI-SERVICES Meeting, Nov. 1999.

10.16 Sertraline and Desmethylsertraline in Serum, Plasma, or Whole Blood for HPLC Analysis Using a 200-mg Clean Screen Extraction Column (ZSDAU020 or ZCDAU020)

1. Prepare sample.
    a. To 1 mL of serum add internal standard, 4 mL of DI H_2O and 2 mL of 0.1 *M* phosphate buffer, pH 6.0.
    b. Mix/vortex. Centrifuge for 10 min at 670*g* and discard pellet
    c. Sample pH should be 6.0 + 0.5.

2. Condition CLEAN SCREEN extraction column.
    1 × 3 mL of CH_3OH; aspirate.
    1 × 3 mL of DI H_2O; aspirate.
    1 × 1 mL of 0.1 *M* phosphate buffer, pH 6.0; aspirate.
    Note: Aspirate at ≤3 in. Hg to prevent sorbent drying.

3. Apply sample.
    Load at 1 mL/min.

4. Wash column.
    1 × 3 mL of DI H_2O; aspirate.
    1 × 1 mL of 0.1 *M* acetic acid; aspirate.
    1 × 3 mL of CH_3OH; aspirate.
    Dry column (5 min at ≥10 in. Hg).

5. Elute.
    1 × 3 mL of CH_2Cl_2–IPA–NH_4OH (78:20:2); collect eluate at 1 mL/min.
    Note: Prepare elution solvent fresh daily. Add IPA–NH_4OH, mix, then add CH_3Cl_2, pH 11.0–12.0.

6. Dry eluate.
    Evaporate to dryness at ≤40°C.

Table 17

Compound	Primary ion[b]	Secondary ion	Tertiary ion	Other
Testosterone TMS	432	301	209	
19-Noretiocholanone-TMS	405	315	225	
Oxymethalone	640	552	462	370, 143
Dehydroepiandosterone-2TMS	432	327	297	
10-Nortestosterone-2TMS	418	287	194	
Oxymethaione metabolite 1	640	552	462	143
Oxymethalone metabolite 2	625	462	370	143
11-β-Hydroxyandosterone	522	417	158	
Methandienone	409	313	281	
19-Norandosterone-2TMS	405	315	225	
a-Hydroxyetiocholanone	504	417		
17-α-Epitestosterone TMS	432	341	327	209
Stanazolol	472	381	342	149

[a]Internal standard.
[b]Quantitation ion.
Source: UCT internal publication.

7. **Quantitate.**
    a. Reconstitute with 200 µL of acetonitrile-DI H_2O (1:3).
    b. Mix/vortex vigorously for 30 s.
    c. Inject 100 µL onto the chromatograph at wavelength 235 nm.
    d. Mobile phase = 0.25 M potassium phosphate, pH 2.7 containing 30% CH_3CN.
    e. Flow rate = 2 mL/min.
8. **HPLC system.**
    Isocratic HPLC using a pump through a C8 HPLC column
    (LC-8 or equivalent HPLC Column) 15 cm × 4.6 mm id coupled to a UV detector set at 235 nm.

10.17 ANABOLIC STEROIDS IN URINE FOR GC OR GC-MS CONFIRMATIONS USING A 200-MG CLEAN SCREEN EXTRACTION COLUMN (ZSDAU020 OR ZCDAU020)

1. **Prepare sample: β-glucuronidase hydrolysis.**
    a. To 5 mL of urine add internal standard(s)a and 2 mL of β-glucuronidase. β-Glucu ronidase: 5000 FU/mL of *Patella vulgata* in 0.1 M acetate buffer, pH 5.0.
    b. Mix/vortex. Hydrolyze for 3 h at 65°C. Cool before proceeding.
    c. Centrifuge for 10 min at 670g and discard pellet.
    d. Adjust sample pH to 6.0 ± 0.5 with approx 700 µL of 1.0 N NaOH.
2. **Prepare CLEAN SCREEN extraction column.**
    1 × 3 mL of CH_3OH; aspirate.
    1 × 3 mL of DI H_2O; aspirate.
    1 × 1 mL of 0.1 M phosphate buffer, pH 6.0; aspirate.
    Note: Aspirate at ≤ in. Hg to prevent sorbent drying.

3. Apply sample.

Load at 1–2 mL/min.

4. Wash column.

1 × 3 mL 10% (v/v) CH_3OH in DI H_2O; aspirate.

Dry column (5 min at ≥10 in. Hg).

1 × 1 mL hexane or hexane-ethyl acetate (50:50); aspirate.

5. Elute anabolic steroids (Choose a, b, c or d).

a. 1 – 3 mL of CH_2Cl_2–IPA–NH_4OH (78:20:2); collect eluate at 1–2 mL/min.

Note: Prepare elution solvent daily. Add IPA–NH_4OH, mix, then add CH_2Cl_2, pH 11.0–12.0.

b. 1 × 3 mL of CH_2Cl_2–IPA (80:20).

c. 1 × 3 mL of ethyl acetate.

d. 1 x 3 mL of CH_3OH.

6. Dry eluate.

Evaporate to dryness at ≤40°C.

7. Derivatize.

a. Add 50 μL of ethyl acetate and 50 μL of MSTFA (with 3% trimethylsilyliodide).

b. Overlay with nitrogen gas and cap. Mix/vortex.

c. React 20 min at 70°C. Remove from heat source to cool.

Note: Do not evaporate MSTFA solution.

8. Quantitate.

a. Inject 1–2 μL onto the chromatograph.

b. Monitor the following ions (GC-MS):

10.18 Extraction of Tear Gas Chloroacetophenone (CS), O-Chlorobenzylidenemalononitrile (CN), and Trans-8-Methyl-N-Vanillyl-6-Nonenamide (OC) from Cloth for GC-MS Analysis Using a 200-mg CLEAN SCREEN Extraction Column (ZSDAU020)

1. Prepare sample.

a. If suspected tear gas is on clothing cut out a portion of the sprayed area and a "negative" control sample. Extract each into hexane.

b. For canisters of suspected tear gas, spray onto a Kimwipe® and extract the sprayed area and a negative control into hexane.

2. Condition CLEAN SCREEN extraction column.

2 × 3 mL of CH_3OH; aspirate.

2 × 3 mL of DI H_2O; aspirate.

1 × 2 mL of 100 mM phosphate buffer, pH 6.0; aspirate.

Note: Aspirate at ≤3 in. Hg to prevent sorbent drying.

3. Apply sample.

Load at 1 mL/min.

4. Wash column.

1 × 3 mL of DI H_2O; aspirate.

1 × 3 mL of hexane; aspirate.

Dry column (5 min at ≥10 in. Hg).

5. Elute analyte.

1 × 1 mL of CH_3OH.

6. Dry eluate.
Evaporate to dryness at ≤40°C.

7. Reconstitute.
Add 200 μL CH₃OH. Mix/vortex. Transfer to GC-MS vial and cap.

8. Quantitative.
Inject 1–2 μL of sample onto the GC-MS.

Gas Chromatography Conditions

SCAN Acquisition: 41 amu–400 amu

Start time: 2.00 min

Column: HP Ultra 1, cross-linked methyl silicone

           12 mm × 0.2 × 0.33 μm film thickness

    GC oven   Initial temperature: 100°C

                     Initial time: 3.00 min

                     Ramp: 17°C/min.

                     Final temperature:305°C

                     Final time = 3.00 min

                     Injection port temperature: 250°C

  Transfer line temperature: 280°C

See Figure 3.

10.19 TRICYCLIC ANTIDEPRESSANTS IN SERUM AND PLASMA FOR GC OR GC-MS CONFIRMATIONS USING A 200-MG CLEAN SCREEN EXTRACTION COLUMN (ZSDAU020 OR ZCDAU020)

1. Prepare sample.
  a. To 1 mL of serum add internal standarda and 2 mL of 0.1 *M* phosphate buffer, pH 6.0.
  b. Mix/vortex. Centrifuge for 10 min at 670*g* and discard pellet.
  c. Sample pH should be 6.0 ± 0.5.

2. Condition CLEAN SCREEN extraction column.
1 × 3 mL of CH₃OH; aspirate.
1 × 3 mL of DI H₂O; aspirate.
1 × 1 mL of 0.1 *M* phosphate buffer, pH 6.0; aspirate.
Note: Aspirate at ≤3 in. Hg to prevent sorbent drying.

3. Apply sample.
Load at 1 mL/min.

4. Wash column.
1 × 3 mL of DI H₂O; aspirate.
1 × 1 mL of 1.0 *M* acetic acid; aspirate.
1 × 3 mL of CH₃OH; aspirate.
Dry column (5 min at ≥ 10 in. Hg).

5. Elute.
1 × 3 mL of CH₂Cl₂–IPA–NH₄OH (78:20:2).
Collect eluate at 1 mL/min or use gravity flow.
Note: Prepare elution solvent fresh daily.
Add IPA–NH₄OH, mix, then add CH₃Cl₂, pH 11.0–12.0.

TIC of DATA: 0924733A.D

Sample prior to
solid phase
extraction procedure

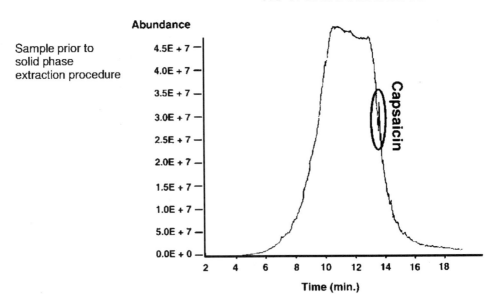

TIC of DATA: 0924733D.D

Sample after
solid phase
extraction procedure

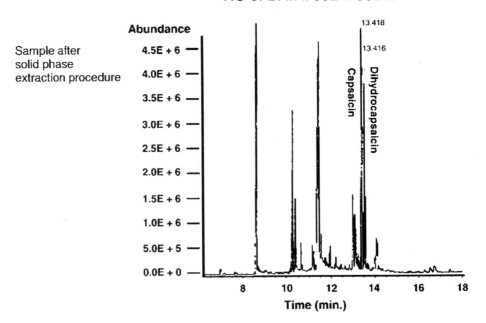

Fig. 3. Tear gas chromatograms.

Table 18
Analytes and Extraction Efficiency

Compound	Retention time (min)	% Recovery	% RSD
Trimipramine ISTD[a]	2.564	100.0%	5.53%
Doxepin	3.048	96.5%	8.04%
Amitriptyline	3.433	98.9%	5.64%
Imipramine	3.865	97.2%	6.09%
Nortriptyline	5.349	88.9%	9.49%
Nordoxepin	5.788	85.0%	5.29%
Desipramine	6.067	85.3%	5.04%
Protriptyline ISTD[a]	6.476	86.3%	5.39%

[a]Internal standards.

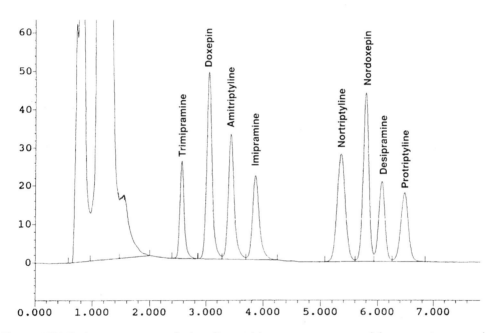

Fig. 4. HPLC chromatogram of tricyclic antidepressant extracted from a urine sample.

6. **Dry eluate.**
   Evaporate to dryness at ≤40°C.
7. **Quantitate.**
   a. Reconstitute with 200 μL of acetonitrile-DI H_2O (1:3). Mix/vortex vigorously for 30 s.
   b. Inject 100 μL onto the chromatograph.

HPLC Conditions
HPLC column: Propylcyano, endcapped 4.6 mm × 150 mm, 5 μm particle size
Column temperature: 30°C
Mobile phase: acetonitrile-buffer-methanol (60:25:15)
   Buffer: 0.01 M K_2HPO_4 adjusted to pH 7.0 with $H_3 PO_4$
Flow rate: 1.75 mL/min

Tips

1. Silica-based HPLC columns are sensitive to pH. To prevent dissolution of the packing, especially at the head of the column, it is best to place a silica column before the injector. This will saturate the mobile phase with silica.

2. Secondary amines bind to glass and polyethylene. Silylation of all surfaces that come in contact with the sample is recommended. Immersion into 5% DMCS in toluene or vapor deposition will deactivate the surface by silylation.

3. To ensure the proper strength of elution solvent, measure the apparent pH of the elution solvent. It should be pH 10.0 or higher. If it is not, add 1%–2% more ammonium hydroxide and check again.
   See Figure 4.

Selected Readings

Abe, J., Asada, A., Fujimori, M., Imaoka, S., and Funae, Y. Binding of lidocaine to plasma proteins resolved by high-performance liquid chromatography. J. Chromatogr. 526:562–568, 1990.

Ahou, F., Krull, I., and Feibush, B. Direct determination of adamantanamine in plasma and urine with automated solid-phase derivatization. J. Chromatogr. 619:93–101, 1993.

Allievi, C., Dostert, P., Strolin Benedetti, M. Determination of free salsolinol concentrations in human urine using gas chromatography-mass spectrometry. J. Chromatogr. 568:271–279, 1991.

Ahnoff, M., and Persson, B. Chromatography of calcium channel blockers. J. Chromatogr. 531:181–213, 1990.

Andrisano, V., Cavrini, V., and Bonazzi, D. HPLC determination of 18 B-glycyrrhetinic and glycyrrhizinic acids in toothpastes after solid-phase extraction. Chromatographia 35:167–172, 1993.

Annan, R., Kim, C., and Martyn, J. Measurement of D-tubocurarine chloride in human urine using solid-phase extraction and reversed-phase high-performance liquid chromatography. J. Chromatogr. 526:228–234, 1990.

Barberi-Heyob, M., Merlin, J., and Weber, B. Determination of 5-fluorouracil and its main metabolites in plasma by high-performance liquid chromatography. J. Chromatogr. 573:247–252, 1992.

Barberi-Heyob, M., Merlin, J., and Weber, B. Analysis of 5-fluorouracil in plasma and urine by high performance liquid chromatography. J. Chromatogr. 581:281–286, 1992.

Bell, R., and Newman, K. Carbohydrate analysis of fermentation broth by high-performance liquid chromatography utilizing solid-phase extraction. J. Chromatog. 732:87–90, 1993.

Bertelloni, S., Baroncelli, G., Benedetti, U., Franchi, G., and Saggese, G. Commercial kits for 1, 25-dihydroxyvitamin D compared with a liquid-chromatographic assay. Clin. Chem. 39:1086–1089, 1993.

Bland, R., Tanner, J., Chem, W., Lang, J., and Powell, J. Determination of albuterol concentrations in human plasma using solid-phase extraction and high-performance liquid chromatography. Pharmaceut. Biomed. Analysis 8:591–596, 1990.

Blanz, J., Rosenfeld, C., Proksch, B. Ehninger, C., and Zeller, K. Quantitation of busulfan in plasma by high-performance liquid chromatography using postcolumn photolysis. J. Chromatogr. 532:429–437, 1990.

Bonnefous, L., Gendre, P., Guillaumont, M., Frederich, A., and Aulagner, G. Determination of six thioguanine nucleotides in human red blood cells using solid phase extraction prior to high performance liquid chromatography. J. Liq. Chromatogr. 15:851–861, 1992.

Bonnefous, L., and Boulieu, R. Comparison of solid phase extraction and liquid-liquid extraction methods for liquid chromatographic determination of diltiazem. J. Liq. Chromatogr. 13:379–380, 1990.

Borvak, J., Kasanicka, J., and Mayer, V. HPLC-monitoring of AZT in HIV-infected patient's plasma: A critical study. Acta Virol. 36:428–434, 1992.

Boulieu, R., Bonnefous, J., and Ferry, S. Solid-phase extraction of diltiazem and its metabolites from plasma prior to high-performance liquid chromatography. J. Chromatogr. 528: 542–546, 1990.

Boukhabza, A., Lugnier, A., Kintz, P., Mangin, P., and Chaumont, A. Simple and sensitive method for monitoring clonazepam in human plasma and urine by high-performance liquid chromatography. J. Chromatogr. 529: 210–216, 1990.

Bozkurt, A., Basci, N., Isimer, A., and Kayaalp, S. Determination of debrisoquine and 4-hydroxydebrisoquine in urine by high-performance liquid chromatography with fluorescence. J. Pharmaceut. Sci. 11:745–749, 1993.

Brownsill, R., Wallace, D., Taylor, A., and Campbell, B. Study of human urinary metabolism of fenfluramine using gas chromatography-mass spectrometry. J. Chromatogr. 562: 267–277, 1991.

Bruns, A., Waldhoff, H., Wilsch-Irrgang, A., and Winkle, W. Automated high performance liquid chromatographic and size exclusion chromatographic sample preparation by means of a robotic workstation. J. Chromatogr. 592:249–253, 1992.

Bwyuktimkin, S., Ekinci, A., Toxunoglu, S., Atmaca, S., and Buyuktimkin, N. Solid phase extraction of 5-hydroxyindole-3-acetic acid from urine and its application to HPLC and spectrophotometric determination. Pharmazie. 46:355–358, 1991.

Campins-Falco, P., Herraez-Hernandez, R., and Sevillano-Cabeza, A. Solid-phase extraction techniques for assay of diuretics in human urine samples. J. Liq. Chromatogr. 14:575–590, 1991.

Caputo, F., Fox, D., Long, G., Moore, C., Mowers, S., Purnel, G. Bonded phase extraction of fentanyls in biological fluids. Internal publication: United Chemical Technologies, Inc.

Castillo, M., and Smith, P. Direct determination of ibuprofen and ibuprofen acyl glucuronide in plasma by high performance liquid chromatography. J. Chromatogr. 614:109–116, 1993.

Chandrashekhar, J., Gaitonde, D., and Pathak, P. Estimation of the analgesic muscle relaxants chlorzoxazone and diazepam in human plasma by reversed-phase liquid chromatography. J. Chromatogr. 528:407–414, 1990.

Chen, Y., Potter, J., and Ravenscroft, P. High-performance liquid chromatographic method for the simultaneous determination of monoethylglycinexylidide and lidocaine. J. Chromatogr. 574:361–364, 1992.

Chen, Y., Potter, J., and Ravenscroft, P. A quick, sensitive high-performance liquid chromatography assay for monoethylglycinexylidide and lidocaine in serum/plasma using solid phase extraction. Ther. Drug Monitor. 14:317–321, 1992.

Chollet, M., and Salanon, M. Determination of ZY 17617B in plasma by solid phase extraction and liquid chromatography with automated pre-column ion exchange chromatography. J. Chromatogr. 593:73–78, 1992.

Christians, U., Braun, F., and Kosian, N. High performance liquid chromatography/mass spectrometry of FK 506 and its metabolites in blood, bile and urine. Transplantat. Proc. 23: 274–279, 1991.

Collins, S., O'Keefe, M., Chen, Y., Potter, J., and Ravenscroft, P. Multi-residue analysis for beta-agonists in urine and liver samples using mixed phase columns with determination by radioimmunoassay. Analyst.119:261–267, 1994.

Colthup, P., Young, G., and Felgate, C. Determination of salmeterol in rat and dog plasma by high-performance liquid chromatography with fluorescence detection. J. Pharmaceut. Sci. 82:323–325, 1993.

Constanzer, L., Hessey, G., and Bayne, W. Analytical method for the quantification of famotidine, an H2-receptor blocker in plasma and urine. J. Chromatogr. 338:438–443, 1985.

Coutant, J., Westmark, P., Nardella, P., Walter, S., and Okerholm, R. Determination of terfenadine and terfenadine acid metabolite in plasma using solid phase extraction and high performance liquid chromatography. J. Chromatogr. 570:139–148, 1991.

Cox, S., Wilke, A., Frazier, D. Determination of adriamycin in plasma and tissue biopsies. J. Chromatogr. 564:322–329, 1991.

Dalbacke, J., and Dahlquist, I. Determination of vitamin B12 in multivitamin-multimineral tablets by high-performance liquid chromatography after solid phase extraction. J. Chromatogr. 541:388–392, 1991.

De Jong, J., Maessen, P., Akkerdaas, A., Cqeung, S., Pinedo, M., and Van Der Vijgh, W. Sensitive method for the determination of daunorubicin and all first known metabolites in plasma and heart by high-performance liquid chromatography. J. Chromatogr. 529:359–368, 1990.

Dikkeschei, L., Wolthers, B., de Ruyter-Buitenhuis, A. Determination of megestrol acetate and cyproterone acetate in serum of patients with advanced breast cancer. J. Chromatogr. 529:145–154, 1990.

Di Pietra, A., Bonazzi, D., and Cavrini, V. Analysis of chlorpropamide, tolbutamide, and their related sulphonamide impurities by liquid chromatography (HPLC). Il Farmaco. 47: 787–797, 1992.

Dixit, V., Nguyen, H., and Dixit, V. Solid-phase extraction of fluoxetine and norfluoxetine from serum with gas chromatography-electron-capture detection. J. Chromatogr. 563: 379–384, 1991.

Ducharme, J., Varin, F., Bevin, D., Donati, F., and Theoret, Y. High-performance liquid chromatography electrochemical detection of vecuronium and its metabolites in human plasma. J. Chromatogr. 573:79–86, 1992.

Eddins, C., Hamann, J., and Johnson, K. HPLC analysis of clenbuterol, a beta blocker in human urine. J. Chromatogr. Sci. 23:308–312, 1985.

El-Yazigi, A., and Wahab, F. Expedient liquid chromatographic analysis of azathioprine in plasma by the use of silica solid phase extraction. Ther. Drug Monit. 14:312–316, 1992.

Farthing, D., Karnes, T., Gehr, T., March, C., Fakhry, I., Sica, D. External standard high-performance liquid chromatographic method for quantitative determination of furosemide in plasma. J. Pharmaceut. Sci. 81:569–571, 1992.

Fernandez, P., Hermida, I., Bermejo, A., Lopez-Rivadul, M., Cruz, A., and Concheiro, L. Simultaneous determination of diazepam and its metabolites in plasma by high-performance liquid chromatography. J. Liq. Chromatogr. 14:587–591, 1991.

Gaillard, Y., Gay-Montchamp, J., and Ollagnier, M. Gas chromatographic determination of meprobamate in serum or plasma after solid-phase extraction. J. Chromatogr. 577: 171–173, 1992.

Gaillard, Y., Gay-Montchamp, J., and Ollagnier, M. Gas chromatographic determination of zopiclone in plasma after solid phase extraction. J. Chromatogr. 619:310–314, 1993.

Garg, V., and Jusko, W. Simultaneous analysis of prednisone, prednisolone and their major hydroxylated metabolites in urine by high-performance liquid chromatography. J. Chromatogr. 567:39–47, 1991.

Gupta, R., and Lew, M. Determination of trazodone in human plasma by liquid chromatography with fluorescence detection. J. Chromatogr. 342:442–446, 1985.

Hansen, A., Poulsen, O., Christenson, J., and Hansen, S. Determination of 1-hydroxypyrene in human urine by high-performance liquid chromatography. J. Analyt. Toxicol. 17:38–41, 1993.

Hattori, H., Yamamoto, S., Iwata, M., Takashima, E., Yamada, T., Suzuki, O. Determination of diphenylmethane antihistaminic drugs and their analogues in body fluids by gas chromatography. J. Chromatogr. 581:213–218, 1992.

He, L., and Stewart, J. A high performance liquid chromatographic method for the determination of albuterol enantiomers in human serum using solid phase extraction and chemical derivatization. Biomed. Chromatogr. 6:291–294, 1992.

Hennig, B., Radler, S., Blaschke, G., and Boos, J. Solid-phase sample preparation of isofamide and dichloroethyl metabolites in biological material. Pharmazie. 47:783–788, 1992.

Hong, W. Application of solid-phase extraction in the determination of U-82217 in rat serum, urine and brain. J. Chromatogr. 629:83–87, 1993.

Hotter, G., Gomez, G., Ramis, I., Bioque, G., Rosello-Catafau, J., and Gelpi, E. Solid phase extraction of prostanoids using an automatic sample preparation system. J. Chromatogr. 307:239–243, 1992.

Huber, R., and Picot, V. Direct injection/HPLC methods for the analysis of drugs in biological samples. Xenobiotica 22:765–774, 1992.

Hubert, P., Ceccato, C., Bechet, I., Sibenaler-Dechamps, R., Maes, P., and Crommen, J. Determination of verapamil and nor-verapamil in human plasma by liquid chromatography: Comparison between a liquid-liquid extraction and solid phase extraction. J. Pharmaceut. Sci. 10:937–942, 1992.

Hussein, Z., Chu, S., and Granneman, G. High-performance liquid chromatographic method for determination of DN-2327, a novel non-benzodiazepine anxiolytic. J. Chromatogr. 613:105–112, 1993.

Igarashi, K., and Castagnoli, N. Determination of the pyridinium metabolite derived from haloperidol in brain tissue, plasma, and urine by high-performance chromatography. J. Chromatogr. 579:277–283, 1992.

Jandreski, M., and Vanderslice, W. Clinical measurement of serum amiodarone and desethylamiodarone by using solid-phase extraction. Clin. Chem. 39:496–499, 1993.

Johnson, K., Kolatkar, V., and Straka, R. Improved selectivity of a high-performance liquid chromatography assay for debrisoquine and its 4-hydroxy metabolite. Ther. Drug Monitor. 12:478–480, 1990.

Kabra, P., and Nzekwe, E. Liquid chromatographic analysis of clonazepam in human serum with solid-phase extraction. J. Chromatogr. 341:383–390, 1985.

Kaiser, S. Sensitive GC/MS assay of cotinine in serum. SOFT Poster, 1997.

Kanazawa, H., Nagata, Y., Matsushima, Y., Takai, N., Vchiyama, H., Nishimura, R., and Takeuchi, H. Liquid chromatography-mass spectrometry for the determination of medetomidine and other anaesthetics in plasma. J. Chromatogr. 631:215–220, 1992.

Knupp, C., Stahoeto, F., Papp, E., and Barbhaiya, R. Quantitation of didanosine in human plasma and urine by high-performance liquid chromatography. J. Chromatogr. 533: 282–290, 1990.

Krailler, R., Adams, P., and Lane, P. Quantitation of doretinal in a topical gel using high performance liquid chromatography with solid phase extraction sample preparation. J. Liq. Chromatogr. 14: 238–239, 1991.

Krishna, R., and Klotz, U. Determination of ivermectin in human plasma by high-performance liquid chromatography. Arzneim Forsch Drug Res. 43:609–611, 1993.

Kristjansson, F. Sensitive determination of buspirone in serum by solid-phase extraction and twodimensional high-performance liquid chromatography. J. Chromatogr. 566: 250–256, 1991.

Kurono, M., Yoshida, K., Arakawa, S., and Naruto, S. Determination of a novel calcium entry blocker, AJ-2615, in plasma using solid-phase extraction and high-performance liquid chromatography. J. Chromatogr. 532:175–180, 1990.

Langner, J., Gan, B., Liu, R., Baugh, D., Chand, P., Weng, J. L., Edwards, C., and Amrik, S. Enzymatic digestion, solid-phase extraction, and gas chromatography/mass spectrometry of derivatized intact oxazepam in urine. Clin. Chem. 37:1595–1600, 1991.

Lave, T., Efthymiopoiu, C., Koffel, J., and Jung, L. Determination of tertatol enantiomers in biological fluids by high-performance liquid chromatography. J. Chromatogr. 572:203–210, 1991.

Leenheers, L., Engel, R., Spruit, W., Meuling, W., and Jongen, M. Determination of methyl 5-hydroxy-2-benzimidazole carbamate in urine by high-performance liquid chromatography. J. Chromatogr. 613:89–94, 1993.

Leneveu, K., Stheneur, A., Bousquet, A., and Roux, R. Automated high-performance liquid chromatographic technique for determining diltiazem and its three main metabolites in serum. J. Liq. Chromatogr. 14:3519–3530, 1991.

Lensmeyter, G., Wiebe, D., and Doran, T. Application of the empore solid-phase extraction membrane to the isolation of drugs from blood. 1. Amiodarone and desethylamiodarone. Ther. Drug Monitor. 13:244–250, 1991.

Lewis, R., Phillips, B., Baldwin, J., Rossi, D., and Narang, P. A sensitive and specific procedure for quantitation of ADR-529 in biological fluids by high-performance liquid chromatography (HPLC) with column switching and amperometric detection. Pharmaceut. Res. 9:101–105, 1991.

Lindberg, C., Jonsson, S., and Paulson, J. Determination of bambuterol, a prodrug of terbutaline, in plasma and urine by gas chromatography/mass spectrometry. Biomed. Environ. Mass 19:218–224, 1990.

Matsubayashi, K., Yoshioka, M., and Tachizawa, H. Simple method for determination of the cephalosporin DQ-2556 in biological fluids by high-performance liquid chromatography. J. Chromatogr. 515:547–554, 1990.

Maya, M., Farinha, A., Lucas, A., and Morais, J. Sensitive method for the determination of phenytoin in plasma, and phenytoin and 5-(4-hydroxyphenol)-5- phenylhydantoin in urine. J. Pharmaceut. Biomed. Analysis 10:1001–1004, 1992.

Mazzi, G., and Schinella, M. Simple and practical high-performance liquid chromatographic assay of proof in human blood. J. Chromatogr. 528:537–541, 1990.

McCarthy, P., Atwal, S., Sykes, A., and Ayres, J. Measurement of terbutaline and salbutamol in plasma by high performance liquid chromatography with fluorescence detection. Biomed. Chromatogr. 7:25–28, 1993.

Michaelis, H. Determination of pyridostigmine plasma concentrations by high-performance liquid chromatography. J. Chromatogr. 534:291–294, 1990.

Michaelis, H., Geng, W., Kahl, G., and Foth, H. Sensitive determination of bupivacaine in human plasma by high-performance liquid chromatography. J. Chromatogr. 527: 201–207, 1990.

Miyauchi, Y., Sano, N., and Nakamura, T. Simultaneous determination of nicotinic acid and its two metabolites in human plasma using solid-phase extraction. Int. J. Vitam. Nutr. Res. 63:145–150, 1992.

Mross, K., Mayer, U., Hamm, K., and Hossfeld, D. High-performance liquid chromatography of lododoxorubicin and fluorescent metabolites in plasma samples. J. Chromatogr. 530:192–199, 1992.

Nicholls, G., Clark, B., and Brown, J. Solid-phase extraction and optimized separation of doxorubicin, epirubicin and their metabolites using reversed-phase chromatography. Pharmaceut. Biomed. Analysis 10:10–12, 1994.

Nichols, J., Charlson, J., and Lawson, G. Automated HPLC assay of fluoxetine and norfluoxetine in serum. Clin. Chem. 40:1312–1316, 1994.

Noguchi, H., Tomita, N., and Naruto, S. Determination of gliclazide in serum by high performance liquid chromatography using solid-phase extraction. J. Chromatogr. 583:266–269, 1992.

Ohkubo, T., Shimoyarna, R., and Sugawara, K. Measurement of haloperidol in human breast milk by high-performance liquid chromatography. Pharmaceut. Sci. 81:947–949, 1992.

Ohkubo, T., Shimoyama, R., and Sugawara, K. High performance liquid chromatographic determination of levomepromazine in human breast milk and serum using solid phase extraction. Biomed. Chromatogr. 7:229–228, 1993.

Papadoyannis, I. A simple and quick solid phase extraction and reversed phase HPLC analysis of sometropane alkaloids in feedstuff and biological samples. Liq. Chromatogr.16:975–998, 1993.

Papadoyannis, I., Zotou, A., and Samanidou, V. Simultaneous reversed-phase gradient HPLC analysis of anthranilic acid derivatives in anti-inflammatory drugs. Liq. Chromatogr. 15:1923–1941, 1992.

Perkins, S., Livesey, J., Escares, E., Belche, J., and Dudley, D. High performance liquid-chromatographic method compared with a modified radioimmunoassay of cotinine in plasma. Clin. Chem. 37:1989–1991, 1992.

Pichini, S., Altied, I., Pacifici, R., Rosa, M., Ottaviani, G., and Zuccaro, P. Elimination of caffeine interference in high-performance liquid chromatographic determination of cotinine in human plasma. J. Chromatogr. 568:267–269, 1991.

Pichini, S., Altied, I., Pacifici, R., Rosa, M., Ottaviani, G., and Zuccaro, P. Simultaneous determination of cotinine and trans-3'-hydroxycotinine in human serum by high-performance liquid chromatography. J. Chromatogr. 577:358–361, 1992.

Picot, V., Doyle, E., and Pearce, J. Analysis of zaprinast in rat and human plasma by automated solid-phase extraction and reversed-phase high performance liquid chromatography. J. Chromatogr. 527:454–460, 1990.

Plomp, T., and Buijs, M. High-performance liquid chromatographic method for the simultaneous determination of pentisomide and its major metabolites. J. Chromatogr. 612:123–135, 1992.

Poirier, J., Lebot, M., and Cheymol, G. Analysis of necainide and its three metabolites in plasma by column liquid chromatography. J. Chromatogr. 534:223–227, 1990.

Qian, M., Finco, T., and Gallo, J. Rapid and simultaneous determination of zidovudine and its glucuronide metabolite in plasma and urine. Pharmaceut. Biomed. Analysis 9:275–279, 1991.

Reid, R., Deakin, A., and Leehey, D. Measurement of naloxone in plasma using high performance liquid chromatography with electrochemical detection. J. Chromatogr. 614:117–122, 1993.

Rop, P., Spinazzola, J., and Brezzon, M. Determination of amineptine and its main metabolite in plasma by high-performance liquid chromatography after solid-phase extraction. J. Chromatogr. 532:351–361, 1990.

Rop, P., Grimaldi, F., Bresson, M., Fornaris, M., and Viala, A. Simultaneous determination of dextromoramide, propoxyphene and nor-propoxyphene in necroptic whole blood. J. Chromatogr. 615:357–364, 1993.

Rouan, M., Campestrini, J., LeClanche, V., Lecaillon, J., and Godbillon, J. Automated microanalysis of carbamazepine and its eposide and trans-diol metabolites in plasma by column liquid chromatography. J. Chromatogr. 573:65–68, 1992.

Rubert, P., and Crommen, J. Automatic determination of indomethacin in human plasma using liquid solid extraction on disposable cartridges in combination with HPLC. Liq. Chromatogr.13:3891–3907, 1992.

Saeed, K., and Becher, M. On-line solid-phase extraction of piroxicam prior to its determination by high-performance liquid chromatography. J. Chromatogr. 567:185–193, 1991.

Sautou, V., Chopineau, J., Terrisse, M., and Bastide, P. Solid-phase extraction of midazolam and two of its metabolites from plasma for high-performance liquid chromatography. J. Chromatogr. 571:298–304, 1991.

Schenck, F., Wagner, R., and Bargo, W. Determination of clorsulon residues in milk using a solid-phase extraction cleanup and liquid chromatographic determination. Liq. Chromatogr. 16:513–520, 1993.

Schwende, F., and Rykert, U. Determination of alentamol hydrobromide, a novel antipsychotic agent, in human blood plasma and urine by high-performance liquid chromatography. J. Chromatogr. 565:488–496, 1991.

Shao, G., Goto, J., and Nambara, T. Separation and determination of propranolol enantiomers in plasma by high-performance liquid chromatography. Liq. Chromatogr. 14:753–763, 1991.

Shintani, H. Solid-phase extraction (SPE) and HPLC analysis of toxic compounds and comparison of SPE and liquid-liquid extraction. J. Liq. Chromatogr. 15:1315–1330, 1992.

Shintani, H., Tsuchiya, T., Hata, Y., and Nakamura, A. Solid phase extraction and HPLC analysis of toxic components eluted from methyl methacrylate dental materials. J. Analyt. Toxicol. 17: 73–78, 1993.

Simmonds, R., Wood, S., and Ackland, J. A sensitive high performance liquid chromatography assay for trospectomycin and aminocyclitol antibiotics in human plasma and serum. Liq. Chromatogr. 16:1125–1142, 1990.

Sioufi, A., Richard, J., Mangoni, P., and Godbillon, J. Determination of diclofenac in plasma using a fully automated analytical system combining liquid-solid extraction with liquid chromatography. J. Chromatogr. 565:401–407, 1990.

Sioufi, A., Sandrenan, N., and Godbillon, J. Determination of 10 alpha-methoxy-9, 10-dihydrolysergol, a nicergoline metabolite, in human urine by high-performance liquid chromatography. Biomed. Chromatogr. 6:9–11, 1992.

Siren, H., Saarinen, M., Hainari, S., Lukkari, P., Riekkola, M. Screening of B-blockers in human serum by ion-pair chromatography and their identification as methyl or acetyl metabolites. J. Chromatogr. 632:215–227, 1993.

Skee, D., Cook, J., and Benziger, D. Determination of a novel steroidal androgen receptor antagonist (WIN 49596) in human plasma using solid-phase extraction. J. Chromatogr. 568:494–500, 1991.

Snell, R. Solid-phase extraction and liquid chromatographic determination of mono-phthalates and phthalide extracted from solution. J. AOAC Int. 76:531–534, 1993.

Soini, H., Tsuda, T., and Novotny, M. Electrochromatographic solid-phase extraction for determination of cimetidine in serum by micellar electrokinetic chromatography. J. Chromatogr. 559:547–558, 1991.

Suss, S., Seiler, W., Hiemke, C., Schollnhammer, G., Wetzel, H., Hillert, A. Determination of benperidol and its reduced metabolite in human plasma by high-performance liquid chromatography. J. Chromatogr. 565:363–373, 1991.

Svensson, C., Nyberg, G., Soomagi, M., and Martensson, E. Determination of serum concentrations of thioridazine and its main metabolites using a solid-phase extraction technique. J. Chromatogr. 529:229–236, 1990.

Szumilo, H., and Dzido, T. Determination of tryptamide and its metabolites with solid phase extraction, TLC, and HPLC in rats. Liq. Chromatogr. 15:337–349, 1992.

Takada, K., Oh-Hashi, M., Yoshikawa, H., and Muranishi, S. Determination of a novel, potent immunosuppressant (FK-506) in rat serum and lymph by high-performance liquid chromatography. J. Chromatogr. 530:212–218, 1990.

Takeda, S., Ono, H., Wakui, Y. Determination of glycyrrhetic acid in human serum by high performance liquid chromatography with ultraviolet detection. J. Chromatogr. 530: 447–451, 1990.

Tan, H., Manning, M., Hahn, M., Hetty, Tan, G., Kotagal, U. Determination of benzyl alcohol and its metabolite in plasma by reversed-phase high-performance liquid chromatography. J. Chromatogr. 568:145–155, 1991.

Tanaka, M., Ono, K., Hakasui, H. Identification of DP1904 and its ESTR glucuronide in human urine and determination of their enantiomeric compositions. Drug Metab. Dispos. 18:698–701, 1990.

Taylor, R., Reid, R., Behrens, R., and Kanfer, I. Multidrug assay method for antimalarials. Pharmaceut. Biomed. Analysis 10:867–871, 1992.

Thienpont, L., Depoureq, G., Nelis, H., and De Leenheer, A. Liquid chromatographic determination of 2-thioxothiazolidine-4-carboxylic acid isolated from urine. Analyt. Chem. 62:2673–2675, 1990.

Thies, R., Cowens, O., Cullis, P., Bally, M., and Mayer, L. Method for rapid separation of liposome-associated doxorubicin from free doxorubicin in plasma. Analyt. Biochem. 188:65–71, 1990.

Torfgard, K., Ahiner, J., and Norlander, B. Simultaneous determination of glyceryl trinitrate and its two dinitrate metabolites in plasma and tissues by capillary gas chromatography. J. Chromatogr. 534:196–201, 1990.

Van Der Horst, A., De Goede, P., Van Diemen, H., Polman, C., Martens, H. Determination of 4-aminopyridine in serum by solid-phase extraction and high-performance liquid chromatography. J. Chromatogr. 574:166–169, 1992.

Vahn, F., Tu, T., Benoit, F., Villeneuve, J., Theoret, Y. High-performance liquid chromatographic determination of spironolactone and its metabolites in human biological fluids. J. Chromatogr. 574:57–64, 1992.

Volmut, J., Matisova, E., and Ha, P. Simultaneous determination of six anti-epileptic drugs by capillary gas chromatography. J. Chromatogr. 527:428–435, 1990.

Volmut, J., Melnik, M., and Matisova, E. Analysis of antiepiletic drugs by capillary gas chromatography with on-column injection. J. High Resolut. Chromatogr. 16:27–31, 1993.

Von Baer, D., Momberg, A., Carrera, M., Arriagada, R., Smyths, M. Liquid chromatography with amperometric detection of some sulphonamides and their N4-acetyl-metabolites in serum and urine. J. Pharmaceut. Biomed. Analysis 9:925 - 928, 1991.

Vu-Duc, T., and Vernay, A. Evaluation of sample treatment procedures for the routine identification and determination at nanogram levels. J. High Resolut. Chromatogr. 13:162–166, 1990.

Wells, T., Hendry, I., and Kearns, G. Measurement of bumetanide in plasma and urine by high-performance liquid chromatography. J. Chromatogr. 570:235–242, 1991.

Whelpton, R., Dudson, P., Cannell, H., and Webster, K. Determination of prilocaine in human plasma samples using high-performance liquid chromatography. J. Chromatogr. 526:215–222, 1990.

Whelpton, R., Hurst, P., Metcalfe, R., and Saunders, S. Liquid chromatographic determination of hyoscine (scopolamine) in urine using solid-phase extraction. Biomed. Chromatogr. 6:198–204, 1990.

Wilhelm, J., Bailey, L., and Shepard, T. Simultaneous determination of phenolphthalein and phenolphthalein glucuronide from dog serum, urine and bile. J. Chromatogr. 578:231–238, 1992.

Wolf, C., Saady, J., and Poklis, A. Determination of gabapentin in serum using solid phase extraction and gas-liquid chromatography. J. Analyt. Toxicol. 20:498–501, 1996.

Yamashita, K., Motohashi, M., and Yashiki, T. Sensitive high-performance liquid chromatographic determination of propranolol in human plasma with ultraviolet detection. J. Chromatogr. 527:196–200, 1990.

Yamashita, K., Motohashi, M., and Yashiki, T. High-performance liquid chromatographic determination of phenylpropanolamine in human plasma and urine. J. Chromatogr. 527:103–114, 1990.

Zhang, H., and Stewart, J. Improved high-performance liquid chromatographic determination of chloroxone and its hydroxy metabolite in human serum. Analyt. Lett. 26:675–687, 1993.

Chapter 11

General Methods for Drug Isolation

The versatility of solid phase extraction (SPE) can be best exhibited by its adaptability to isolate a wide variety of different drugs using a general method. This chapter highlights applications that separate a wide variety of drugs and metabolites. Table 1 summarizes a partial listing of those drugs that have been isolated by the CLEAN SCREEN DAU SPE column.

Table 1
Drugs that Have Been Isolated Using the CLEAN SCREEN DAU Extraction Column

Acepromazine	Etorphine	Naproxen
Acetaminophen	Etorphine-3-glucuronide	Nicotine
Amantadine	Fentanyl	Nordiazepam
Amitriptyline	Floxin	Nubain
Amitriptyline metabolite	Fluoxetine	Oxybutynin
Amphetamine	Furosemide	Oxycodone
Apomorphine	Glutethimide	Pemoline
Azaperone	Glutethimide metabolite	Pentazocine
Azaperone-5-glucuronide	Glycopyrrolate	Phencyclidine
Barbiturates	Hordenine	Phenethylamine
Benzocaine	Hydrocortisone	Phentermine
Benzoic acid	Hydromorphone	Phenylbutazone
Benzoylecgonine	Ibuprofen	l-Phenylcyclohexone
Benztropine	Imipramine	Phenylpropanolamine
Buspirone	Imipramine metabolite	Phenytoin
Caffeine	Indomethacin	Primidone
Carbamazepine	Ketamine	Procaine
Carisoprodol	Lidocaine	Propionylpromazine
Chlordiazepoxide	Loxapine	Propoxyphene
Chloroquine	Mazindol	Propoxyphene metabolite
Chlorpheniramine	Meclizine	Propranolol

From: *Forensic Science and Medicine:*
Forensic and Clinical Applications of Solid Phase Extraction
Edited by: M. J. Telepchak, T. F. August, and G. Chaney © Humana Press Inc., Totowa, NJ

Chlorpromazine
Chlorpropamide
Clenbuterol
Clonazepam
Cocaine
Codeine
Cotinine
Cresol
Cyclobenzaprine
Dextromethorphan
Dextrophan
Diazepam
Dihydrocodeine
Diltiazem
Diphenhydramine
Dipyrone
Doxepin
Doxepin metabolite
Doxylamine
Ecgonine
Ethacrynic acid

Mefenamic acid
Meperidine
Meprobamate
Methadone
Methadone metabolite
Methamphetamine
Methylbenzoate
Methylecgoninine
Methyl p-aminobenzoate
Methylphenidate
Methyl salicylate
Methylparaben
Methyprylon and metabolite
Metolazone
Morphine
Morphine-3-glucuronide
N-N-Diethyltryptamine
Nalorphine-3-glucuronide
Naloxone

Propylparaben
Quinidine
Quinine
Salbutamol
Salicylic acid
Strychnine
Temazepam
Terbutaline
Tetracaine
THC and metabolite
Theophylline
Thiopental
Thioridazine
Timolol
Tranylcypromine
Trifluoperazine
Trimethoprim
Trimipramine
Verapamil
Verapamil metabolite

Courtesy of the Philadelphia Medical Examiner's Office, using Forensic Drug Extraction Method 11.7.

11.1 Therapeutic and Abused Drugs in Urine: Manual Method for Acid Neutral Drugs for GC-MS Confirmations Using a 200-mg CLEAN SCREEN Extraction Column (ZSDAU020 or ZCDAU020)

1. **Prepare sample.**
   a. To 5 mL of urine add internal standard(s) and 2 mL of 0.1 *M* phosphate buffer, pH 6.0.
   b. Mix/vortex.
   c. The sample pH should be 6.0 ± 0.5. Adjust pH accordingly with 0.1 *M* monobasic or dibasic sodium phosphate.
2. **Condition CLEAN SCREEN extraction column.**
   1×3 mL of CH_3OH; aspirate.
   1×3 mL of DI H_2O; aspirate.
   1×1 mL of 0.1 *M* phosphate buffer, pH 6.0; aspirate.
   Note: Aspirate at ≤ 3 in. Hg to prevent sorbent drying.
3. **Apply sample.**
   Load at 1–2 mL/min.
4. **Wash column.**
   1×3 mL of DI H_2O; aspirate.
   1×1 mL of 0.1 *M* acetic acid; aspirate.
   Dry column (5 min at ≥ 10 in. Hg).
   1×2 mL of hexane; aspirate.

Table 2

Step		Source	Destination	mL	mL/min	Liq. chk
1.	Condition	MeOH	Org.	3	12.	No
2.	Condition	H_2O	Aq.	3	12	No
3.	Condition	pH 6.0	Aq.	1	12	No
4.	Load	Sample	Bio.	5	1.2	No
5.	Load	Sample	Bio.	2.2	1.2	No
6.	Purge—cannula	H_2O	Cannula	6	30	No
7.	Purge—cannula	MeOH	Cannula	6	30	No
8.	Rinse	H_2O	Aq.	3	12	No
9.	Rinse	HAc	Aq.	1	12	No
10.	Dry	Time = 5 min				
11.	Rinse	Hexane	Bio.	2	12.	No
12.	Dry	Time = 3 min				
13.	Collect	Elute	Fract1	6	2.0	No
14.	Rinse	H_2O	Aq.	6	12	No
15.	Rinse	MeOH	Aq.	6	12	No
15.	Purge—cannula	H_2O	Cannula	6	12	No
16.	Purge—cannula	MeOH	Cannula	6	12	No

Load cannula depth = 0   Mix volume = .5
Mix cannula depth = 0   Mix speed = 0.30
Mix cycles = 2   Reagent mix cycles = 2

5. Elute acidic and neutral drugs.
    1 × 3 mL of hexane-ethyl acetate (50:50); collect eluate at ≤5 mL/min.
6. Dry eluate.
    a. Evaporate to dryness at ≤40°C.
    b. Reconstitute with 100 μL of ethyl acetate.
7. Quantitate.
    Inject 1–2 μL onto the chromatograph.
Source: UCT internal publication.

11.2 Therapeutic and Abused Drugs in Urine: Automated Method for Acid Neutral Drugs for GC or GC-MS Confirmations Using a 200-mg CLEAN SCREEN Extraction Column (CSDAU203 or CCDAU203)

1. Prepare sample.
    a. To 5 mL of urine add internal standard(s) and 2 mL of 0.1 *M* phosphate
        buffer, pH 6.0.
    b. Mix/vortex.
    c. The sample pH should be 6.0 ± 0.5. Adjust pH accordingly with 0.1 *M* monobasic
        or dibasic sodium phosphate.

11.2.1 Settings for RapidTrace Analysis of Acid/Neutral Drugs

Table 3

Reagent Setup

No.	Reagent	Abbreviation	Sip speed
1	Water	H_2O	30
2	Methanol	MeOH	30
3	Hexane	Hex	30
4	0.1 *M* Acetic acid	HAc	30
5	Hexane-Ethyl acetate (50:50)	Elute	15
6	Methylene chloride	MeCl	30
7	Phosphate buffer, pH 6.0	pH 6.0	30
8	Mixing vessel	Mixer	15
9	Sample	Sample	15

Column air push volume = 2
Column air push volume speed multiplier = 2

Table 4

No.	Waste	Abbreviation
1	Aqueous	Aq.
2	Organic solvent	Org.
3	Biohazardous	Bio.

2. **Place into the RapidTrace sample rack.**
   Follow the RapidTrace procedure described on procedure described in Section 11.2.1.
3. **Remove extracted sample from the RapidTrace.**
4. **Dry eluate.**
   a. Evaporate to dryness at ≤40°C.
   b. Reconstitute with 100 µL of ethyl acetate.
5. **Quantitate.**
   Inject 1–2 µL onto the chromatograph.

Source: UCT internal publication.

11.3 BASIC DRUGS FOR HPLC ANALYSIS USING 200-MG CLEAN SCREEN® EXTRACTION COLUMN (ZSDAU020 OR ZCDAU0202)

1. **Prepare sample.**
   a. To 5 mL of urine add internal standard(s) and 2 mL of 0.1 *M* phosphate buffer, pH 6.0.
   b. Mix/vortex.
   c. The sample pH should be 6.0 ± 0.5. Adjust pH accordingly with 0.1 *M* monobasic or dibasic sodium phosphate.

2. Condition CLEAN SCREEN extraction column.

1 × 3 mL of CH_3OH; aspirate.

1 × 3 mL of DI H_2O; aspirate.

1 × 1 mL of 0.1 M phosphate buffer, pH 6.0; aspirate.

Note: Aspirate at ≤3 in. Hg to prevent sorbent drying.

3. Apply sample.

Load at 1–2 mL/min.

4. Wash column.

1 × 3 mL of DI H_2O; aspirate.

1 × 1 mL of 0.1 M acetic acid; aspirate.

1 × 3 mL of methanol; aspirate.

Dry column (5 min at ≥10 in. Hg).

5. Elute bases.

1 × 2 mL of CH_3OH–NH_4OH (98:2).

Collect eluate at 1–2 mL/min.

Note: Prepare elution solvent daily.

6. Extract.

a. To eluate add 2.0 mL of DI H_2O and 500 µL of methylene chloride.

b. Mix/vortex.

c. Centrifuge at 670g for 10 min.

d. Transfer organic (lower) layer to a clean test tube.

7. Evaporate.

Evaporate to dryness at ≤40°C using a TurboVap or equivalent evaporator.

8. Quantitate.

Reconstitute in mobile phase and inject onto the HPLC.

Source: UCT internal publication.

11.4. BASIC DRUGS IN HUMAN URINE: AUTOMATED PROCEDURE FOR HPLC ANALYSIS USING A 200-MG CLEAN SCREEN EXTRACTION COLUMN (CSDAU203 OR CCDAU203)

1. Prepare sample.

a. To 5 mL of urine add internal standard(s) and 2 mL of 0.1 M phosphate buffer, pH 6.0.

b. Mix/vortex.

c. The sample pH should be 6.0 ± 0.5. Adjust pH accordingly with 0.1 M monobasic or dibasic sodium phosphate.

2. Place sample onto the RapidTrace.

Follow the procedure described in Section 11.4.1.

3. Remove sample from RapidTrace.

4. Extract.

a. To eluate add 2.0 mL of DI H_2O and 500 µL of methylene chloride.

b. Mix/vortex.

c. Centrifuge at 670g for 10 min.

d. Transfer organic (lower) layer to a clean test tube.

5. Evaporate.

Evaporate to dryness at ≤40°C using a TurboVap or equivalent apparatus.

6. Quantitate.

Reconstitute in mobile phase and inject onto the HPLC.

Source: UCT internal publication.

11.4.1 Settings for RapidTrace Analysis of Basic Drugs

Table 5

Step		Source	Destination	mL	mL/min	Liq. chk
1.	Condition	MeOH	Org.	3	12.	No
2.	Condition	H_2O	Aq.	3	12.	No
3.	Condition	pH 6.0	Aq.	1	12.	No
4.	Load	Sample	Bio.	5	1.2	No
5.	Load	Sample	Bio.	2.2	1.2	No
6.	Purge—cannula	H_2O	Cannula	6	30.	No
7.	Purge—cannula	MeOH	Cannula	6	30.	No
8.	Rinse	H_2O	Aq.	3	12.	No
9.	Rinse	HAc	Aq.	2	12.	No
10.	Rinse	MeOH	Aq.	3	12	No
11.	Dry	Time = 5 min				
12.	Collect	Elute	Fract1	3	1.0	No
13.	Rinse	H_2O	Aq.	6	12	No
14.	Rinse	MeOH	Aq.	6	12	No
15.	Purge—cannula	H_2O	Cannula	6	30	No
16.	Purge—cannula	MeOH	Cannula	6	30	No

Load cannula depth = 0   Mix volume = 0.5
Mix cannula depth = 0   Mix speed = 3.0
Mix cycles = 2   Reagent mix cycles = 2

Table 6

Reagent Setup

No.	Reagent	Abbreviation	Sip speed
1.	Water	H_2O	30
2.	Methanol	MeOH	30
3.	Hexane	Hex	30
4.	0.1 *M* Acetic acid	HAc	30
5.	MeCl: 2–IPA–NH_4OH (78:20:2)	Elute	15
6.	Methylene chloride	MeCl	30
7.	Phosphate buffer, pH 6.0	pH 6.0	30
8.	Mixing vessel		15
9.	Sample		15

Column air push volume = 2
Column air push volume speed multiplier = 2

Table 7

No.	Waste	Abbreviation
1.	Aqueous	Aq.
2.	Organic solvent	Org.
3.	Biohazard	Bio.

11.5 THERAPEUTIC AND ABUSED DRUGS IN WHOLE BLOOD: MANUAL METHOD FOR EMIT SCREENING USING A 200-MG CLEAN SCREEN EXTRACTION COLUMN (ZSDAU020 OR ZCDAU020)

1. **Prepare sample.**
   a. To 1 mL of blood add 4 mL of H_2O ($5.0 \leq pH \leq 7.0$).
   b. Mix/vortex. Let stand for 5 min to lyse red blood cells.
   c. Centrifuge for 10 min at $670g$ and discard pellet.
   d. Add 2 mL of 0.1 M phosphate buffer, pH 6.0. Mix/vortex.
   e. Sample pH should be 6.0 ± 0.5. Adjust pH accordingly with 0.1 M monobasic or dibasic sodium phosphate.
2. **Condition CLEAN SCREEN extraction column.**
   1 × 3 mL of methanol; aspirate.
   1 × 3 mL of DI H_2O; aspirate.
   1 × 1 mL of 0.1 M phosphate buffer, pH 6.0; aspirate.
   Note: Aspirate at ≤ 3 in. Hg to prevent sorbent drying.
3. **Apply sample.**
   Load at 1–2 mL/min.
4. **Wash column.**
   1 × 3 mL of DI H_2O.
   1 × 1 mL of 0.1 M acetic acid; aspirate.
   Dry column (5 min at ≥ 10 in. Hg).
   1 × 2 mL of hexane; aspirate.
5. **Elute acidic and neutral drugs.**
   1 × 3 mL of hexane-ethyl acetate (50:50).
   Collect eluate at ≤ 5 mL/min.
6. **Wash column.**
   1 × 3 mL of methanol; aspirate.
   Dry column (5 min at ≥ 10 in. Hg).
7. **Elute basic drugs.**
   Prepare elution solvent daily.
   1 × 3 mL of CH_2Cl_2–IPA–NH_4OH (78:20:2); collect eluate at 1–2 mL/min.
   Note: Elute into tubes containing the acidic and neutral drugs.
8. **Dry eluate; combine eluates (steps 5 and 7).**
   Evaporate to a volume 100 µL using a TurboVap or equivalent evaporator at $\leq 40°C$.
9. **Reconstitute.**
   Add 900 µL of DI H_2O (sample volume is now its original 1.0 mL).
10. **Analyze by EMIT.**
    Process according to urine drug screening methods provided for EMIT or other automated analyzers.

Source: UCT internal publication.

11.6 THERAPEUTIC AND ABUSED DRUGS IN WHOLE BLOOD: AUTOMATED METHOD FOR EMIT SCREENING USING A 200-MG CLEAN SCREEN EXTRACTION COLUMN (CSDAU203 OR CCDAU203)

1. **Prepare sample.**
   a. To 1 mL of blood add 4 mL of H_2O ($5 \leq pH \leq 7.0$).
   b. Mix/vortex. Let stand for 5 min to lyse red blood cells.
   c. Centrifuge for 10 min at 670g and discard pellet.
   d. Add 2 mL of 0.1 M phosphate buffer, pH 6.0. Mix/vortex.
   e. Sample pH should be 6.0 ± 0.5. Adjust pH accordingly with 0.1 M monobasic or dibasic sodium phosphate.
2. **Add sample to the RapidTrace module for analysis.**
   Follow the procedure described in Section 11.6.1.
3. **Remove combined eluates.**
   Combine fract 1 + fract 2.
4. **Dry eluate—evaporate.**
   Evaporate to a volume of 100 μL using a TurboVap or equivalent evaporator at ≤40°C.
5. **Reconstitute.**
   Add 900 μL of DI H_2O (sample volume is now its original 1.0 mL).
6. **Analyze by EMIT.**
   Process according to urine drug screening methods provided for EMIT or other automated analyzers.

Source: UCT internal publication.

11.6.1 Settings for RapidTrace Analysis of Abused Drugs in Whole Blood

Table 8

Step		Source	Destination	mL	mL/min	Liq. chk
1.	Condition	MeOH	Aq.	3	12	No
2.	Condition	H_2O	Aq.	3	12	No
3.	Condition	pH 6.0	Aq.	1	12	No
4.	Load	Sample	Bio.	4	1	No
5.	Load	Sample	Bio.	3.2	1	No
6.	Purge—cannula	H_2O	Cannula	6	12	No
7.	Purge—cannula	MeOH	Cannula	6	12	No
8.	Rinse	H_2O	Aq.	3	12	No
9.	Rinse	HAc	Aq.	1	12	No
10.	Dry	Time = 5 min				
11.	Rinse	Hexane	Org.	2	12	No
12.	Collect	MeCl	Fract1	6	2.0	No
13.	Rinse	MeOH	Org.	3	12	No
14.	Dry	Time = 2 min				
15.	Collect	Elute 2	Fract2	3	2.0	No

16.	Rinse	H_2O	Aq.	6	12	No
17.	Rinse	MeOH	Aq.	6	12	No
18.	Purge—cannula	H_2O	Cannula	6	30	No
19.	Purge—cannula	MeOH	Cannula	6	30	No

Load cannula depth = 0   Mix volume = 0.5
Mix cannula depth = 0   Mix speed = 0.30
Mix cycles = 2   Reagent mix cycles = 2

Table 9

Reagent setup

No.	Reagent	Abbreviation	Sip speed
1.	Water	H_2O	30
2.	Methanol	MeOH	30
3.	Hexane	Hexane	30
4.	0.1 *M* acetic acid	HAc	30
5.	CH_2Cl_2–IPA—NH_4OH (78:20:2)	Elute 2	15
6.	Methylene chloride	MeCl	30
7.	0.1 *M* Phosphate buffer, pH 6.0	pH 6.0	30
8.	Hexane-ethyl acetate (50:50)	Elute 1	15
9.	Mixing vessel	Mixer	30
10.	Sample	Sample	15

Column air push volume = 2
Column air push volume speed multiplier = 2

Table 10

No.	Waste	Abbreviation
1.	Aqueous	Aq.
2.	Organic solvent	Org.
3.	Biohazardous	Bio.

11.7 THERAPEUTIC AND ABUSED DRUGS IN SERUM, PLASMA, OR WHOLE BLOOD: MANUAL METHOD FOR GC OR GC OR GC-MS CONFIRMATIONS USING A 200-MG CLEAN SCREEN EXTRACTION COLUMN (ZSDAU020 OR ZCDAU020)

1. Prepare sample.
  a. To 1 mL of sample add internal standard(s) and 4 mL of DI H_2O (5.5 ≤ pH ≤ 5.7).
  b. Mix/vortex and let stand 5 min.
  c. Centrifuge for 10 min at 670*g* and discard the pellet.
  d. Add 2 mL of 0.1 *M* phosphate buffer, pH 6.0.
  e. Mix/vortex.

    f. Sample pH should be 6.0 ± 0.5. Adjust pH accordingly with 0.1 M monobasic or dibasic sodium phosphate.

2. Condition CLEAN SCREEN extraction column.

    1 × 3 mL of methanol; aspirate.

    1 × 3 mL of DI H_2O; aspirate.

    1 × 1 mL of 0.1 M phosphate buffer, pH 6.0; aspirate.

    Note: Aspirate at ≤3 in. Hg to prevent sorbent drying.

3. Apply sample.

    Load at 1–2 mL/min.

4. Wash column.

    1 × 3 mL of DI H_2O; aspirate.

    1 × 1 mL of 0.1 M acetic acid; aspirate.

    Dry column (5 min at ≥10 in. Hg).

    1 × 2 mL of hexane; aspirate.

5. Elute acidic and neutral drugs.

    1 × 3 mL hexane - ethyl acetate (50:50); collect eluate at ≤5 mL/min.

6. Dry eluate.

    Evaporate to dryness at ≤40°C. Reconstitute with 100 μL of ethyl acetate.

7. Quantitate acid/neutral drugs (see note a).

    Inject 1–2 μL onto the chromatograph.

8. Wash column.

    1 × 3 mL of methanol; aspirate.

    Dry column (5 min at ≥10 in. Hg).

9. Elute basic drugs.

    a. 1 × 3 mL CH_2Cl_2–IPA–NH_4OH (78:20:2); Collect eluate at 1–2 mL/min.

    Note: Prepare elution solvent daily.

    b. Add isopropanol to the NH_4OH, then add methylene chloride.

    c. The pH of this solution should be approx 11.0.

10. Dry eluate.

    a. Evaporate to dryness at ≤40°C using a TurboVap or equivalent evaporator.

    b. Take care not to overheat or overevaporate.

    c. Certain compounds are heat-labile, such as amphetamines and phencyclidine.

    d. Reconstitute with 100 μL of methanol.

11. Quantitate Basic Drugs.

    Inject 1–2 μL onto the chromatograph.

12. Notes.

    a. Fraction 1 (acid/neutrals) and fraction 2 (bases) can be combined.

    b. A keeper solvent, such as dimethyl formamide (DMF), can be used to prevent the volatilization of amphetamines and phencyclidine. Use 30–50 μL of high-purity DMF in the sample (fraction 1) before evaporation.

    c. A 0.1 M methanolic hydrochloric acid solution has been used to prevent volatization by the formation of the hydrochloric salt of the drugs.

Source: UCT internal publication.

11.8 THERAPEUTIC AND ABUSED DRUGS IN SERUM, PLASMA, OR WHOLE BLOOD: AUTOMATED METHOD FOR GC OR GC-MS CONFIRMATIONS USING A 200-MG CLEAN SCREEN EXTRACTION COLUMN (CSDAU203 OR CCDAU203)

1. **Prepare sample.**
   a. To 1 mL of sample add internal standard(s) and 4 mL of DI H_2O ($5 \leq pH \leq 7$).
   b. Mix/vortex and let stand 5 min.
   c. Centrifuge for 10 min at $670g$ and discard pellet.
   d. Add 2 mL of 0.1 M phosphate buffer, pH 6.0.
   e. Mix/vortex.
   f. Sample pH should be 6.0 ± 0.5. Adjust pH accordingly with 0.1 M monobasic or dibasic sodium phosphate.

2. **Load samples onto the RapidTrace module.**
   Follow the procedure described Section of 11.8.1.

3. **Remove eluted samples from the RapidTrace.**
   a. Fraction 1 represents the acid and neutral drugs extracted from the sample.
   b. Fraction 2 represents the basic drugs extracted from sample.
   c. The fractions can be combined or evaporated separately.

4. **Dry acid/neutral drug eluate (fraction 1).**
   a. Evaporate to dryness at ≤40°C.
   b. Reconstitute with 100 μL of ethyl acetate.

5. **Quantitate.**
   Inject 1–2 μL onto the chromatograph.

6. **Dry basic elute (fraction 2).**
   a. Evaporate to dryness at ≤40°C using a TurboVap or equivalent evaporator.
   b. Take care not to overheat or overevaporate.
   c. Certain compounds are heat-labile, such as amphetamines and phencyclidine.
   d. Reconstitute with 100 μL of methanol.

7. **Quantitate.**
   Inject 1–2 μL onto the chromatograph.

8. **Notes:**
   a. Fraction 1 (acid/neutrals) and fraction 2 (bases) can be combined.
   b. A keeper solvent, such as DMF, can be used to prevent the volatilization of amphetamines and phencyclidine. Use 30–50 μL of high-purity DMF in the sample (fraction 1) before evaporation.
   c. A 0.1 M methanolic hydrochloric acid solution has been used to prevent volatiliza tion by the formation of the hydrochloric salt of the drugs.

Source: UCT internal publication.

11.8.1 Settings for RapidTrace Analysis of Therapeutic and Abused Drugs in Whole Blood

Table 11

Step		Source	Destination	mL	mL/min	Liq. chk
1.	Condition	MeOH	Aq.	3	12	No
2.	Condition	H₂O	Aq.	3	12	No
3.	Condition	pH 6.0	Aq.	1	12	No
4.	Load	Sample	Bio.	5	1	No
5.	Load	Sample	Bio.	2.2	1	No
6.	Purge—cannula	H₂O	Cannula	6	12	No
7.	Purge—cannula	MeOH	Cannula	6	12	No
8.	Rinse	H₂O	Aq.	3	12	No
9.	Rinse	HAc	Aq.	1	12	No
10.	Dry	Time = 5 min				
11.	Rinse	Hexane	OrgSol	2	12	No
12.	Collect	MeCl	Fract1	6	2.0	No
13.	Rinse	MeOH	Org	3	12	No
14.	Dry	Time = 2 min				
15.	Collect	MeCl	Fract2	3	2.0	No
16.	Rinse	H₂O	Aq.	6	12	No
17.	Rinse	MeOH	Aq.	6	12	No
18.	Purge—cannula	H₂O	Cannula	6	30	No
19.	Purge—cannula	MeOH	Cannula	6	30	No

Load cannula depth = 0   Mix volume = 0.5
Mix cannula depth = 0   Mix speed = 30
Mix cycles = 2   Reagent mix cycles = 2

Table 12

Reagent setup

No.	Reagent	Abbreviation	Sip speed
1.	Water	H₂O	30
2.	Methanol	MeOH	30
3.	Hexane	Hexane	30
4.	0.1 *M* Acetic acid	HAc	30
5.	CH₂CL₂–IPA–NH₄OH (78:20:2)	Elute 2	15
6.	Methylene chloride	MeCl	30
7.	0.1 *M* phosphate buffer. pH 6.0	pH 6.0	30
8.	Hexane-ethyl acetate (50:50)	Elute 1	15
9.	Mixing vessel	Mixer	30
10.	Sample	Sample	15

Column air push volume = 2
Column air push volume speed multiplier = 2

Table 13

No.	Waste	Abbreviation
1.	Aqueous	Aq.
2.	Organic solvent	Org.
3.	Biohazardous	Bio.

11.9 FORENSIC DRUG ANALYSIS: MANUAL METHOD FOR GC OR GC-MS USING A 200-MG CLEAN SCREEN EXTRACTION COLUMN (ZSDAU020 OR ZCDAU020)

1. **Prepare sample.**
   Urine:
   To 5 mL of urine add 150–300 μL of 1.0 *M* acetic acid to adjust sample pH to between 4.8 and 5.5.
   Whole blood:
   a. To 2 mL of blood add 8 mL of DI H_2O. Mix/vortex and let stand 5 min.
   b. Add 150–300 μL of 1.0 *M* acetic acid to adjust sample pH to between 4.8 and 5.5.
   c. Centrifuge for 10 min at 2000 rpm and discard pellet.
   Tissue:
   a. Homogenize 1 part tissue with 3 parts of DI H_2O.
   b. Centrifuge for 10 min at 2000 rpm and discard pellet.
   c. Transfer 10 mL of supernatant to a clean tube.
   d. Add 150–300 μL of 1.0 *M* acetic acid to adjust sample pH to between 4.8 and 5.5.
2. **Condition CLEAN SCREEN extraction column.**
   1 × 3 mL of CH_3OH; aspirate.
   1 × 3 mL of DI H_2O; aspirate.
   1 × 1 mL of 0.1 *M* acetic acid; aspirate.
   Note: Aspirate at ≤3 in. Hg to prevent sorbent drying.
3. **Apply sample.**
   Load at 1–2 mL/min.
4. **Wash column.**
   1 × 3 mL of 0.1 *M* phosphate buffer (pH 6.0); aspirate.
   1 × 1 mL of 0.1 *M* acetic acid; aspirate.
   Dry column (5 min at ≥10 in. Hg).
   1 × 3 mL of hexane; aspirate.
5. **Elute acidic and neutral drugs (fraction 1).**
   2 × 2 mL of CH_2Cl_2; collect eluate at ≤5 mL/min.
   Evaporate to dryness at ≤40°C.
6. **Extract and analyze fraction 1.**
   a. Add 1 mL of hexane and 1 mL of CH_3OH–H_2O (80:20). Mix/vortex.
   b. Centrifuge to separate layers. Aspirate and discard hexane (upper) layer.
   c. Evaporate again to dryness at ≤40°C.
   d. Reconstitute with 100 μL of ethyl acetate and inject 1–3 μL onto the chromatograph.
7. **Wash column.**
   1 × 2 mL of methanol; aspirate.
   Dry column (5 min at ≥10 in. Hg).

8. Elute basic drugs (fraction 2).

1 × 2.0 mL of methanol-ammonium hydroxide (98:2); collect eluate at 1–2 mL/min.

Note: Prepare elution solvent daily.

9. Extract and analyze fraction 2.

a. Add 3.0 mL of DI H_2O and 250 μL of chloroform to eluate. Mix/vortex 30 s.

b. Centrifuge to separate phases. Aspirate and discard aqueous (upper) layer.

c. Inject 1–2 μL of the chloroform layer onto the chromatograph.

Source: UCT internal publication.

11.10 Abused Drugs in Canine or Equine Urine: Manual Method Using 500-mg XtrackT Extraction Column (XRDAH515)

1. Prepare sample.

Enzymatic hydrolysis of glucuronides:

a. To 5 mL of urine add internal standard(s) and 2 mL of β glucuronidase 5000 FU/mL of *Patella vulgata* in 1.0 *M* acetate buffer, pH 5.0.

b. Mix/vortex. Hydrolyze at 65°C for 3 h.

c. Cool before proceeding.

Base hydrolysis of glucuronides:

a. To 2 mL of urine add internal standard(s) and 100 μL of 10 *N* NaOH.

b. Mix/vortex. Hydrolyze at 60°C for 20 min.

c. Cool before proceeding.

Combine hydrolysates.

a. Combine both hydrolysis products with 5 mL of 0.1 *M* phosphate buffer, pH 6.0.

b. Adjust sample pH to 6.0 ± 0.5 with 0.5 *M* phosphoric acid.

2. Condition XtrackT extraction column.

1 × 5 mL of CH_3OH; aspirate.

1 × 5 mL of DI H_2O; aspirate.

1 × 3 mL of 0.1 *M* phosphate buffer, pH 6.0; aspirate.

Note: Aspirate at ≤3 in. Hg to prevent sorbent drying.

3. Apply sample.

Load at 1–2 mL/min.

4. Wash column.

1 × 3 mL of 0.1 *M* phosphate buffer, pH 6.0; aspirate.

1 × 2 mL of 1.0 *M* acetic acid; aspirate.

Dry column (5 min at ≥10 in. Hg).

1 × 2 of mL hexane; aspirate.

5. Elute acidic and neutral drugs.

1 × 4 mL of methylene chloride; collect eluate at ≤5 mL/min.

6. Elute steroids.

2 × 4 mL of ethyl acetate; collect eluate at ≤5 mL/min.

7. Wash column.

1 × 5 mL of methanol; aspirate

8. Elute basic drugs.

1 × 5 mL of methylene chloride-isopropanol-ammonium hydroxide (78:20:2).

Note: Prepare elution solvent fresh daily

9. Dry eluate.
   a. Evaporate to dryness at ≤40°C.
   b. Reconstitute with 100 μL of ethyl acetate.
10. Quantitate.
   Spot onto TLC plate or inject 1–2 μL onto the chromatograph

Source: UCT internal publication.

Chapter 12

Chemical Derivatization

12.1 INTRODUCTION

Sensitive, specific, reliable detection and quantification of drugs in biological matrices is often required for compounds that do not chromatograph well. The presence of active hydrogen groups (i.e., hydroxyl, thiol, carboxylic acid, amine, and amide groups) on compounds creates sites for the hydrogen bonding of the stationary phase, often resulting in poor peak shape and sites for absorption of the molecule to other surfaces. In addition, the metabolism of many drugs creates more polar functional groups (e.g., glucuronides) and lowers the lipophilicity of these molecules.

The primary use of derivatization is to modify the functional groups on the analyte to promote chromatography (Table 1). Alteration of active sites on the molecule by derivatization can lead to increased volatility, improved selectivity, and enhanced detectability.

Table 1
Goals of Chemical Derivatization

1. Make compounds more suitable for analysis.
   - Change the volatility and/or thermal stability
2. Improve chromatographic efficiency.
   - Change retention times
   - Reduce or eliminate peak tailing
   - Improve peak shape, resolution, and symmetry
3. Improve detectability.
   - Generate more abundant ions
   - Ions are free of interferents
   - Increase sensitivity and reproducibility
4. Simplify the picture.
   - Chemical derivatization procedures should be robust and simple.

From: *Forensic Science and Medicine:*
Forensic and Clinical Applications of Solid Phase Extraction
Edited by: M. J. Telepchak, T. F. August, and G. Chaney © Humana Press Inc., Totowa, NJ

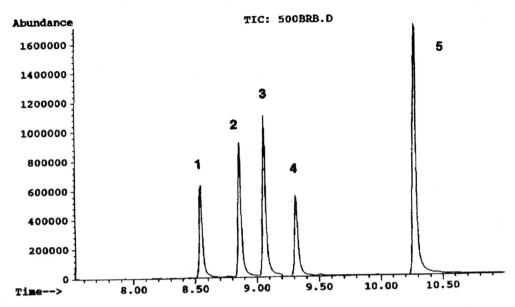

Fig. 1. Chromatography of barbiturates. The figure represents the separation of underivatized barbiturates on a capillary column. All the peaks show "tailing" at the back edge of each compound. The improvement of peak shape is the primary reason that we perform chemical derivatization. Barbiturates are derivatized by alkylation with trimethylanilium hydroxide (TMPAH) to form their methyl derivatives. Improved peak shape allows for better quantitation and lower limits of detection.

The goal of derivatization is to find simple ways to eliminate active sites on molecules. The reaction of compounds and the subsequent addition of more chemical structures to compounds improves the chromatography, thermal and chemical stability, and detectability characteristics of our analytes. Improvements of peak shape also lead to better detection limits and quantitation. Figures 1 through 3 illustrate the advantages of chemical derivatization.

12.1.1 Which Chemical Groups Derivatize?

Active sites on molecules are usually due to the presence of a single hydrogen atom that is combined with oxygen, nitrogen, or sulfur. It is hypothesized that this atom can cause nonspecific and nonpredictive binding to chromatographic supports and to surfaces. This is the primary reason for peak tailing and surface adsorption.

Our efforts in derivatization have been directed to react with this site to produce groups that have high atomic mass (higher mass ions), less adsorption (no free hydrogen groups), and better volatility (improved peak shape).

Figures 4 and 5 simplify the identification of which chemical groups can derivatize. Figure 4 shows chemical groups that can be derivatized; Figure 5 shows chemical groups that do not derivatize. The presence of the single hydrogen atom is a key site for derivatization. The only tricky group will be the keto-enol group found on opiate rings, where the resonance of the double bond plays a role if the group can derivatize (Figure 6). There can be other active sites on the molecule to derivatize. In addition, more than one derivatizable site may be present on a molecule (Figure 7).

A

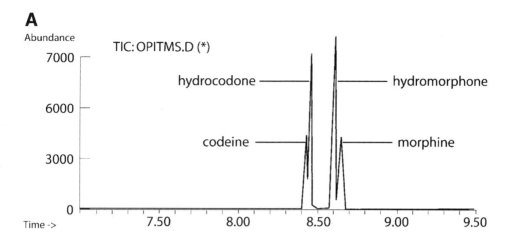

B

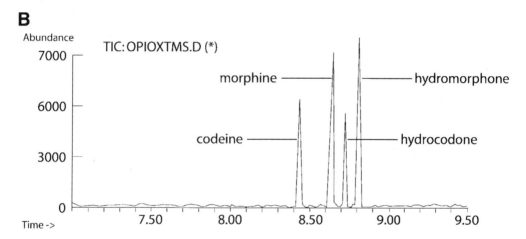

Fig. 2. Chromatography of opiate deriviatives. The figure illustrates, by the use of oxime-TMS derivatives, that separation of the primary opiates (morphine and codeine) from the semisynthetic opiates (hydrocodone and hydromorphone) can be accomplished easily. This separation shows that by selective derivatization many problems associated with the chromatography of these and other compounds can be overcome.

12.1.2 Using Nonderivitizable Sites to Your Advantage

AU: Page out of order or change head numbers? Correct table and figure numbers?

Critical to this example is that the absence of sites to derivatize often helps in the separation of the parent drug from polar metabolites. The formation of polar metabolites often adds more groups to be derivatized. As groups are added to the molecule the molecular mass increases, improving the mass fragmentation and confirmation of a specific drug (Figure 8).

It is necessary to be aware of certain assumptions made when using chemical derivatization (Table 2).

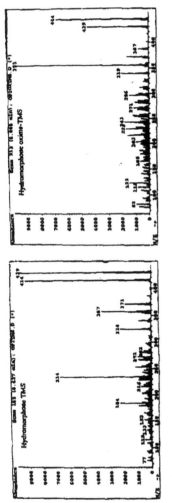

Derivatized Drug	Retention Times		Major Ions in Spectra	
	TMS	HOX-TMS	TMS	HOX-TMS
Codeine	8.43	8.43	371*,356,343,234	371*, 356, 343, 234
Morphine	8.67	8.67	429, 414, 401, 236*	429, 414, 401, 236*
Hydrocodone	8.47	8.77	371*, 356, 313, 234	386*, 371, 329, 297
Hydromorphone	8.63	8.86	429*, 414, 371, 357	444, 429, 355*, 339
Oxycodone	8.65	9.07	459*, 444, 368, 312	474*, 459, 401, 385
Oxymorphone	8.84	9.14	517*, 502, 412, 355	532*, 517, 459, 287

Fig. 3. Mass fragmentation patterns. This figure represents how we can improve on the mass fragmentation patterns of our analytes of interest by different chemical derivatization reactions. For example, hydromorphone, by the addition of hydroxylamine in addition to the derivatization with BSTFA with 1% TMCS, forms an oxime-TMS derivatives that has higher mass values for spectral ions. This reduces the chances of interfering ions from endogenous sources. Besides improving the mass fragmentation of these compounds, the chromatography is baseline-resolved and away from the parent molecules. (Codeine and morphine are separated from their metabolites hydrocodone and hydromorphone and the semisynthetic opiate oxycodone.) Improving the separation and having higher mass spectral ions will make the identification and quantitation of these agents easier and more accurate.

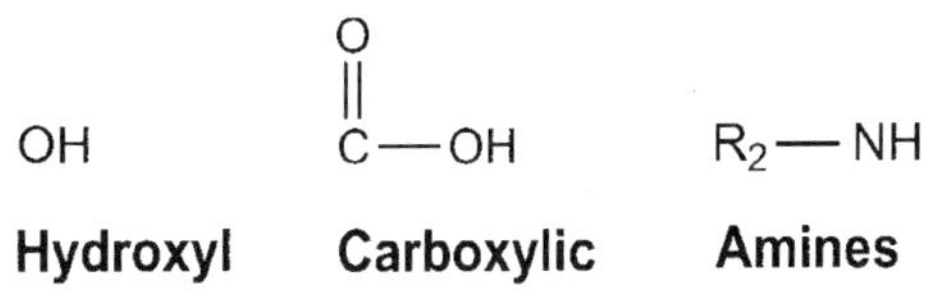

OH

O
‖
C—OH

R₂—NH

Hydroxyl **Carboxylic** **Amines**

Fig. 4. Chemical groups that can derivatize.

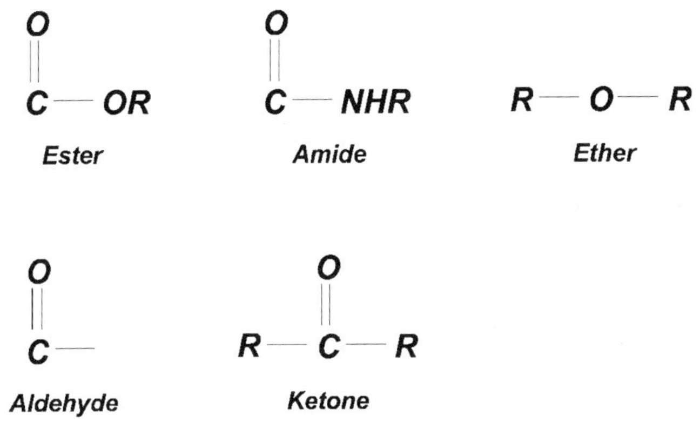

O
‖
C—OR

Ester

O
‖
C—NHR

Amide

R—O—R

Ether

O
‖
C—

Aldehyde

O
‖
R—C—R

Ketone

Fig. 5. Chemical groups that do not derivatize.

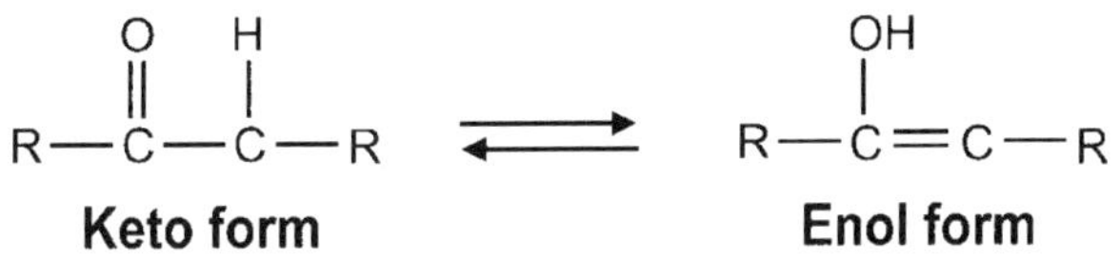

O   H
‖ |
R—C—C—R   ⇌   R—C=C—R   OH
                         |

Keto form   **Enol form**

Fig. 6. Chemical groups that could derivatize.

GHB

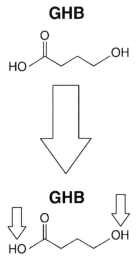

Fig. 7. Multiple sites for derivatization can occur on an analyte. Can, and where will, this drug derivatize?

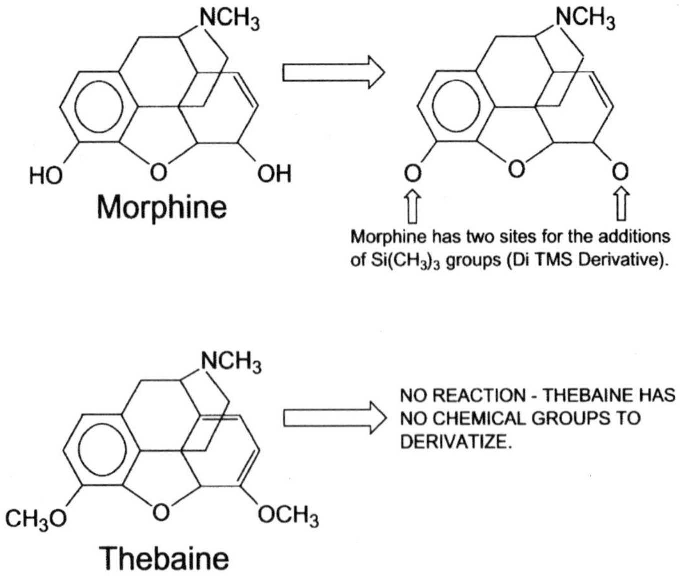

Fig. 8. Opiate derivatization. The mixture of drugs that derivatize and those that do not derivatize often lends to the chromatographic separation of drug-metabolite mixtures.

Table 2
Assumption for Chemical Derivatization

- A single derivative should be formed for each drug.
- The derivatization reaction should be simple and rapid, and should occur under mild conditions.
- The derivative is stable in the reaction medium.
- The derivative is formed in a reproducible manner with a high yield.
- Quantitatively, the calibration curve is linear.

Chemical derivatization reactions for most analytes have been characterized into three types:

silylation, alkylation, and acetylation. A brief description of each reaction is listed in the following sections.

12.2 SILYLATION

Silylation is the introduction of a silyl group into a molecule, usually to substitute active hydrogen (Table 3). Active hydrogens are present on acids, alcohols, thiols, amines, amides, enolizable ketones, and aldehydes.

Silylation refers to addition of a trimethylsilyl, $Si(CH_3)_3$ group, or TMS, into the analyte. Silylation reactions account for more than 85% of all derivatization reactions done using gas chromatography.

Table 3
Ease of Silylation

Alcohols	**Easiest**
Primary > Secondary > Tertiary	
Phenols	
Carboxylic acids	
Amines	
Primary > Secondary	
(Tertiary DO NOT REACT)	
Amides	**Difficult**

Replacement of active hydrogen by a silyl group reduces the polarity of the compound and decreases hydrogen bonding. The silyl derivative is more volatile and the stability is enhanced because the number of reactive sites has been reduced. Silyl derivatives have been observed to have greater thermal stability and enhanced detection owing to improvements in the peak shape.

Silyl reactions are influenced by the solvent system and the addition of a catalyst. Nonpolar solvents such as hexane, diethyl ether, and toluene can be used; however, more polar solvents are preferred. Acetonitrile, DMF, DMSO, pyridine, and THF are favored in these reactions because they tend to facilitate the production of reaction products.

Pyridine is commonly referred to as the universal silylation catalyst and acts as an HCl acceptor for reactions using chlorosilanes. Some reactions are facilitated by the use of pyridine; however, some reactions become slower in pyridine. In addition, side reactions have been observed in pyridine reaction mixtures. DMF is used for steroids and other large molecules. DMSO is used for reacting tertiary alcohols and other molecules with a limited solubility in other solvents. The mixing of insoluble reactants or use of a co-solvent, such as dioxane, has been employed to overcome solubility issues.

Catalysts such as trimethylchlorosilane (TMCS) and *t*-butyldimethylchlorosilane (TBDMCS) are added to improve the hydrolytic stability of the reaction mixture and increase the reactivity (especially for hindered hydroxyls and secondary amines).

Most silyl reactions require heat to facilitate the reaction. It is critical to determine the reaction time and temperature when developing derivatization procedures. Silyl reagents are moisture sensitive and must be kept sealed to prevent moisture deactivation. Usually a 10- to 50-fold excess of derivatization reagent can be used to consume any residual moisture in the sample.

Many silyl reagents are flammable, and those containing active chlorine atoms form HCl in the presence of water. Silyl reagents react readily with active hydrogens; therefore, they cannot be used with stationary GC phases that possess these groups (such as glycol phases).

Direct injection of the reaction mixture of silylation reagent and analyte is usually performed.

A list of the commonly used silylation reagents is given in Table 4.

Table 4
Commonly Used Silylation Reagents Relative Strength of the Silylation Reagents

BSTFA + TMCS > BSTFA > BSA > MSTFA > TMCS > HMDS

N,O-bis (trimethylsilyl) trifluoroacetamide (BSTFA)
Most commonly used silylation reagent that is normally combined with TMCS.
Byproducts of the reaction (trimethylsilyltrifluoroacetamide and trifluoroacetamide) are
   volatile.
The TMS group on the nitrogen is most active however, both TMS groups react.
Trimethylchlorosilane (TMCS)
TMCS is similar to HMDS in its effectiveness as a silylation reagent when used alone.
This reagent has a pronounced effect when combined with other silylation reagents as a
   catalyst.
N,O-bis (trimethylsilyl)acetamide (BSA)
Very similar to BSTFA in its reactivity; however, its byproducts are not as volatile as BSTFA.
TMCS is often used with BSA as a catalyst.
N-methyl-N-trimethylsilyltrifluoroacetamide (MSTFA)
MSTFA has similar silylation donating power as BSA. MSTFA produces very volatile
   byproducts that can be removed in the solvent delay. Hydrochloride salts of amine can be
   directly silylated.
Hexamethyldisilazane (HMDS)
HMDS is the most widely known silylation reagent. Used alone its activity is slow and has
   very weak silylation properties. By combining this with TMCS it becomes a fast and
   quantitative reagent.
N-(tert-butyldimethylsilyl-N-methyltrifluoroacetamide) (MTBSTFA)
This reagent reacts with alcohols, phenols, thiols, primary and secondary amines, and
   carboxylic acids, forming stable *tert*-butyldimethylsilyl derivatives. These derivatives are
   more stable than TMS derivatives.
The disadvantage is that the products are more sterically hindered than TMS derivatives. The
   product can be injected directly into the GC-MS.

12.3 ACYLATION

Acylation reactions occur when an alcohol, thiol, or amine (only primary or secondary) is reacted with an acid anhydride. This reaction forms an ester and, depending
on the derivatization reagent, acid or imidazole byproducts. The primary use of this
reaction is to make derivatives that have higher and more stable masses for GC-MS
detection or to create derivatives that are sensitive to other GC detectors, such as
electron capture
   detection (ECD) or flame ionization detection (FID).

There are two different types of acylation reagents: acid anhydride and acyl-
imidazole. These are discussed below.

12.3.1 Acyl Acid Anhydrides

The reaction is:

R_1 (OH)	+	$(R_2CO)_2O$	$\rightarrow$	R_2COOR_1	+	R_2 COOH
Alcohol		Acyl anhydride		Ester product		Carboxylic acid derivatives

Table 5
Perfluoro Acid Anhydrides

$$\underset{R-C-O-C-R}{\overset{\displaystyle O \qquad O}{\overset{\displaystyle \| \qquad \|}{}}}$$

R	Name	Mol wt	BP
CF_3	Trifluoroacetic acid anhydride (TFAA)	210.0	39.5–40.5°C
C_2F_5	Pentafluoropropionic acid anhydride (PFAA)	310.0	74°C
C_3F_7	Heptafluorobutyric acid anhydride (HFAA)	410.0	106–107°C

Active groups for this reaction include OH, SH, and NH and the products for these reactions are esters, thioesters, and amides. The acidic byproducts of the acid anhydride reactions must be removed before injection onto the chromatographic system. This is usually accomplished by evaporation of the reaction mixture to dryness and then reconstitution using a suitable solvent.

Agents such as 2,2,3,3,3-pentafluoro-1-propanol have been added to the acid anhydride reaction mixture to yield higher molecular weight products (Table 5). PFAA is commonly used for the derivatization of opiates and benzoylecgonine. HFAA has been used for phencyclidine and amphetamines and TFAA is used for the detection of methamphetamines.

12.3.2 Acyl-Imdazole

The reaction is:

$$R_1(OH) \quad + \quad R_2CO(C_3H_4N_2) \quad \rightarrow \quad R_2COOR_1 \quad + \quad C_3H_4N_2$$
Alcohol Acyl imidazole Ester product Imidazole

Active groups for this reaction include OH, SH, and NH and the products for these reactions are esters, thioesters, and amides (Table 6).

Advantages of this reaction are:

- Produces no acid byproducts that have to be removed before chromatography. The principal byproduct is imidazole, which is relatively inert.
- Ideal for flame ionization detection (FID) and electron capture detection (ECD).
- Can be used in bifunctional derivatization where hydroxyl groups are derivatized with TMSI followed by derivatization of the amines with HFBI.
- Exchange reactions can occur where TMS derivatives are replaced with HFBI derivatives.

Table 6
Perfluoroacylimidazole Derivatives

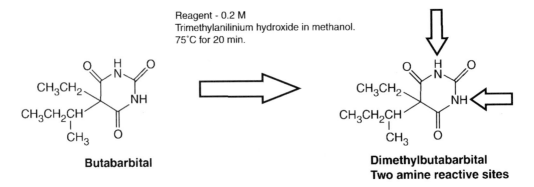

R	Name	Mol wt	BP
CF_3	Trifluoroacetylimidazole (TFAI)	164.08	38–40°C/14 mm
C_2F_5	Pentafluoropropionylimidazole (PFPI)	214.10	38–40°C/14 mm
C_3F_7	Heptafluorobutyrylimidazole (HFBI)	264.10	57–58°C/14 mm

Reagent - 0.2 M
Trimethylanilinium hydroxide in methanol.
75°C for 20 min.

Butabarbital

**Dimethylbutabarbital
Two amine reactive sites**

Fig. 9. The alkylation of butabarbital using TMPAH.

12.4 ALKYLATION

In alkylation, a reactive hydrogen such as amine or hydroxyl is replaced by an alkyl group. This process eliminates hydrogen bonding, thereby improving peak shape and increasing volatility. The adding group can improve the sensitivity of the analyte; for example, addition of halogens increases the sensitivity of certain detectors such as electron capture. Compounds that can be subjected to alkylation reactions include carboxylic acids, alcohols, thiols, phenols, primary and secondary amines, and amides (Figure 9).

Common reactions include:

- Alkyl iodide—reflux with methyl iodide in dry acetone with potassium carbonate.
- Methylation using TMPAH (barbiturates).
- Diazomethane alkylation reaction of carboxylic acids and phenols.

Table 7
Selected Properties of Derivatization Reagents

A. Silylation Reagents

Name	Abbreviation	Mol wt	BP
N,O-bis (trimethylsilyl) acetamide	BSA	203.4	71–73°C
N,O-bis (trimethylsilyl) trifluoroacetamide	BSTFA	257.4	40°C/12 mm
N,O-bis (trimethylsilyl) trifluoroacetamide with 1% trimethylchlorosilane	BSTFA with 1% TMCS		
Hexamethyldisilazane	HMDS	161.4	
Tetramethylchlorosilane	TMCS	108.7	
Trimethylsilylimidazole	TMSI	140.26	99°C/14 mm
N-Methyl-*N*-trimethyl trifluoroacetamide	MSTFA	199.1	70°C/75 mm
N-Methyl-*N*-trimethyl trifluoroacetamide with 1% trimethylchlorosilane	MSTFA with 1% TMCS		
Tert-butyldimethylchlorosilane	TBDMCS	150.7	125°C
N-tert-butyldimethylsilyl-*N*-methyltrifluoroacetamide	MTBSTFA	241.3	168–170ºC
N-tert-butyldimethylsilyl-*N*-methyltrifluoroacetamide with tert-butyldimethylchlorosilane	MTBSTFA with 1% tBDMCS		
Dimethylchlorosilane	DMCS	94.62	

B. Alkylation reagents

Name	Abbreviation	Mol wt	BP	Comments
0.2 *M* Trimethylanilinium hydroxide in methanol	TMPAH			Used for methyl derivatives of barbiturates and phenytoin
Pentafluorobenzyl bromide	PFBBR	260.9	174–175°C	HPLC applications for UV detection
14% Boron trifluoride in methanol	BF3/methanol			carboxylic acids to methylesters

C. Acetylation reagent

Name	Abbreviation	Mol wt	BP
Trifluoroacetic acid anhydride	TFAA	210.0	39.5–40.5°C
Pentafluorpropionic acid anhydride	PFAA	310.0	74°C
Petafluoropropionic anhydride	PFPA		
Heptafluorobutyric acid anhydride	HFAA	410	106–107°C
Heptafluorbutyric anhydride	HFBA		
Trifluoroacetylimidazole	TFAI	164.08	38–40°C/14 mm

Pentaflurorpropionylimidazole	PFPI	214.10	38–40°C/14 mm
Heptafluorobutyrylimidazole	HFBI	264.10	57–58°C/14 mm
N-Methyl-bis(trifluoroacetamide)	MBTFA	223.0	123–124°C

D. Other reagents

Name	Abbreviation	Mol wt	BP	Applications
2,2,3,3,3-Pentafluoro-1-propanol	PFPOH	150.05	80°C	Additive to Acylation reaction
Acetonitrile	ACN	41.05	81.6°C	Solvent
Dimethylformamide	DMF	73.09	153°C	Solvent
Dimethylsulfoxide	DMSO	78.13	189°C	Solvent
Pyridine		79.10	115.2°C	Solvent
Tetrahydrofuran	THF	72.10	66.0°C	Solvent

Table 8
Guide to Derivatization Reactions

Class name	Derivatization reagent	Conditions	Reference
Amphetamines	TFAA	40°C for 15 min	1
	PFAA	75°C for 15 min	
	HFAA	60°C for 40 min	
	4CB	50°C for 15 min	2
Barbiturates (0.2 *M* in methanol)	TMPAH	75°C for 20 min	3
Benzodiazepines	BSTFA with 1% TMCS	70°C for 20 min	4
Flunitrazepam	MTBSTFA with 1% TBDMCS	90°C for 20 min	5
Cannabinoids	BSTFA with 1% TMCS	70°C for 20 min	6
Cocaine and metabolites (benzoylecgonine)	BSTFA with 1% TMCS	70°C for 20 min	7
LSD	BSTFA with 1% TMCS	70°C for 20 min	8
Opiates—oxime TMS	Hydroxylamine and MSTFA	85°C for 20 min	9
Propyl	Propionic anhydride	40°C for 60 min	10

REFERENCES

[1]Thompson, W., and Dasgupta, A. Microwave induced rapid preparation of fluoro derivatives of amphetamine, methamphetamine and 3, 4-dimethylenedioxymethamphetamine for GC-MSD confirmation. Clin. Chem. 40:1703–1706, 1994.

[2]Thurman, E., Pedersen, M., Stout, R., and Martin, T. Distinguishing sympathomimetic amines from amphetamine and methamphetamine in urine by gas chromatpgraphy/mass spectroscopy. J. Analyt. Toxicol. 16:19–28, 1992.

[3]Joern, W. Unexpected volatility of barbiturate derivatives: An extractive alkylation procedure for barbiturates and benzoylecgonine. J. Analyt. Toxicol. 18:423–427, 1994.

[4]Moore, C., Long, G., and Marr, M. Confirmation of benzodiazepines in urine as trimethylsilyl derivatives using gas chromatography-mass spectroscopy. J. Chromatogr. B (Biomed. Appl.) 655:132–137, 1994.

[5]El Sohly, M., Feng, S., Salamone, S., and Wu, R. A sensitive GC-MS procedure for the analysis of flunitrazepam and its metabolite in urine. J. Analyt. Toxicol. 21:61–67, 1997.

[6]Baker, T., Harry, J., Russell, J., and Myers, R. Rapid method for the GC-MS confirmation of 11 nor-9-carboxy Δ9 tetrahydocannabinol in urine. J. Analyt. Toxicol. 8:255–259, 1984.

[7]Moore, C., Brown, S., Negrusz, A., Tebbett, J., Meyer, W., Jain, L. Determination of cocaine and its major metabolite, benzoylecgonine, in amniotic fluid, umbilical cord, blood, umbilical cord tissue and neonatal urine: A case study. J. Analyt. Toxicol. 17:62–65, 1993.

[8]Paul, B., Mitchell, J., Burbage, R., Moy, M., Sroka, R. Gas chromatographic electron impact mass fragmentometric determination of lysergic acid diethylamide in urine. J. Chromatogr. 529:103–112, 1990.

[9]Jones, C., Chaney, G., and Mastorides, S. Simultaneous analysis of opiates in the urine by SPE and GC-MS with stabilization of the keto-opiates by conversion to the oxime derivatives. J. Analyt. Toxicol. 21:86–92, 1997.

[10]Soper, J. A single step GC procedure for quantitation of 6-monoacetyl morphine coupled with simultaneous quantitation and/or detection of 14 additional opiate compounds following derivatization with propionic anhydride. Proc. Am. Acad. of Forensic Sci. 2:215–216, 1996.

Appendix A: Glossary

Analyte
: The compound of interest for analysis; sometimes called an *isolate*.
Bed volume. The volume of liquid required to fill the spaces and pores in an SPE sorbent bed. Also the theoretical amount of solvent required to wash a completely unretained component through the bed. Usually the bed volume of functionalized silica is approx 120 µL/100 mg of sorbent.

Bimodal interactions
: Interactions that occur between the analyte and sorbent; in this case more than one chemical mechanism of attachment is occurring.

Breakthrough
: The process of the drug passing through the column unretained. This occurs when the analyte is too weakly attached or the column capacity has been exceeded. Breakthrough occurs during the loading and wash phases of the procedure.

Buffer
: An aqueous solvent system containing a mixture of a weak acid-conjugate base (or weak base-conjugate acid) that resists pH change in spite of the addition of moderate amounts of acid or base. Buffers have a certain finite capacity that can be exceeded.

Capacity
: The ability of the sorbent to retain a given compound under certain condition (solvent environment). The capacity of a given sorbent is related to the analyte and the matrix environment.

Conditioning
: Solvation or the addition of solvents (especially water) to the surface of a SPE material. This process sets up the sorbent for retaining the analyte of interest.

Counter-ion
: Used in ion-exchange chromatography, this is a group that has a higher affinity for the ion-exchange surface and usually replaces the analyte attached to the ion exchanger.

Eluate
: The solution that has passed through the sorbent bed containing both solvent and analyte of interest or interfering substance.

Eluent
: The solvent mixture used to remove the analyte of interest or interfering substance from the sorbent bed.

Elution
: The process of passing the eluent through a prepared sorbent bed with the final result of isolating the analyte or removal of an interfering substance. This solvent mixture disrupts the isolate-sorbent interaction.

Fines
: Silica particles that are much smaller than the average particle size, which are generated from the handing or processing of the silica (i.e., mixing of the

From: *Forensic Science and Medicine:*
Forensic and Clinical Applications of Solid Phase Extraction
Edited by: M. J. Telepchak, T. F. August, and G. Chaney © Humana Press Inc., Totowa, NJ

	reaction mixture and column packing by machine). These particles act to block the flow of solvents through the pores of the silica.
Functional group	A chemical group that is affixed onto a surface such as silica that imparts properties that can be used to retain analytes on sorbents. Functional groups include ionic groups, such as anion or cation exchangers (e.g., benzene sulfonate, a strong cation group), hydrophobic groups (such as C18, C8) and the like.
Interaction	The attraction or repulsion between two chemical species in a specific chemical environment.
Interferent	An undesired component in the sample matrix. This is usually removed by our sample preparation procedure.
Isolate	This term has the same meaning as "analyte." A compound that is to be isolated from the sample.
Linear velocity	The velocity of a solvent through a sorbent bed, expressed as mm/s. The linear velocity is not affected by column dimensions and is used when discussing mass transfer efficiency.
Matrix	The substance in which the analyte is found. For example, biological matrices are urine, blood, plasma, etc. Environmental matrices are soil, water, oil, and air. The matrix is critical in sorbent extraction because the retention of an isolate on a sorbent is strongly influenced by the chemistry of the matrix.
Mechanism	The nature of the chemistry leading to isolation or interference retention. Mechanisms include nonpolar, polar, ion-exchange, covalent, etc.
Miscibility	The ability to dissolve into each other. For example, water and alcohols are miscible but water and hexane are not miscible. In SPE it is necessary to pass and dry columns containing water before adding hexane to the column.
Mixed mode	The term used to describe the retention of an analyte by two or more retention mechanisms.
Nonpolar	A commonly used mechanism in sorbent extraction that uses van der Waals interactions. These interactions are between two molecules of a nonpolar nature. An example of a nonpolar sorbent is C18.
Normal phase	Chromatographic system in which the stationary phase is polar and the mobile phase is nonpolar.
Packed bed	Another word used to describe the sorbent in a cartridge.
Phase	The functional group on the sorbent—for example, C18, C2, etc.
pH	Chemical term for the negative log of the hydrogen ion concentration. A high pH means pH > 7.0 and denotes basic conditions. A low pH means pH < 7.0 and denotes acidic conditions. Sorbent extractions are usually run in a pH range of 3.0–8.0.
pK_a	Chemical term to describe the pH where half of the compound present is ionized and half non-ionized (neutral). If the pK_a is known, then placing the compound in a pH of 2.0 pH units above acid or below base will completely ionize the compound. A listing of pK_a values is given in Appendix G.
Polar	A commonly used mechanism in sorbent extraction using dipole moments. For example, unbonded silica is a very polar sorbent because of the high content of silanol groups on the surface.
Protein binding	A characteristic of a chemical compound to attach or adhere to a protein or other biological substrate by hydrogen, ionic, or hydrophobic interaction. Changing the pH, denaturing the protein, or precipitating the protein may be needed to release the analyte from its protein-bound state.

Retention   The quality that attaches an analyte to a sorbent so that the species is immobilized. The degree of attachment is referred to as the strength of attachment and is dependent on the interaction between the functional group on the surface of the sorbent and the analyte and the ionic and polar environment present.

Reverse
phase   Chromatographic system in which the stationary phase is nonpolar and the mobile phase is polar. This is the most common separation mechanism used for the isolation of drugs and other substances from various matrices.

Selectivity   The quality to which the separation mechanism discriminates between chemical species relative to other compounds in the sample (i.e., the matrix).

Solvation   The treatment or conditioning of the sorbent bed prior to sample application. This process conditions and makes the functional groups assume a more active position with respect to their orientation in space. The solvation of a sorbent surface is a critical step to make the sorbent chemistry function. An improperly solvated sorbent will retain nothing.

Solvent   A liquid phase involved in sorbent extraction. The solvent may be an organic solvent, buffer, water, and so on. The matrix solvent is referred to as the principal character of the matrix. For example, water is the principal matrix solvent of serum.

Sorbent   A generic term used to describe a solid functionalized silica stationary phase.

Sorbent bed   The size of material that is used in an SPE column. Usually it is held between two polyethylene frits or embedded into a disk material.

Appendix B: Reagents

Acetic acid, glacial (CH₃COOH): 17.4 *M*
Ammonium hydroxide (NH⁴OH): concentrated (14.8 *M*)
β-Glucuronidase: lyophilized powder from limpets (*Patella vulgata*)
Dimethylformamide (DMF): silylation grade
Hydrochloric acid (HCl): concentrated (12.1 M)
N,O-bis(Trimethylsilyl)trifluoroacetamide (BSTFA) with 1% trimethylchlorosilane (TMCS)
Pentafluropropionic acid anhydride (PFAA or PFPA)
Phosphoric acid (H₃PO₄): concentrated (14.7 M)
Sodium acetate trihydrate (NaCH₃COO·3H₂O): FW 136.08
Sodium borate decahydrate (Na₂B₄O₇·10H₂O): FW 381.37
Sodium hydroxide (NaOH): FW 40.00
Sodium phosphate dibasic, anhydrous (Na₂HPO₄): FW 141.96
Sodium phosphate monobasic, monohydrate (NaH₂PO₄·H₂O): FW 137.99

NOTES

1. Storage of organics in some plastic containers may lead to plasticizer contamination of the solvent or solvent mixture; this may interfere with analyte quantitation.
2. Good laboratory practice dictates that all who handle or are potentially exposed to reagents, solvents, and solutions used or stored in the laboratory should familiarize themselves with manufacturers' recommendations for chemical storage, use, and handling, and also the familiar with an appropriate Material Safety Data Sheet (MSDS).

From: *Forensic Science and Medicine:*
Forensic and Clinical Applications of Solid Phase Extraction
Edited by: M. J. Telepchak, T. F. August, and G. Chaney © Humana Press Inc., Totowa, NJ

Appendix C: Preparation of Solutions and Buffers

1.0 *M* Acetic acid:

To 400 mL of DI H_2O add 28.6 mL of glacial acetic acid. Dilute to 500 mL with DI H_2O.
Storage: 25°C in glass or plastic.
Stability: 6 mo.

0.1 *M* Acetic acid:

Dilute 40 mL of 1.0 *M* acetic acid to 400 mL with DI H_2O. Mix.
Storage: 25°C in glass or plastic.
Stability: 6 mo.

0.1 *M* Acetate buffer, pH 4.5:

Dissolve 2.93 g of sodium acetate trihydrate in 400 mL of DI H_2O; add 1.62 mL of glacial acetic acid. Dilute to 500 mL with DI H_2O. Mix.
Adjust pH to 4.5 ± 0.1 with 0.1 *M* sodium acetate or 0.1 *M* acetic acid.
Storage: 25°C in glass or plastic
Stability: 6 mo. Inspect daily with use for contamination.
A precipitate or cloudy solution may indicate bacterial growth.

1.0 *M* Acetate buffer, pH 5.0:

Dissolve 42.9 g of sodium acetate trihydrate in 400 mL of DI H_2O; add 10.4 mL of glacial acetic acid. Dilute to 500 mL with DI H_2O. Mix.
Adjust pH to 5.0 ± 0.1 with 1.0 *M* sodium acetate or 1.0 *M* acetic acid.
Storage: 25°C in glass or plastic.
Stability: 6 mo. Inspect daily with use for contamination.

0.1 *M* Acetate buffer, pH 5.0:

Dilute 40 mL of 1.0 M acetate buffer to 400 mL with DI H2O. Mix.
Storage: 25°C in glass or plastic
Stability: 6 mo.

From: *Forensic Science and Medicine:*
Forensic and Clinical Applications of Solid Phase Extraction
Edited by: M. J. Telepchak, T. F. August, and G. Chaney © Humana Press Inc., Totowa, NJ

7.4 *M* Ammonium hydroxide:

To 50 mL of DI H$_2$O add 50 mL of concentrated NH$_4$OH. Mix.
Storage: 25°C in glass or fluoropolymer plastic.
Stability: Dependent on storage condition.

β-Glucuronidase, 5000 Fishman U/mL:

Dissolve 100,000 Fishman U of lyophilized powder with 20 mL of acetate buffer 1 *M* (pH 5.0).
Storage: –5°C in plastic.
Stability: Several days; prepare daily for best results.

0.1 *M* Hydrochloric acid:

To 400 mL of DI H$_2$O add 4.2 mL concentrated HCl. Dilute to 500 mL with DI H$_2$O. Mix.
Storage: 25°C in glass or plastic.
Stability: 6 mo.

Methanol-ammonium hydroxide (98:2):

To 98 mL CH3OH add 2 mL of concentrated NH$_4$OH. Mix.
Storage: 25°C in glass or fluoropolymer plastic.
Stability: 1 d.

Methylene chloride-isopropanol-ammonium hydroxide (78:20:2):

To 40 mL of IPA add 4 mL of concentrated NH$_4$OH. Mix. Add 156 mL of CH$_2$Cl$_2$. Mix.
Storage: 25°C in glass or fluoro polymer plastic.
Stability: 1 d.
Order of mixing critical.

0.1 *M* Phosphate buffer, pH 6.0:

Dissolve 1.70 g of Na$_2$HPO$_4$ and 12.14 g of NaH$_2$PO$_4$ H$_2$O in 800 mL of DI H$_2$O. Dilute to 1000 mL using DI H$_2$O. Mix.
Adjust pH to 6.0 ± 0.1 with 0.1 *M* monobasic sodium phosphate (lowers pH) or 0.1 *M* dibasic sodium phosphate (raises pH).
Storage: 5°C in glass
Stability: 1 mo. Inspect daily with use for contamination.

0.5 *M* Phosphoric acid:

To 400 mL of DI H$_2$O add 17.0 mL of concentrated phosphoric acid. Dilute to 500 mL with DI H$_2$O. Mix.
Storage: 25°C in glass or plastic.
Stability: 6 mo.

1.0 *M* Sodium acetate:

Dissolve 13.6 g of sodium acetate in 90 mL of DI H$_2$O. Dilute to 100 mL with DI H$_2$O. Mix.
Storage: 25°C in glass or plastic.
Stability: 6 mo.

0.1 *M* Sodium acetate:

Dilute 10 mL of 1.0 *M* sodium acetate to 100 mL with DI H$_2$O. Mix.
Storage: 25°C in glass or plastic.
Stability: 6 mo.

0.1 *M* Sodium borate:

Dissolve 3.81 g of $Na_2B_4O_7 \cdot 10\ H_2O$ in 90 mL of DI H_2O.
Dilute to 100 mL with DI H_2O. Mix.
Storage: 25°C in glass or plastic.
Stability: 6 months.

0.1 *M* Sodium phosphate dibasic:

Dissolve 2.84 g of Na_2HPO_4 in 160 mL of DI H_2O. Dilute to 200 mL using DI H_2O. Mix.
Storage: 5°C in glass.
Stability: 1 mo. Inspect daily with use for contamination.

0.1 *M* Sodium phosphate, monobasic:

Dissolve 2.76 g $NaH_2PO_4 \cdot H_2O$ in 160 mL DI H_2O. Dilute to 200 mL with DI H_2O. Mix.
Storage: 5°C in glass.
Stability: 1 mo. Inspect daily with use for contamination.

0.1 *M* Sulfuric acid:

To 400 mL of DI H_2O add 5.6 mL of concentrated H_2SO_4. Dilute to 500 mL with DI H_2O. Mix.
Storage: 25°C in glass or plastic.
Stability: 6 mo.

Appendix D: Milliequivalent and Millimole Calculations

Definitions

mole	=	gram molecular weight of a substance (molar weight)
millimole (mol)	=	milligram molecular weight of a substance (a millimole is 1/1000 of a mole)
equivalent weight	=	gram weight of a substance that will combine with or replace 1 gram (1 mole) of hydrogen; an equivalent weight can be determined by dividing the molar weight of a substance by its ionic valence
milliequivalent (mEq)	=	milligram weight of a substance that will combine with or re place 1 milligram (1 millimole) of hydrogen (a milliequivalent is 1/1000 of an equivalent)

Calculations

moles $\quad = \quad \dfrac{\text{weight of a substance (grams)}}{\text{molecular weight of that substance (grams)}}$

millimoles $\quad = \quad \dfrac{\text{weight of a substance (milligrams)}}{\text{molecular weight of that substance (milligrams)}}$

equivalents	=	moles × valence of ion
milliequivalents	=	millimoles × valence of ion

moles $\quad = \quad \dfrac{\text{equivalents}}{\text{valence of ion}}$

millimoles $\quad = \quad \dfrac{\text{milliequivalents}}{\text{valence of ion}}$

millimoles	=	moles × 1000
milliequivalents	=	equivalents × 1000

Note: Use of equivalents and milliequivalents is valid only for those substances that have fixed ionic valences (e.g., sodium, potassium, calcium, chlorine, magnesium, bromine, etc.). For substances with variable ionic valences (e.g., phosphorus), a reliable equivalent value cannot be determined. In these instances, one should calculate millimoles (which are fixed and reliable) rather than milliequivalents.

From: *Forensic Science and Medicine:*
Forensic and Clinical Applications of Solid Phase Extraction
Edited by: M. J. Telepchak, T. F. August, and G. Chaney © Humana Press Inc., Totowa, NJ

Appendix E: Selected Solvent Polarity and Property Scale

Solvent	Adsorptive energy	Boiling point (°C)	Viscosity
Fluoroalkanes	–0.25	45–55	
n-Pentane	0.00	36	0.23
Hexane	0.00	69	0.33
Isooctane	0.01	99	0.3
Petroleum ether	0.01	175–240	0. 3
n-Decane	0.04	174	0.92
Cyclohexane	0.04	81	1.00
Cyclopentane	0.05	49	0.47
1-Pentene	0.08	30	
Carbon disulfide	0.15	46	0.37
Carbon tetrachloride	0.18	77	0.97
Amyl chloride	0.26	108	0.43
Butyl chloride	0.26	77	0.47
Xylene	0.26	138–144	0.62–0.81
Isopropyl ether	0.28	69	0.37
Isopropyl chloride	0.29	35	0.33
Toluene	0.29	111	0.59
n-Propyl chloride	0.30	47	0 35
Chlorobenzene	0.30	132	0.80
Benzene	0.32	80	0.65
Ethyl ether	0.38	35	0.23
Ethyl sulfide	0.38		0.45
Chloroform	0.40	61	0.57
Methylene chloride	0.42	40	0.44
Methyl-isobutylketone	0.43	117	
Tetrahydrofuran	0.45	65	0.35

(continued)

From: *Forensic Science and Medicine:*
Forensic and Clinical Applications of Solid Phase Extraction
Edited by: M. J. Telepchak, T. F. August, and G. Chaney © Humana Press Inc., Totowa, NJ

Table (*Continued*)

Solvent	Adsorptive energy	Boiling point (°C)	Viscosity
Ethylene dichloride	0.49	84	0.79
Methylethylketone	0.51	80	0.3
Acetone	0.56	57	0.32
Dioxane	0.56	101	1.54
Ethyl acetate	0.58	77	0.45
Methyl acetate	0.60	57	0.37
Amyl alcohol	0.61	138	4.1
Dimethyl sulfoxide	0.62	189	2.24
Diethyl amine	0.63	56	0.38
Nitromethane	0.64	101	0.67
Acetonitrile	0.65	82	0.37
Pyridine	0.71	115	0.94
Butyl cellusolve	0.74	192	
Isopropanol, *n*-propanol	0.82	83	2.3
Ethanol	0.88	79	1.20
Methanol	0.95	65	0.60
Ethylene glycol	1.11	198	19.9
Acetic acid	Large	118	1.26
Water	Larger	100	1.0
Salts and buffers	Very large	100+	

Appendix F: Buffers for Solid Phase Extraction

Buffer	Group or name	pK$_a$	pH range
Phosphate	pK$_a$1	2.1	1.5–2.7
	pK$_a$2	7.2	6.6–7.8
	pK$_a$3	12.3	11.7–12.9
Citrate	pK$_a$1	3.1	2.5–3.7
	pK$_a$2	4.7	4.1–5.3
	pK$_a$3	5.4	4.8–6.0
Formate[a]		3.8	3.2–4.4
Acetate[a]		4.8	4.2–5.4
MES	2-(*N*-Morpholino)ethanesulfonic acid	6.1	5.5–6.7
Bis-tris	*bis*-(2-Hydroxyethyl)amino *tris*(hydroxymethyl) methane	6.5	5.8–7.2
PIPES	Piperazine-*N,N-bis* (2-ethanesulfonic acid)	6.8	6.1–7.5
BES	*N,N* bis(2-Hydroxyethyl)-2-aminoethanesulfonic acid	7.1	6.4–7.8
MOPS	3-(*N*-Morpholino)propanesulfonic acid	7.2	6.5–7.9
HEPES	*N*-(2-Hydroxethyl)piperazine-*N*-ethanesulfonic acid	7.5	6.8–8.2
Tris	Tris (hydroxymethyl)aminomethane	8.3	7.7–8.9
Ammonia[a]		9.2	8.6–9.8
Borate		9.2	8.6–9.8
Diethylamine[a]		10.5	9.9–11.1

[a]Volatile buffers can be evaporated.

From: *Forensic Science and Medicine:*
Forensic and Clinical Applications of Solid Phase Extraction
Edited by: M. J. Telepchak, T. F. August, and G. Chaney © Humana Press Inc., Totowa, NJ

Appendix G: pK$_a$ Reference for Solid Phase Extraction

(pK$_a$ Values are Given for Protonated Species)

A

Acenocoumarol	4.7
Acepromazine	9.3
Acetaminophen	9.5
Acetanilid	0.5
Acetarsone 3.7, 7.9, 9.3	
Acetazolamide	7.2
Acetic acid	4.8
Acetohexamide	6.6
Acetylcysteine	9.0
Acetylmethodol	8.3
Acetylsalicylic acid	3.5
Aconitine	8.1
Acriflavine	9.1
Alfentanil	6.5
Allobarbital	7.5
Allopurinol	0.2
Allylamine	10.7
Allylbarbituric acid	7.6
Alphaprodine	8.7
Alprenolol	9.6
Alprostadil	6.3
Amantidine	10.1
Amidopyrine	5.0
Aminodarone	5.6
p-Aminobenzoic acid	2.4, 4.9
Aminocaproic acid	4.4, 10.8
Aminopyrine	5.0
Aminosalicylic acid	1.7, 3.9

Amitriptyline	9.4
Ammonia	9.3
Amobarbital	7.9
Amoxapine	7.6
Amphetamine	9.8
Ampicillin	2.7, 7.3
Anileridine	3.7, 7.5
Aniline	5.6
Antazoline	2.5, 10.0
Antipyrine	2.2
Apomorphine	7.2, 8.9
Aprobarbital	7.8
Arecoline	7.6
Arsthinol	9.5
Ascorbic acid	4.2, 11.6
Aspirin	3.5
Atenolol	9.6
Atropine	9.7
Azatadine maleate	9.3
Azathioprine	8.2

B

Baclofen	3.9, 9.6
Barbital	7.8
Barbituric acid	4.0
Bendroflumethiazide	8.5
Benzilic acid	3.0
Benzocaine	2.8
Benzoic acid	4.2
Benzphetamine	6.6

From: *Forensic Science and Medicine:*
Forensic and Clinical Applications of Solid Phase Extraction
Edited by: M. J. Telepchak, T. F. August, and G. Chaney © Humana Press Inc., Totowa, NJ

Benzquinamide	5.9
Benztropine	10.0
Benzylamine	9.3
Benzylmorphine	8.1
Betaine	1.8
bis-Coumacetic acid	3.1, 7.8
Bromazepam	2.9, 11.0
Bromodiphenhydramine	8.6
Bromothen	8.6
8-Bromotheophylline	5.5
Brompheniramine maleate	3.59, 9.12
Brucine	2.3, 8.0
Bujormin	1 1.3
Bupivicaine	8.1
Buprenorphine	8.5, 10.0
Bupropion	8.0
Butalbital	7.6
Butethal	8.1
Butorphanol	8.6
Butylparaben	8.4
Butyric acid	4.8

C

Caffeine	0.6, 14.0
Camphoric acid	4.7
Captopril	3.7, 9.8
Carbachol	4.8
Carbamazepine	7.0
Carbenicillin	2.6, 2.7
Carbinoxamine maleate	9.2
Carbonic acid	6.4, 10.4
Cephalexin	2.5, 5.2, 7.3
Cephradine	2.5, 7.3
Chloral hydrate	10.0
Chlorambucil	1.3, 5.8
Chloramphenicol	5.5
Chlorazepate	3.5, 12.5
Chlorcyclizine	7.8
Chlordiazepaxide	4.8
Chlormethiazole	3.2
Chloropheniramine	9.2
Chlorphentermine	9.6
Chloroprocaine	9.0
Chloroprothixene	8.8
Chloroquin	8.1
8-Chlorotheophylline	5.3
Chlorpromazine	9.3
Chlorpropamide	4.8
Chlorthen	8.4

Chlorothiazide	6.7, 9.5
Chlorthalidone	9.4
Cimetidine	7.09
Cinchonidine	4.2, 8.4
Cinchonine	4.0, 8.2
Cinnamic acid	4.5
Citric acid	3.1, 4.8, 6.4
Clindamycin	7.5
Clofibrate	2.95
Clomipramine	9.5
Clonazepam	1.5, 10.5
Clonidine	8.3
Cloxacillin	2.7
Cocaine	8.4
Codeine	7.9
Colchicine	1.7, 12.4
m-Cresol	10.1
o-Cresol	10.3
Cyanide	9.1
Cyanic acid	3.8
Cyclizine	2.4, 7.7
Cyclobarbitone	7.6
Cyclobenzaprine	8.47
Cyclopentamine	3.5
Cyclopentolate	7.9
Cycloserine	4.5, 7.4
Cyclothiazide	10.7
Cyproheptidine	9.3
Cytarbine (60% MeOH)	4.35

D

Dantrolene	7.5
Dapsone	1.3, 2.5
Demaxepam	4.5, 10.6
Deserpidine	5.67
Desipramine	1.5, 10.2
Dextromethorphan	8.3
Diamorphine	7.6
Diazepam	3.3
Diazoxide	8.5
Dibenzapine	8.5
Dibucaine	8.5
Dichlorphenamide	7.4, 8.6
Dichloracetic acid	1.3
2,4-Dichlorophenoxyacetic acid	3.3
Dicloxacillin	2.8
Dicumerol	4.4, 8.0, 8.9
Dicyclomine	9.0
Diethanolamine	8.9

Diethylamine	11.0
Diethylcarbamazine	7.7
Diflunisal	3.3
Dihydrocodeine	8.8
Dihydroergotamine	6.9
Dihydromorphine	8.6
Dihydrostreptomycin	7.8
3,5-Diiodo-L-thyrosine	2.5, 6.5, 7.5
Dimethadione	6.1
Dimethylamine	10.7
Dimethylamphetamine	9.8
Dimethylbarbituric acid	7.1
Dimethylhydantoin	8.1
Diphenhydramine	9.0
Diphenoxylate	7.1
Dipipanone	8.5
Disopyramide	8.4
Dixyrazine	7.8
Dolbutamine	9.4
Dopamine	8.8
Dothiepin	2.8, 7.4
Doxepin	9.0
Doxorubicin	8.2, 10.2
Doxycycline	3.5, 7.7, 9.5
Doxylamine	4.4, 9.2
Doxylamine succinate	5.8, 9.3
Droperidol	7.6

E

Ecgonine	2.8, 11.1
Emetine	7.4, 8.3
Ephedrine	9.6
Epinephrine	8.5, 9.5
Ergometrine	6.8
Ergotamine	6.3
Erythromycin	8.8
Ethacrynic acid	3.5
Ethambutol	6.3, 9.5
Ethanolamine	9.5
Ethopropuzine	4.8
Ethosuximide	9.3
Ethotoin	8.5
Ethoxolamine	2.2, 7.4
Ethylamine	10.7
Ethylbarbituric acid	4.4
Ethyl-bis-coumacetate	3.1
Ethylenediamine	6.8, 9.9
Ethylmorphine	8.2
Ethylnoradrenaline	8.4

Ethylparaben	8.4
Ethylphenylhydantoin	8.5
Etidocaine	7.7
Etodolac	4.65
Etomidate	4.2
Etorphine	1.9, 7.4
β-Eucaine	9.4
Eugenol	9.8

F

Fencamiamine	8.7
Fenclofenac	5.5
Fendosal	3.1
Fenfluramine	9.1
Fenprofen calcium	4.s
Fentanyl	8.43
Flecainide	9.3
Flucloxacillin	2.7
Flucytosine	2.9, 10.7
Flunitrazepam	1.8
Flupromazine	9.2
Flurazepam	1.9, 8.2
Fluroacetate	2.6
Fluorouracil	8.0, 13.0
Fluphenazine	3.9, 8.1
Fluriprofen	4.2
Folic acid	4.7, 6.8, 9.0
Formic acid	3.7
Fumaric acid	3.0, 4.4
Furosemide	4.7
Fusidic acid	5.4

G

Gadodiamide	5.5–7.0
Gallic acid	3.4
Gentamycin	8.2
Glibenclamide	5.3
Gliclazine	5.8
Glipizide	5.9
Gluconic acid	3.6
Glucuronic acid	3.2
Glutamic acid	4.3
Glutarimide	1.4
Glutethimide	9.2
Glyburide	5.3
Glycerophosphoric acid	1.5, 6.2
Glycine	2.4, 9.8
Glycolic acid	3.8
Guanethidine	9.0, 12.0

Guanidine	3.6
Guanoxan	12.3

H

Haloperidol	8.3
Harmine	7.6
Heptobarbital	7.4
Heroin	7.8
Hexachlorophene	5.7
Hexitine	8.3
Hexobarbital	8.3
Hexylcaine	9.1
Hippuric acid	3.6
Histamine	9.9, 6.0
Homatropine	9.9
Hydantoin	9.1
Hydralazine	0.5, 7.1
Hydrochlorothiazide	7.9, 9.2
Hydrocodone	8.9
Hydrocortisone hemisuccinic acid	5.1
Hydroflumethazide	8.9, 10.7
Hydrogen Peroxide	11.3
Hydromorphone	8.2
Hydroxyamphetamine	9.6
p-Hydroxybenzoic acid	4.6
Hydroxylamine	6.0
Hydroxyquinoline	5.0, 9.9
Hydroxyzine	2.6, 7.0
Hyoscine	7.6

I

Ibuprofen	4.4, 5.2
Idoxuridine	8.3
Imidazole	7.0
Imipramine	9.5
Indapamide	8.8
Indomethacin	4.5
Iocetamic acid	4.1, 4.25
Iopanoic acid	4.8
Iophenoxic acid	7.5
Iprindole	8.2
Isocarboxazid	10.4
Isomethadone	8.1
Isoniazid	1.9, 3.5, 10.8
Isophthalic acid	3.6
Isoprenalin	8.6, 10.1
Isoproterenol	8.7
Isoxsuprine	8.0, 9.8
Itraconazole	3.7

K

Kannamycin	7.2
Ketamine	7.5
Ketobemidone	8.7
Ketorolac	3.5

L

Labetalol	7.4, 8.7
Lactic acid	3.9
Leucovorin	3.1, 4.8, 10.4
Levallorphan	4.5, 6.9
Levamisole	8.0
Levarterenol	8.7, 9.8
Levodopa	2.3, 8.7, 9.7, 13.4
Levomepromazine	9.2
Levorphanol	8.9
Levulinic acid	4.6
Lidocaine	7.9
Lincomycin	7.5
Liothyronine	8.4
Loperimide	8.6
Lorazepam	1.3, 11.5
Loxapine	6.6
Lysergic acid	3.4, 6.3
Lysergic acid diethylamide	7.8

M

Malamic acid	3.6
Maleic acid	3.5, 5.1
Malic acid	3.5, 5.1
Malonic acid	2.8
Mandelic acid	3.4
Maprotiline	10.5
Mazindol	8.6
Mecamylamine	11.2
Mechlorethamine	6.1
Meclizine	3.1, 6.2
Medazepam	6.2
Mefenamic acid	4.2
Mepuzine	9.3
Meperidine	8.7
Mephentermine	10.3
Mephenytoin	8.1
Mepivacaine	7.6
Mephobarbital	7.7
Mercaptopurine	7.6
Metarminol	8.6
Metazoline	9.7
Metformin	2.8, 11.5

Methacillin	2.8	Neostigmine	12.0
Methacycline	3.1, 7.6, 9.5	Nicotinamide	3.3
Methadone	8.3	Nicotine	6.2, 11.0
Methamphetamine	9.5	Nicotinemethiodide	3.2
Methapyrilene	3.7, 8.9	Nicotinic acid	2.0, 4.8
Methaqualone	2.5	Nikethamide	3.5
Metharbital	8.2	Nitrazepam	3.2, 10.8
Methazolamide	7.3	Nitrofurantoin	7.2
Methclothiazide	9.4	Nitrofurazone	10.0
Methenamine	4.9	Nitromethane	1.0
Methidilazine	7.5	8-Nitrotheophylline	2.1
Methohexital	8.3	Noradrenalin	8.6, 9.8, 12.0
Methotrexate	4.3, 5.5	Norcodeine	5.7
Methotrimeprazine	9.2	Nordiazepam	3.5, 12.0
Methoxamine	9.2	Norfloxacin	6.34, 8.75
Methoxyacetic acid	3.5	Norhexabarbital	7.9
Methylamine	10.6	Normethadone	9.2
1-Methylbarbituric acid	4.4	Normorphine	9.8
Methyldopa	2.2, 10.6, 9.2, 12.0	Norparamethadione	6.1
n-Methylephedrine	9.3	Nortrimethadione	6.2
Methylhexylamine	0.5	Nortriptylene	9.7
Methylhydroxybenzoate	8.4	Noscapine	6.2
Methylparaben	8.4		

O

Methylphenidate	8.8	Opipramol	3.8
Methyprylon	12.0	Orphenadrine	8.4
Methylsergide	6.6	Oxalic acid	1.2, 4.2
Methylthiourea	8.2	Oxamic acid	2.1
Metoclopramide	0.6, 9.3	Oxaprozin	4.3
Metopon	8.1	Oxazepam	1.7, 11.6
Metoprolol	9.7	Oxedrine	9.3, 10.2
Metolazone	9.7	Oxphenbutazone	4.5
Metronidazole	2.5	Oxprenolol	9.5
Mexiletine	8.4	Oxybutynin	6.96
Mianserin	7.1	Oxycodone	8.5
Midazolam	6.2	Oxymorphone	8.5, 9.3
Minocycline	2.8, 5.0, 7.8, 9.5	Oxytetracycline	3.3, 7.3, 9.1
Minoxidil	4.6		

P

Molindone	6.9	Papaverine	5.9
Monochloracetic acid	2.9	Pargyline	6.9
Morphine	8.0, 9.6	Pemoline	10.5

N

		Penicillamine	1.8, 7.9, 10.5
Nafcillin	2.7	Penicillin G	2.8
Nalidixic acid	1.0, 6.0	Pentachlorophenol	4.8
Nalorphine	7.8	Pentozocine	8.5, 10.0
Naloxone	7.9	Pentobarbital	8.0
Naphazoline	10.9	Pentoxifylline	0.3
Naproxen	4.2	Perphenazine	7.8
Nefopam	9.2		

Phenacetin	2.2	Propylhexedrine	10.7
Phencyclidine	8.5	Propylparaben	8.4
Phendimetrazine	7.6	Propylthiouracil	7.8
Phenformin	2.7, 11.8	Propoxyphene	6.3
Phenindiamine	8.3	Pseudoephedrine	9.9
Pheniramine	4.2, 9.3	Pyridine	5.2
Phenmetrazine	8.5	Pyridoxine	2.7, 5.0, 9.0
Phenobarbital	7.5	Pyrilamine	4.0, 8.9
Phenol	9.9	Pyrimethamine	7.2
Phenolphthalein	9.7	Pyrobutamine	8.8
Phenoxyacetic acid	3.1	Pyruvic acid	2.5
Phenoxybenzamine	4.4	**Q**	
Phentermine	10.1	Quinacrine	8.0, 10.2
Phenylbutasone	4.7	Quinidine	4.3, 8.3
Phenylephrine	8.9	Quinine	4.2
Phenylethylamine	9.8	**R**	
Phenylpropanolamine	9.4	Ranitidine	2.7, 8.2
Phenylpropylmethylamine	9.9	Reserpine	6.6
Phenytoin	8.3	Resorcinol	6.2
Phentolamine	7.7	Riboflavin	1.7, 10.2
Phentoloxamine	9.1	Rifampicin	1.7, 7.9
Pholcodine	8.0, 9.3	Rimiterol	8.7, 10.3
Physostigmine	2.0, 8.1	Rolitetracycline	7.4
Picric acid	0.4	**S**	
Pilocarpine	1.6, 7.1	Saccharic acid	3.0
Pimozide	7.3	Saccharin	1.6
Pindolol	9.7	Salbutemol	9.3, 10.3
Piperazine	5.7, 10.0	Salicylamide	8.1
Piperidine	11.2	Salicylic acid	3.0, 13.4
Piroxicam	1.8, 5.1	Salsalate	3.5, 9.8
Plasmoquin	3.5, 10.1	Scopolamine	8.2
Practolol	9.5	Secobarbital	8.0
Pralidoxime chloride	8.0	Serotonin	9.1, 9.8
Prazepam	2.7	Sodium chromoglycate	2.5
Prazosin	6.5	Sorbic acid	4.8
Prilocaine	7.9	Sotolol	8.3, 9.8
Primaquin	8.7	Strychnine	2.5, 8.2
Probarbital	8.0	Succinic acid	4.2, 5.6
Probenecid	3.4	Succinimide	9.6
Procaine	9.0	Suientanil	8.01
Procainamide	9.2	Sulfadiazine	6.5
Procarbazine	6.8	Sulfamethizole	5.5
Prochloroperazine	3.6, 7.5	Sulfamerazine	7.1
Promazine	9.4	Sulfamethazine	7.4
Promethazine	9.1	Sulfanilamide	10.4
Propuienone	9.0	Sulfapyridine	8.4
Propionic acid	4.9	Sulfasalazine	0.6, 2.4, 9.7, 11.8
Propranol	9.5		
i-Propylamine	10.6		

Sulfisoxazole	5.0
Sumatriptan	4.21, 5.65, 9.63, >12.0

T

Talbutal	7.8
Tamoxifen	8.85
Temazepam	1.6
Tataric acid	3.0, 4.5
Terazosin	7.04
Terbutaline	8.7, 10.0, 11.0
Tetracaine	8.2
Tetracycline	3.3, 7.7, 9.5
Tetrahydrocannabinol	10.6
Thebaine	8.2
Theobromine	0.7, 8.8
Theophylline	0.7, 8.8
Thiamine	4.8, 9.0
Thiamylal	7.3
Thioacetic acid	3.3
Thioglycolic acid	3.6
Thioguanine	8.1
Thiopental	7.5
Thioridazine	9.5
Thonzylamine	3.1, 8.8
l-Thyronine	9.6
Thyroxine	6.4
Tobramycin	6.7, 8.3, 9.9
Tocainide	7.7
Tolazoline	10.5
p-Toluidine	5.3
Tolazamide	3.5, 5.7
Tolbutamide	5.3
Tolmectin	3.5
Tranylcypromine	8.2
Triampterene	6.2
Trichloracetic acid	0.9
Trichlormethiazide	8.6

Trifluoperazine	4.1, 8.4, 9.4
Trifluopromazine	9.4
Trimethoprim	7.2
Tripelennamine	4.2, 8.7
Triprolidine	3.6, 9.3
Tropicamide	5.2
Tubocurarine	8.1, 9.1
Tyramine	9.5, 10.8

U

Urea	0.2
Uric Acid	5.4, 10.3

V

Valproic acid	4.8
Vanillic acid	4.5
Vanillin	7.4
Vincristine	5.0, 7.4

W

Warfarin	5.1

X

Y

Yohimbine	7.13

Z

Zomepriac	4.5

REFERENCES

1. Wilson, Gisvold, Doerge. Textbook of Organic and Pharmaceutical Chemistry, 7th ed. 1977.
2. United States Dispensing Information, 1996.
3. Clarks Isolation and Identification of Drugs, The Pharmaceutical Press, 1986.

Appendix H: RapidTrace®
Operating Guide

Daily Operation Checklist

The following is a list of details that, if monitored on a daily basis, will maintain your Zymark RapidTrace modules in good working order.

1. Preparing the Workstation

Check your reagents to determine that:
1. They are the correct reagents for the procedure you are going to run.
2. The reagents are fresh.
3. You have enough reagents to run the desired number of samples.
4. Each reagent is on the correct numbered line.

- Make sure the waste reservoirs are empty.
- Purge the reagent lines before running the workstation whenever it has not been used for 10 h or more, and whenever the reagents are changed.
- Check that all sample tubes are clean and you have the correct number of sample and collection tubes needed to run your procedures.
- Check that all SPE columns are new, are the correct type for your procedure, and that you have as many as you need to run your samples.

If necessary, perform a post-run cleanup at the end of the day when you have run SPE procedures on your RapidTrace workstation.

2. Cleaning the RapidTrace Modules

We recommend the following post-run cleanup as a routine maintenance procedure to use in addition to the Purge and Clean Cannula steps, which serve as a standard operational procedure to use between sample runs. Cleaning your modules will remove any proteins that have built up in your fluid path. You may need more or less cleaning depending on the samples and solvents used on your modules.

From: *Forensic Science and Medicine:*
Forensic and Clinical Applications of Solid Phase Extraction
Edited by: M. J. Telepchak, T. F. August, and G. Chaney © Humana Press Inc., Totowa, NJ

Cleaning Reagents Questions and Answers

Why should I run a cleanup procedure on my RapidTrace?

To prevent protein buildup in your system, "cleaning reagents" are used to clean the entire fluid path. Water is used after the cleaning reagent to wash the cleaning reagents out of the fluid path. The fluid path cleanup consists of steps to clean all parts of the fluid path with which the sample comes in contact: the cannula, 12-port valve, syringe, wash station, and lines.

Who should run this procedure?

This procedure should be done by anyone running biological samples.

How often should I run this procedure?

The number of samples run and the sample matrix should determine frequency of fluid path cleanup. The greater the number of samples, the more frequently fluid path cleanup should be performed. In addition, the more protein contained in the sample matrix, the more frequently the fluid path cleanup should be performed.

What about protein in my samples?

Protein content is highest in plasma samples, while a serum sample typically contains half that amount of protein.

What if I have urine as a sample matrix?

Urine samples in a healthy individual contain very little, if any, protein. Zymark recommends that cleanup be done at least on a weekly basis and more frequently if large numbers of plasma samples are run.

Is there anything else I should know?

If the RapidTrace is going to sit idle for a number of days, it is critical that cleanup be done before the modules sit unused.

Procedure for Cleaning

Note: Your biological and organic wastes may contain proteins, so these waste lines are important to clean.

Set up your sample rack as follows:

1. Place two sample tubes in the first two positions of the rack and the cleaning procedure assigned to these two samples.

2. Place 7.5 mL of 2 N sodium hydroxide (NaOH) into your first sample tube and 2 N nitric acid (HNO_3) into your second test tube.

3. Place two empty cartridges with spacers in the positions for samples 1 and 2 in the turret. The empty cartridges with spacers come in your startup kit.

4. Using the described reagent setup and cleanup procedure, run the method listed below.

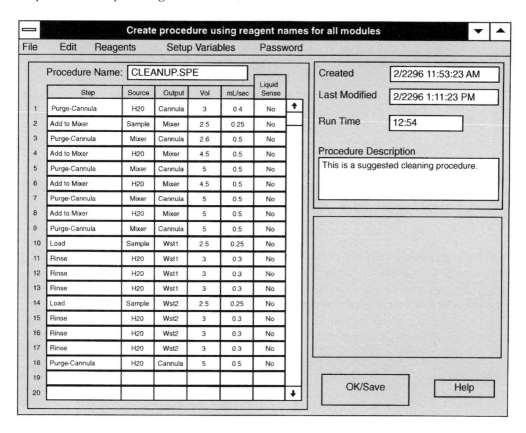

5. In the Setup Racks screen, assign the procedure to samples 1 and 2. While the test is running, check that you have no leaks in the fluid path and that you are not pulling in air once your lines are primed. The lines should be fully primed by the start of the second sample. If you have leaks, retighten fittings.

Understanding the Cleanup Procedure

Step number	Step	Purpose
1	Purge—cannula	Initial water cleaning of cannula, syringe, 12-port valve, and associated lines to remove any residual sample matrix from last samples run.
2	Add to mixer	Adds the cleaning reagent to the mixing vessel.
3	Purge—cannula	Cleaning of cannula, syringe, 12-port valve, and associated lines with sample (cleaning reagent) from the mixing vessel to remove protein buildup.
4–9	Add to mixer	Washing of mixing vessel to remove residual cleaning reagent to purge–cannula.
10	Load	Loads the cleaning reagent through the cannula, lines, and 12-port valve to the syringe. The sample is then directed back through the 12-port valve through the SPE column to waste.

(continued)

Understanding the Cleanup Procedure (continued)

Step number	Step	Purpose
11–13	Rinse	Water is used to rinse the fluid path just used to load the sample through the SPE column.
14	Load	Loads the cleaning reagent through the cannula, lines, and 12-port valve to the syringe. The sample is then directed back through the 12-port valve through the SPE column to waste.
15–17.	Rinse	Water is used to rinse the fluid path just used to load the sample through the SPE column.
18.	Purge—cannula	Final water purge of the fluid path to ensure that all remaining cleaning reagent has been washed out of the system.

For a most efficient cleanup, we recommend that biological waste be limited to one of the three available was lines. Be sure that your fluid path cleanup procedure uses that waste line. If your procedures typically segregate organic waste, good cleanup practice is to run a cleanup routine on that waste line. Edit the cleanup procedure to duplicate steps 10–13 for the organic waste lines, as they may contain proteins as well. The cleanup procedure on the previous page cleans waste line 1. Be sure your procedure contains adequate cleaning steps for all waste lines that come in contact with organic or biological waste.

Waste Test

Use the procedure below, using appropriate reagents, to test for leaks in your waste lines. While the test is running, check for leaks in the waste fluid path and retighten fittings as necessary.

Line: Purge

Whenever changing solvents or using different solvents, follow the procedure below as a general guideline to purge solvent lines and to check for the integrity of the solvent lines. Retighten or replace any leaking fitting as needed.

RapidTrace Initialization Steps

The following list outlines the steps that the RapidTrace performs once it is turned on.

	Create procedure using reagent names for all modules									
File	Edit	Reagents	Setup Variables	Password						

Procedure Name:	waste.spe					Created	10/5/98 2:23:05 PM

	Step	Source	Output	Vol	mL/sec	Liquid Sense
1	Condition	Reag1	Waste1	6	.7	No
2	Condition	Reag2	Waste2	6	.7	No
3	Condition	Reag3	Waste3	6	.7	No
4						
5						
6						
7						
8						

Last Modified

Run Time

Procedure Description

This procedure checks the integrity of the waste fluid paths.

1. The "Run" light is illuminated.
2. The rack is scanned twice. This locates the shuttle "Home" position, and confirms that the rack is present and correctly positioned on the shuttle. In addition, the rack is checked for sample and fraction tubes. If the "Start" button was pressed to initiate the run, the sensors would check to see if the rack is magnetically coded and reads the code.

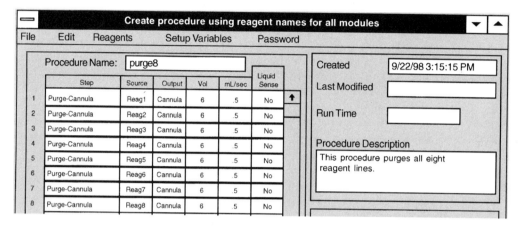

3. The rack is positioned so the cannula wash station is located under the cannula.
4. The cannula is moved down into the cannula wash station.
5. If the syringe is not at the Home position (0 mL), the 12-port valve is positioned at the cannula, and the syringe is homed to 0 mL. Once the syringe is at the "Home" position, the 12-port valve is positioned to draw from the mixing vessel, and the syringe draws a full stroke, the 12-port valve moves to the "Cannula" position and dispenses the syringe volume through the cannula wash station.
6. Next, the 12-port valve moves to the "Vent" position, and the syringe draws a full stroke, then the 12-port valve moves to the "Cannula" position and dispenses the syringe volume through the cannula waste station.
7. The turret moves to position 1.
8. The column plunger goes down into the "Lock" position.
9. The column plunger moves back up to the "Home" position.
10. The turret returns to the "Home" position.
11. The cannula moves up to the "Home" position.
12. The rack is shuttled to the "Out" position.
13. The "Run" light goes off.

RapidTrace Troubleshooting Guide

Once the Warm Start is completed, the hardware should be checked to ensure that it is ready to run the desired procedure.

Item	Check to see	Solution
Power light	Green light is on.	Turn RapidTrace on.
Run light	Run light is off.	Run in progress, wait until run completed or stop run.
Error light	Error light is off.	Go to ERROR RECOVERY

(continued)

(Continued from page 339)

Item	Check to see	Solution
		Window and use STATUS? Correct the error.
Module ID	Each module has a unique module identification number.	Correct so each module has a unique number.
Syringe	At HOME position	Go to ERROR RECOVERY and move the syringe to the HOME position. HOME position is when the plunger is at the bottom of the syringe, 0 mL.
	Clean, no liquid on top of the syringe plunger	If the syringe is not clean, run the recommended cleanup procedure. If the syringe still looks dirty, or there is liquid on top of the syringe, call Zyline* to arrange to have the syringe replaced.
Cannula	At HOME position	Go to ERROR RECOVERY and move the cannula to UP position.
	Clean	Run the recommended cleanup procedure.
	O-ring intact	Replace O-ring.
Rack	In the HOME position	Go to ERROR.
RECOVERY and home position for shuttle to be RapidTrace		Use SHUTTLE OUT to the shuttle. (HOME the Shuttle is for the extending from the housing by about 4 cm).
SPE COLUMN PLUNGER RECOVERY and UP PLUNGER	At UP position	Go to ERROR. Use COLUMN PLUNGER to home the SPE column.
Cleanup	Clean	Run the recommended procedure.
	O-ring intact	Replace the O-ring.
	Nut is screwed on tightly on the column plunger assembly.	
	Teflon tubing is connected to the top of the SPE column plunger. Refer to fluid path diagram in the RapidTrace manual to connect the Teflon tubing.	
Shuttle	Moves smoothly	Contact Zyline.*

Additional Comments about RapidTrace Methods
a. Protein precipitation
All the methods listed in this book close with a cannula purge with water, then methanol. If you are running a large amount of serum or blood samples, follow at the end of day with a waste test. This will prevent protein precipitating in the lines.
b. Cross-contamination
When one performs SPE on the RapidTrace, prior to the elution, reagents and samples go directly through the SPE column and down into the waste line. At the time of elution, the tip of the SPE drops into a test tube and a drop forms at the tip of the column, essentially contaminating the tip of the column. Then, if you do a rinse, the tip contaminates the O-ring of the aqueous waste line. When your second sample is processed the column tip is contaminated by the first sample when the aqueous waste line is used. It is recommended that each RapidTrace procedure use only two waste lines: aqueous and organic. Place bleach in the aqueous waste container to deactivate any biological proteins. All post-elution rinses should be placed into waste 3. This essentially prevents this cross-contamination problem.

---

*Zyline: The Zymark Corporation has a special department that handles all RapidTrace problems and questions. The phone number for the Zyline is (508) 435-9761.

PREPARING THE RAPIDTRACE FOR SHIPPING

Biohazardous substances are routinely present in your RapidTrace instrument. To protect yourself and minimize the risks to others the following procedure should be followed whenever a RapidTrace unit is shipped out.

1. Run the standard cleaning procedure.
   a. Clean. SPE for two samples: the first sample is 8 mL of 2 N NaOH, the second sample 8 mL of 2 N HNO$_3$.
   b. Use the empty 1–3-mL SPE columns and spacers (provided in the startup kit) in turret positions 1 and 2.
2. Pull all reagent lines out of the reagents and put them into a beaker of water. Run a procedure to purge all lines.
3. Pull all reagent lines out of the water beaker and run the procedure to purge all lines.
4. Pull all reagent lines into a beaker of methanol. Run a procedure to purge all lines.
5. Pull all reagent lines out of the methanol beaker and run the procedure to purge all lines. This will run the lines dry with the last reagent inside each fluid path being methanol.
6. To prepare the RapidTrace(r) for shipping: Go into Error Recovery. Make sure there is a rack in the RapidTrace with a sample tube in position.
   • Send rack to shuttle wash (Shuttle Wash, send).
   • Send turret to any position (Turret, 1, send).
   • Select column plunger-squash column (Column plunger, squash, send). Be ready to turn power switch in the back of the unit off when tip of plunger is just above shutter.
   • Move shutter manually to clear path for cannula. (Reach in through the left side and pull the shutter left.)
   • Move cannula manually into wash. (Push down on the cannula gear shaft until cannula is inside wash station.)
   • Pull sample rack out of the shuttle.

Appendix I: Further Reading

BIOCHEMISTRY

[1]Anderson, L., Cummings, J., and Smyth, J. Rapid and selective isolation of radio labeled inositol phosphates from cancer using solid-phase extraction. Chromatogr. 574:150–155, 1992.

[2]Becker, D., Galili, N., and Degani, G. GC/MS-identified steroids and steroid glucuronides in the gonads and holding water of *Trichogaster trichopterus*. Comp. Biochem. Physiol. 103B:15–19, 1992.

[3]Bioque, G., Tost, D., Closa, D., Rosello-Catatu, Ramis, J., Cabrer, F. Concurrent C-18 solid phase extraction of platelet activating factor (PAF) and arachidonic acid metabolites. Liq. Chromatogr. 15:1249–1250, 1992.

[4]Brooks, M., Tessler, D., and Soderstrom, D. A rapid method for the simultaneous analysis of chlorpyrifos, isofenphos, carbaryl, iprodione and triadimefon in groundwater by solid phase extraction. Chromatogr. Sci. 28:487–492, 1990.

[5]Carmona, G., Baum, I., and Schindler, C. Plasma butyrylcholinesterase activity and cocaine half-life differ significantly in rhesus and squirrel monkeys. Life Sci. 11:939–943, 1992.

[6]Causon, R., and McDowell, R. Sample pretreatment techniques for the bioanalysis of peptides. Controll. Release. 21:37–48, 1992.

[7]Chiba, H., Ho, Y., and Matsuno, K. Determination of urinary 18-hydroxycortisol by isocratic normal phase high-performance liquid chromatography. Chromatogr. 613:132–136, 1993.

[8]Coene, J., Van Den, E., Eeckhout, E. Gas chromatographic determination of alkyl lysophospholipids after solid-phase extraction from culture media. Chromatogr. 612:2126–2128, 1993.

[9]Crowe, T., and Jacobsen, D. Rapid solid phase extraction of dopamine, serotonin and their acidic metabolites for high-performance liquid chromatography. Liq. Chromatogr. 15:221–230.

[10]Doehl, J., and Greibrokk, T. Determination of prostaglandins in human seminal fluid by solid-phase extraction with pyridinium dichromate derivatization. J. Chromatogr. 529:21–32, 1990.

[11]Goto, J. Gas chromatographic-mass spectrometric determination of 4- 6-hydroxylated bile acids in human urine with negative ion chromatography. Chromatogr. 574:1–7, 1992.

[12]Harmenberg, J., Cox, S., and Akesson-Johnsson, A. High-performance liquid chromatography of deoxyribonucleoside thriphosphates. Chromatogr. 508:75–79, 1990.

From: *Forensic Science and Medicine:*
Forensic and Clinical Applications of Solid Phase Extraction
Edited by: M. J. Telepchak, T. F. August, and G. Chaney © Humana Press Inc., Totowa, NJ

[13]Henden, T., Strand, H., Borde, E. Measurements of leukotrines in human plasma by solid phase extraction and high performance liquid chromatography. Prostagland. Leukotr. 49:851–854, 1993.

[14]Janero, D., Yarwood, C., and Thakkar, J. Application of solid-phase extraction on anion exchange cartridges to quantify 5-nucleotidase activity. Chromatogr. 573:207–218, 1992.

[15]Legrand-Defretin, V., Juste, C., Henry, R., and Corring, T. Ion-pair high performance liquid chromatography of bile salt conjugates: Application to pig bile. Lipids. 26:578–583, 1991.

[16]McCormick, R. Solid phase extraction procedure for DNA purification. Analyt. Biochem. 181:66–74, 1989.

[17]Minegishi, A., and Ishizaki, T. Rapid and simple method for the simultaneous determination of 3,4 dihydroxyphenylacetic acid, 5-hydoxyindole-3 methoxyphenylacetic acid in human plasma. J. Chromatogr. 308:55–63, 1984.

[18]Niwa, T., Fujita, K., Goto, J., Nambara, T. Separation and characterization of ursodeoxycholate 7-N-acetylglucosamides in human urine by high-performance liquid chromatography. J. Liq. Chromatogr. 16:2531–2540, 1993.

[19]Penka-Davidson, V., and Traiger, G. Determination of *P*-methylthiobenzamide and *P*-methylthiobenzamide-*S*-oxide from rat plasma using solid phase extraction. J. Chromatogr. 567:213–220, 1991.

[20]Pratt, D., Daniloff, Y., Duncan, A., and Robins, S. Automated analysis of the pyridinium crosslinks of collagen in tissue and urine using solid-phase extraction and reversed phase high performance liquid chromatography. Analyt. Biochem. 207:168–175, 1992.

[21]Renberg, L., and Jurgen-Hoffman, K. Determination of a renin inhibitor in plasma by solid-phase extraction using acetone as protein binding displacer. Pharmaceut. Biomed. 10:959–983, 1992.

[22]Riufta, A., Mucha, I., and Vapaatalo, H. Solid-phase extraction of urinary 11 dehydrothromboxane B2 for reliable determination with radioimmunoassay. Analyt. Biochem. 202:299–305, 1992.

[23]Rissler, K., Katlein, R., Cramer, H. Recovery of substance P and related C-terminal fragments on solid-phase extraction cartridges. J. Chromatogr. 612:150–155, 1993.

[24]Salvadod, M., Dolara, P., Bertini, E., and Coppi, C. Analysis of mutagenic activity in human urine after concentration of different resins and high performance liquid chromatography. Toxicol. Lett. 45:241–249, 1989.

[25]Schmid, R. Specific extraction of glycosolated amino acid from protein hydrolysates using boronic acid derivatized silica gel. Proceedings of the Second International Symposium on Sample Preparation and Isolation Using Bonded Silicas, p.15. Philadelphia, 1985.

[26]Serhan, C. High performance liquid chromatography separation and determination of lipoxins. Methods Enzymol. 187:167–175, 1990.

[27]Shi, M., and Ellin, R. Mechanism of solid phase extraction of nanogram levels of pyridostigmine from plasma. Proceedings of the Second International Symposium on Sample Preparation and Isolation Using Bonded Silicas, p. 33. Philadelphia, 1985.

[28]Shintani, H. Solid phase extraction and high performance liquid chromatographic analysis of a toxic compound from Y-irradiated polyurethane. J. Chromatogr. 600:93–97, 1992.

[29]Sugahara, K., and Kodama, H. Liquid chromatography-mass spectrometry for simultaneous analysis of iminodipeptides containing an *N*-terminal or *C*-terminal. Chromatography 565:408–415, 1991.

[30]Vesterqvist, O., and Green, K. Development of a GC-MS method for quantitation of 2, 3-dinor-6-keto PGF and determination of the urinary excretion rates in healthy humans under normal conditions and following drugs. Prostaglandins 28:139–154, 1994.

[31]Van Boxiaer, J., and De Leenleer, A. Solid phase extraction technique for gas chromatographic profiling of acylcarnitines. Clin. Chem. 39:1911–1915, 1993.

[32]Van de Heijning, B., Koekkoek-Van den Herik, I., Ivanyi, T. Solid-phase extraction of plasma vasopressin: evaluation, validation and application. Chromatography. 565:159–171, 1991.

[33]Wilson, R., Henderson, R., Burkow, I., Sargent, J. The enrichment of *N*-3 polyunsaturated fatty acids using aminopropyl solid phase extraction columns. Lipids 28:51–54, 1993.

ENVIRONMENTAL

[1]Butlerman, A., Vreuls, J., Ghijsen, R., and Brinkman, U. Selective and sensitive detection of organic contaminants in water samples by on-line trace enrichment-gas chromatography mass spectrometry. J. High Resolut. Chromatogr. 16:397–403, 1993.

[2]Andrews, J., and Good, T. Trace enrichment of pesticides using bonded-phase sorbents. Am. Lab. 14:70–75, 1994.

[3]Angerer, J., Horsch, B. Determination of aromatic hydrocarbons and their metabolites in human blood and urine. J. Chromatogr. 580:229–255, 1992.

[4]Bagheri, J., Vreuls, J., Ghijsen, R., and Brinkman, U. Determination of triazine herbicides in surface and drinking waters by off-line combination of liquid chromatography and gas chromatography. Chromatographia 34:5–9, 1992.

[5]Burkhard, L., Durham, E., and Lukasewcyz, M. Identification of nonpolar toxicants in effluents using toxicity-based fractionation with gas chromatography/mass spectroscopy. Analyt. Chem. 63:277–283, 1991.

[6]Cai, Z., Ramanujam, V., Giblin, D., Gross, M., and Spalding, R. Determination of atrazine in water at low and sub parts per trillion levels by using solid-phase extraction. Analyt. Chem. 65:2370–2373, 1993.

[7]Caldwell, K., Ramanujam, V., Cai, Z., Gross, M. Herbicide trace analysis by high resolution fast atom bombardment mass spectrometry. Analyt. Chem. 65:2372–2375, 1993.

[8]Canals, A., Fortenza, R., and Cerda, V. The routine determination of PCBs in waste automotive engine oils. Chromatographia 34:35–40, 1993.

[9]Carabias, R., Gonzolo, M., Moran, M., Mendez, J Sensitive method for the determination of organophosphorus pesticides in fruits and surface waters by high-performance liquid chromatography. J. Chromatogr. 607:37–45, 1992.

[10]Chang, R., Jarman, W., and Hennings, J. Sample cleanup by solid-phase extraction for the ultratrace determination of polychlorinated dibenzo-*P*-dioxins. Analyt. Chem. 85:2420–2423, 1992.

[11]Chladek, E., and Marano, R. Use of bonded phase silica sorbents for the sampling of priority pollutants in wastewaters. J. Chromatogr. Sci. 22:313–320, 1984.

[12]Cotsaris, E., and Nicholson, B. Low-level determination of formaldehyde in water by high performance liquid chromatography. Analyst 188:265–268, 1993.

[13]Dalbacke, J., Dalquist, I., and Persson, C. Determination of warfarin in drinking water by high performance liquid chromatography after solid phase extraction. J. Chromatogr. 507:381–387, 1992.

[14]De Kok, A., Hiemstra, M., and Brinkman, U. Low nanogram per milliliter level determination of twenty *N*-methylcarbamate pesticides and twelve of their polar metabolites in surface water. J. Chromatogr. 623:265–276, 1992.

[15]Di Corcia, A., Samperi, R., Marcomini, A., and Stelluto, S. Graphitized carbon black extraction cartridges for monitoring polar pesticides in water. Analyt. Chem. 65:907–912, 1993.

[16]Durhan, E., Lukasewycz, M., and Baker, S. Alternatives to methanol-water elution of solid phase extraction columns for the fractionation of high log low organic compounds in aqueous environmental samples. J. Chromatogr. 629:67–74, 1993.

[17]Fingler, S., Drevenkar, V., Tkalcevic, B., and Smit, Z. Levels of polychlorinated biphenyls, organochlorine pesticides, and chlorophenols in the Kupa River water and in drinking waters. Bull. Environ. Contam. Toxicol. 49:805–812, 1992.

[18]Font, G., Manes, J., Molto, J., and Pico, Y. Solid-phase extraction in multi-residue pesticide analysis of water. J. Chromatogr. 642:135–161, 1993.

[19]Fujita, I., Ozasa, Y., Tobino, T., and Sugimura, T. Determination of sodium linear alkylbenzene sulfonate in river waters by high-peformance liquid chromatography and solid phase extraction. Chem. Pharmaceut. Bull. 38:1425–1427, 1990.

[20]Fuoco, R., Colombini, M., and Samcova, E. Individual determination of ortho and non-ortho substituted polychlorobiphenyls (PCBs) in sediments by high performance liquid chromatography. Chromatographia 36: 1993.

[21]Gundel, A., Mahanama, K., and Daisey, J. Fractionation of polar organic extracts of airborne particulate matter using cyanopropyl bonded silica in solid-phase extraction. J. Chromatogr. 629:75–82, 1993.

[22]Hong, J., Eo, Y., Rhee, J., Kim, T., Kim, K. Simultaneous analysis of 25 pesticides in crops using gas chromatography and their identification by gas chromatography-mass spectroscopy. J. Chromatogr. 639:261–271, 1993.

[23]Howard, A., and Taylor, L. Quantitative supercritical fluid extraction of sulfonylurea herbicides from aqueous matrices via solid phase extraction. Chromatographia. 30:374–392, 1992.

[24]Huhnerfuss, H., and Kallenborn, R. Chromatographic separation of marine organic pollutants. J. Chromatogr. 580:191–214, 1992.

[25]Ikeda, K., Migliorese, K., and Curtis, H. Analysis of nitrosamines in cosmetics. J. Soc. Cosmet. Chem. 41:284–333, 1990.

[26]Klafenback, P., and Holland, P. Analysis of sulfonylurea herbicides by gas-chromatography II. Determination of chlorsulfuron and metsulfuronmenthyl in soil and water samples. Agric. Food Chem. 41:396–401, 1993.

[27]Lorger, B., and Smith, J. Multiresidue method for the extraction and detection of organophosphate pesticides. Food Chem. 41:303–307, 1993.

[28]Meyer, M., Mills, M., and Thurman, E. Automated solid-phase extraction of herbicides from water for gas chromatographic-mass spectrometric analysis. J. Chromatogr. 629:55–59, 1993.

[29]Mills, M., and Thurman, E. Mixed mode isolation of triazine metabolites from soil and aquifer sediments using automated solid-phase extraction. Analyt. Chem. 60:1985–1990, 1992.

[30]Orti, D., Hill, R., Liddle, J., Needham, L., Vickers, L. High performance liquid chromatography of mycotoxin metabolites in human urine. J. Analyt. Toxicol. 10:41–45, 1986.

[31]Ngan, F., and Ikesaki, T. Determination of nine acidic herbicides in water and soil by gas chromatography using an electron-capture detector. J. Chromatogr. 537:385–395, 1991.

[32]Page, M., and French, M. N-methylcarbonate determination of N-methylcarbamate insecticides in vegetables, fruits, and foods using solid phase extraction cleanup. AOAC Int. 75:1073–1074, 1991.

[33]Poziomek, E. Solid-phase extraction and solid-state spectroscopy for monitoring water pollution. Analyt. Lett. 24:1913–1920, 1991.

[34]Redondo, M., Ruiz, M., Boluda, R., Font, G. Determination of pesticides in soil samples by solid phase extraction disks. Chromatographia. 36:187–190, 1993

[35]Rostad, C., Pereira, W., Ratcliff, S. Bonded-phase extraction column isolation of organic compounds in groundwater at a hazardous waste site. Analyt. Chem. 56:2856–2860, 1993.

[36]Saady, J., and Poklis, A. Determination of chlorinated hydrocarbon pesticides by solid phase extraction and capillary GC with electron capture detection. J. Analyt. Toxicol. 14:301–304, 1991.

[37]Schad, H., Schafer, F., Weber, L., and Seidel, H. Determination of benzene metabolites in urine of mice by solid-phase extraction and high-performance liquid chromatography. J. Chromatogr. 593:147–151, 1992.

[38]Schwartz, T., and Stalling, D. Chemometric comparison of polychlorinated biphenyl residues and toxicologically active polychlorinated biphenyl congeners. Arch. Environ. Contam. Toxicol. 20:183–199, 1991.

[39]Shepherd, T., Carr, J., Duncan, D., Pederson, D. C-18 Extraction of atrazine from small water sample volumes. J. AOAC Int. 75: 581–583, 1991.

FOOD AND FOOD ADDITIVES

[1]Barker, S., and Walker, C. Chromatographic methods for tetracycline analysis in foods. J. Chromatogr. 624:195–209, 1992.

[2]Bello, A. Rapid isolation of the sterol fraction in edible oils using a silica cartridge. J. AOAC Int. 75:1120–1123, 1992.

[3]Bobbit, D., Ng, K. Chromatographic analysis of antibiotic materials in food. J. Chromatogr. 624:153–170, 1992.

[4]Boison, J. Chromatographic methods of analysis for penicillins in food-animal tissues and their significance in regulatory procedures. J. Chromatogr. 624:171–194, 1992.

[5]Busto, O., Valero, Y., Guasch, J., and Borrull, F. Solid phase extraction applied to the determination of biogenic amines in wines by HPLC. Chromatographia. 38:571–578, 1994.

[6]Calull, M., Marce, R., Borrull, F. Determination of carboxylic acids, sugars, glycerol and ethanol in wine and grape must by ion-exchange high-performance liquid chromatography. J. Chromatogr. 592: 215–222, 1992.

[7]Calull, M., Marce, R., Sanchez, G., and Borrull, F. Determination of additives in wine by high performance liquid chromatography. J. Chromatogr. 607:339–347, 1992.

[8]Cartoni, G., Ciogioli, G., and Pontelli, L. Separation and identification of free phenolic acids in wines by high-performance liquid chromatography. J. Chromatogr. 537:83–90, 1991.

[9]Coulibaly, K., Jeon, I. Solid phase extraction of less volatile flavor compounds from ultrahigh-temperature processed milk. Agric. Food Chem. 40:612–616, 1992.

[10]Fenton, M. Chromatographic separation of cholesterol in foods. J. Chromatogr. 624:369–388, 1992.

[11]Finger, A., Khur, S., Engelhardt, U. Chromatography of tea constituents. J. Chromatogr. 624:293–315, 1992.

[12]Fodor-Csorba, K. Chromatographic methods for the determination of pesticides in foods. J. Chromatogr. 624:353–367, 1992.

[13]Horie, M., Saito, K., Hoshino, Y., Nose, N., Nakazawa, H., and Yamane, Y. Simultaneous determination of residual synthetic antibacterials in fish by high-performance liquid chromatography. J. Chromatogr. 538:484–491, 1991.

[14]Horie, A., Saito, K., Hoshino, Y., Nose, N., and Nakazawa, H. Simultaneous determination of sulfonamides in honey by liquid chromatography. J. AOAC Int. 75:786–789, 1992.

[15]Mingues-Mosquera, M., Gandul-Rojas, B., and Gallardo-Guerrero, M. Rapid method of quantification of chlorophylls and carotenoids in virgin olive oil by high-performance liquid chromatography. J. Agric. Food. 40:60–63, 1992.

[16]Pensabene, J., Fiddler, W., and Gates, R. Solid-phase extraction method for volatile nitrosamines in hams processed with elastic rubber netting. J. AOAC Int. 75:438–441, 1992.

[17]Pizollo, A., and Polesello, S. Chromatographic determination of vitamins in foods. J. Chromatogr. 624:103–152, 1992.

[18]Schenck, F., and Hennessy, M. Determination of dinocap in apples, grapes, and pears using a solid phase extraction cleanup and HPLC-UV detection. Liq. Chromatogr. 16: 755–766, 1993.

[19]Shaikhm B., and Moats, W. Liquid chromatographic analysis of antibacterial drug residues in food products of animal origin. J. Chromatogr. 643:369–378, 1993.

[20]Takatsuki, K., and Kikuchi, T. Gas chromatographic-mass spectrometric determination of six sulfonamide residues in egg and animal tissues. Analyt. Chem. 73:886–888, 1990.

[21]Tomas-Barberan, F. A., Ferreres, F., Blazquez, M. A., Garcia-Viguerra, C., Tomas-Lorente, F. High-performance liquid chromatography of honey flavonoids. J. Chromatogr. 634:41–46, 1993.

[22]Unruh, J., Piotrowski, E., Schwartz, D., Barford, R. Solid-phase extraction of sulfamethazine in milk with quantitation at low PPB levels using thin-layer chromatography. J. Chromatogr. 519:179–187, 1990.

[23]Vadukul, N. Determination of maleic hydrazide in onions and potatoes using solid-phase extraction and anion-exchange high-performance liquid chromatography. Analyst. 116:1369–1372, 1991.

[24]Vidal-Valverde, C., and Reche, A. Reliable system for the analysis of riboflavin in foods by high performance liquid chromatography and UV detection. Liq. Chromatogr. 13:2089–2101, 1990.

PLANTS

[1]Albrecht, J., and Schafer, H. Comparison of two methods of ascorbic acid determination in vegetables. Liq. Chromatogr. 13:633–640, 1990.

[2]Amelio, M., Rizzo, R., and Varazini, F. Determination of sterols, erythrodiol, uvaol and alkanols in olive oils using combined solid phase extraction, high performance liquid chromatography. Chromatography 606:179–185, 1992.

[3]Buszewski, B., Kawka, S., Suprynowicz, Z., Wolski, T. Simultaneous isolation of rutin and esculin from plant material and drugs using solid-phase extraction. J. Pharmaceut. Biomed. Analysis 11:211–215, 1993.

[4]Charuet, N., Rho, D., and Archambault, J. Solid-phase extraction and fluorimetric detection of benzophenanthridine alkaloids from *Sanguinaria Ccanadensis*. J. Chromatogr. 519:99–107, 1990.

[5]Chortyk, O., and Chamberlain, W. The application of solid phase extraction to the analysis of tobacco-specific nitrosamines. Chromatogr. Sci. 29:522–527, 1991.

[6]Neff, W., Zeitoun, M., and Weisleder, D. Resolution of lipolysis mixtures from soybean oil by a solid-phase extraction procedure. J. Chromatogr. 589:353–357, 1992.

[7]Nisperos-Carriedo, M., Buslig, B., and Shaw, P. Simultaneous detection of dehydroascorbic and some organic acids in fruits and vegetables by HPLC. Agric. Food Chem. 40:112–113, 1992.

[8]Wiegrebe, H., and Wichtl, M. High-performance liquid chromatographic determination of cardenolides in digitalis leaves after solid-phase extraction. J. Chromatogr. 630:402–407, 1993.

[9]Wigfield, Y., and Lacroix, M. Determination of N-nitrosodimethylamine in thiram formulations using steam distillation followed by solid phase extraction. Bull. Environ. Contam. Toxicol. 49:827–833, 1992.

VETERINARY

[1]Arts, C., van Baak, M., and den Hartog, J. Control system for detection of illegal use of naturally occurring steroids in calves. Chromatography 564:429–444, 1991.

[2]Els, A., Daeseleire, I., De Guesquire, A., van Peteghem, C. Multiresidue analysis of anabolic agents in muscle tissue and urines of cattle by GC-MS. J. Chromatogr. Sci. 30:409–414, 1992.

[3]Gaspar, P., and Maghuin-Rogister, G. Rapid extraction and purification of diethylstilbesterol in bovine urine hydrolysates using reversed-phase C-18 columns. Chromatography 328:413–416, 1985.

[4]Hansen-Moller, J. Determination of indolic compounds in pig back fat by solid phase extraction and gradient high-performance liquid chromatography. Chromatography 624:479–490, 1992.

[5]Heebner, E., Fox, D., Phillips, T. Improved removal of water soluble interferences from racing greyhound urine. Proceedings of the 9th International Conference of Racing Analysts and Veterinarians. New Orleans, 1992.

[6]Heinz-Wemer, H., and Schulz, R. Detection of diuretics in horse urine by GC/MS. J. Analyt. Toxicol. 16:194–198, 1992.

[7]Heinz-Wemer, H., Schulz, R., and Friedrich, A. Detection of methandienone (methandrostenolone) and metabolites in horse urine by gas chromatography-mass spectroscopy. J. Chromatogr. 577:195–203, 1992.

[8]Hooijerink, H., Schilt, R., Haasnoot, W., and Courtheujn, D. Determination of clenbuterol in urine of calves by high performance liquid chromatography. Pharmaceut. Biomed. Analysis 9:485–492, 1992.

[9]Horspool, J., and McKellar, Q. Determination of short-chaine fatty acids in equine caecal liquor by ion exchange high performance liquid chromatography after. Biomed. Chromatogr. 5:202–206, 1991.

[10]Hurst, W., and Young, J., Jr. The use of bonded silica extraction columns in the isolation of ampicillin from animal serum. Proceedings of the Second Analytichem International Symposium, p. 27. Philadelphia, 1985.

[11]Medina, M., and Unruh, J. Solid-phase clean-up and thin-layer chromatographic detection of veterinary aminoglycosides. J. Chromatogr. 663:127–135, 1995.

[12]Moore, C. Solid-phase cation exchange extraction of basic drugs from the urine of racing greyhounds. Forensic Sci. Soc. 30:123–129, 1990.

[13]Moore, C., Tebbett, I., Kalita, S., Artememko, M. Rapid extraction and detection of mazindol in horse urine. Pharmaceut. Biomed. Analysis 8:445–448, 1990.

[14]Murphey, L., and Olsen, G. A stereospecific microassay for the determination of morphine 6-glucuronide and other active morphine metabolites in the neonatal guinea pig. J. Liq. Chromatogr. 16:2545–2561, 1993.

[15]Nelis, H., Vandenbranden, J., Verhaeghe, B. Liquid chromatographic determination of ampicilllin in bovine and dog plasma by using a tandem solid phase extraction method. Antimicrob. Agents Chemother. 36:1606–1610, 1992.

[16]Pierce, T., Murray, A., and Hope, W. Determination of methadone and its metabolites by high performance liquid chromatography following solid-phase extraction in rat plasma. Chromatogr. Sci. 30:443–447, 1992.

[17]Renner, G., and Hopfer, C. Metabolic studies on pentachlorophenol in rats. Xenobiotica 20:573–582, 1990.

[18]Ruprecht, R., Sharpe, A., Jaenisch, R., and Trites, D. Analysis of 3-azido-3-deoxythymidine levels in tissues and milk by isocratic high-performance liquid chromatography. J. Chromatogr. 528:371–383, 1990.

[19]Sapp, R., and Davidson, S. Determination of roxarsone in feeds using solid phase extraction and liquid chromatography with ultraviolet detection. J. AOAC Int. 76:956–961, 1993.

[20]Singh, A., Ashraf, M., Granley, K., Mishra, V., Kao, M. M., and Gordon, B. Screening and confirmation of drugs in horse urine by using a simple column extraction procedure. J. Chromatogr. 473:215–226, 1989.

[21]Uboh, C., Rudy, J., Railing, F., Enright, J. M., Shoemaker, J. M., Kikler, M. C., Shellenberger, J. M., Kemecsie, Z., Das, D. N. Postmortem tissue samples: An alternative to urine and blood for drug analysis in racehorses. J. Analyt. Toxicol. 19:307–315, 1995.

[22]Van Rhien, J., and Tuinstra, L. Automated determination of aflatoxin B1 in cattle feed by two-column solid-phase extraction with one-line high-performance liquid chromatography. J. Chromatogr. 592:265–269, 1992.

[23]Voogt, P., Lambert, J., Granneman, J., and Jansen, M. Confirmation of the presence of Bestradiol-17B in sea star *Asterias rubens* by GC-MS. Comp. Biochem. Physiol. 101B:13–16, 1992.

[24]Walsh, J., Walker, L., and Webber, J. Determination of tetracyclines in bovine and porcine muscle by high-performance liquid chromatography using solid phase chromatography. Chromatogr. 596:211–216, 1992.

[25]Yongmanitchai, W., and Ward, O. Separation of lipid classes from *Phaeodactylum Tricornutum* using silica cartridges. Phytochemistry 31:3405–3409, 1992.

Index

f, figure
t, table

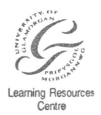